浙江省普通本科高校"十四五"重点教材

中医跨文化传播

Communicating TCM Across Cultures

主编　徐宁骏　黄在委

U0221702

ZHEJIANG UNIVERSITY PRESS
浙江大学出版社
·杭州·

图书在版编目（CIP）数据

中医跨文化传播 / 徐宁骏，黄在委主编. — 杭州：
浙江大学出版社，2024.6. — ISBN 978-7-308-25076-4

Ⅰ. R2-05

中国国家版本馆 CIP 数据核字第 2024DM0572 号

中医跨文化传播
Communicating TCM Across Cultures

徐宁骏　黄在委　主编

责任编辑	殷晓彤
责任校对	陈　宇
封面设计	杭州浙信文化传播有限公司
出版发行	浙江大学出版社
	（杭州市天目山路148号　邮政编码310007）
	（网址:http://www.zjupress.com）
排　　版	杭州晨特广告有限公司
印　　刷	浙江省邮电印刷股份有限公司
开　　本	710mm×1000mm　1/16
印　　张	24.5
字　　数	630千
版 印 次	2024年6月第1版　2024年6月第1次印刷
书　　号	ISBN 978-7-308-25076-4
定　　价	99.00元

《中医跨文化传播》
编委会

主　编：

徐宁骏　（浙江中医药大学）　　　黄在委　（浙江中医药大学）

副主编（按姓氏笔画排序）：

方继良　（中国中医科学院广安门医院）　宓芬芳　（浙江中医药大学）

严暄暄　（湖南中医药大学）　　　徐春南　（浙江中医药大学）

张红霞　（浙江中医药大学）　　　林　敏　（浙江中医药大学）

陈云慧　（成都中医药大学）

编　委（按姓氏笔画排序）：

丁　颖　（湖南中医药大学）　　　周志焕　（天津中医药大学）

王　彤　（南京中医药大学）　　　郝建军　（湖北中医药大学）

王凌之　（浙江中医药大学）　　　侯跃辉　（广东外语外贸大学）

孔冉冉　（山东中医药大学）　　　袁　芳　（浙江中医药大学）

乔丽娟　（浙江中医药大学）　　　唐　路　（浙江中医药大学）

刘海舟　（江西中医药大学）　　　梁世伟　（浙江中医药大学）

刘雁云　（湖北中医药大学）　　　宿哲骞　（长春中医药大学）

许华琳　（浙江中医药大学）　　　扈李娟　（浙江中医药大学）

李　颖　（成都中医药大学）　　　谢苑苑　（浙江中医药大学）

李兰兰　（天津中医药大学）　　　谭秀敏　（天津中医药大学）

宋　梅　（南昌医学院）　　　　　戴晓东　（上海师范大学）

张　洁　（南京中医药大学）

学术秘书：

江秀云　（浙江中医药大学）

编写说明

单元结构

Objectives：章节目标，用英语简单列举本章的学习要点和关键要素。

Key Terms：关键词，供学生预习复习本章核心概念。

Quotes：中英双语名言、摘录（摘自时政文件、中外名人名言等），供学生课前预习使用，为课上分析理解课文内容做好热身准备。

Text A and Text B：主文章，配有课前讨论、难词解析、课后思辨阅读讨论题目。每章配有案例分析、调查报告、翻译练习等活动。

Further Reading：扩展文章，配有与本章主题相关的进一步阅读和研究文献，供师生选读。

Summary：配有总结性的章节小结，供学生复习之用。

Checklist：学习进度，供学生检验学习效果之用

教学建议

本书共有5篇14章，建议每章2课时。教师可根据本校每学期实际教学课时确定教学任务。建议采用线上线下结合的教学方式。所有章节内容均配有慕课，可布置学生进行课前线上视频学习。课堂上可采用生生讲解、师生讨论、生生问答、小组辩论等形式开展。课后除了巩固性的任务之外，还可进行跨文化实践。

学习内容、学时分配和教学形式建议

学习内容	学时分配	教学形式
章节目标	—	慕课学习、小组学习
名言摘录		
主文章（一）		
阅读讨论、汇报	1	小组讨论与汇报、师生点评
主文章（二）	—	慕课学习、小组学习
思辨阅读讨论	0.5	小组讨论与演讲、写作、教师点评
翻译、案例分析	0.5	小组讨论与汇报、教师点评
扩展文章	—	慕课自主学习
合计	2	

前　言

中医是中华民族的瑰宝，千百年来守护着中华儿女的健康，为世界生命科学提供原创智慧，在防治传染病，治疗疑难杂症、罕见病等方面发挥重要作用。"人类卫生健康共同体""治未病""辨证论治""天人合一"等中国人熟知的词汇、中医药术语、中医文化等已经在世界各地得到传播。世界卫生组织权威文件《国际疾病分类手册（第11版）》首次将起源于古代中国且当前在中国、日本、韩国和其他国家普遍使用的传统医学病证进行了分类。这不仅有助于世界各国人民认识中医，还能促进中医的自身发展。

但我们也看到，自西医传入中国，中西医科学之争、中医存废之争一直延续至今。其根源在于西方科学慢慢在中国生根发芽之后，人们习惯于以西方的科学标准诠释和衡量中国本土的一切，包括中医。殊不知，中医和西医原本就源自两个不同的文化体系，硬生生地相互适应，最终可能是两败俱伤。因此，如何从跨文化传播的角度审视中医国际化，是当前亟需解决的问题，也是本书的核心目标。

《中医跨文化传播》作为全国第一本融合跨文化交际和中医文化国际传播的高等学校教材，旨在通过理论讲解、模拟展示、案例分析、实际操练、角色扮演等方式，理论与实践双轨并举，适当穿插编者真实见闻，融知识性、学术性、趣味性、可操作性为一体，打造独一无二的中医跨文化传播模式。编写老师主要来自全国各大中医院校，既有多年从事中西医实践的"老"医生，也有扎实掌握跨文化理论和具有丰富训练实操经验的跨文化从业人员，还有海外留学归国、多年从事孔子学院管理和教学及外语教育的优秀中青年教师。他们将从中医跨文化传播的关键要素、实际操作、域外中医的发展、跨文化障碍和突破途径、未来趋势等五方面展开设计和内容编写，既有高屋建瓴式的诸如"一带一路"等国家政策的外语解读，又有心系中国传统文化和中医核心价值体系、胸怀天下健康的抱负，将中医跨文化传播置于提升全球人民健康福祉的大环境，为培养具有国际化视野和全球化意识的世界公民作出贡献。

本书适合本科生、研究生、来华留学生、出国留学生、在职（中）医护人员，以及对中医药文化和跨文化传播感兴趣的社会人士。只要具备中等水平的英语能力

(如通过大学英语四级)和一定的恒心和毅力便可在(中医)跨文化传播的知识海洋中自由遨游。经过数月的理论学习和互动实践,读者将在知识、情感、行动和道德四个维度上均有提升,在英语听、说、读、写、译等技能方面,在中国传统文化、中医核心价值体系和跨文化传播基础知识与实践方面,在人格养成和素养提高方面均有突破。

在本书编写过程中,我们得到了成都中医药大学、广东外语外贸大学、湖北中医药大学、湖南中医药大学、江西中医药大学、南昌医学院、南京中医药大学、山东中医药大学、上海师范大学、天津中医药大学、长春中医药大学、浙江中医药大学、中国中医科学院等单位领导的关心和指导,在此一并致谢。

徐宁骏　黄在委
2024年4月于浙江中医药大学

慕课二维码

Contents

Part Three   Messages

Part Four   Health

─────────────── **Part Five** **Action** ───────────────

Part One
Foundations

Chapter 1

Rationale of TCM Interculturalization

Chapter Objectives

After reading this chapter, you should be able to:

◆ Provide reasons, with evidence, as to why it is important to study intercultural communication and TCM interculturalization.

◆ Describe possible limitations of studying intercultural communication.

◆ Summarize the history of TCM interculturalization.

─[**Key Terms**]─────────────────────────────────

traditional Chinese medicine (TCM)

benefits of promoting TCM globalization

career boost

communicating TCM across cultures

communication

community engagement

COVID-19

culture

deglobalization

intercultural communication

Memory of the World Register

personal growth

TCM cultural ambassador

TCM culture facilitator

TCM globalization

TCM interculturalization

ICD-11

Quotes

"The unprecedented level of interconnection and interdependence among countries binds them into a global community of shared future. Guided by this vision, China's international development cooperation in the new era has a more profound philosophical basis and clearer goals, which lead to more concrete actions." (当今世界, 各国相互联系、相互依存日益紧密, 人类越来越成为你中有我、我中有你的命运共同体。新时代的中国国际发展合作, 以推动构建人类命运共同体为引领, 精神内涵更加丰富, 目标方向更加清晰, 行动实践更有活力。)

——2021年1月10日《新时代的中国国际发展合作》

"How shall I talk of the sea to the frog, if he has never left the pond? How shall I talk of the frost to the bird of the summer land if he has never left the land of his birth? And how shall I talk of life with the sage if he is a prisoner of his doctrine?" (井蛙不可以语于海者, 拘于虚也; 夏虫不可以语于冰者, 笃于时也; 曲士不可以语于道者, 束于教也。)

——庄子(公元前369—前286年)

"If there is one lesson from the past 100 years, it is that we are doomed to co-operate. Yet we remain tribal." (若观百年之历程, 所得一诚曰: 吾辈当通力合作。然而今人仍存部族之心。)

——Martin Wolf

Before reading this section, please consider the following questions:

1. How much do you know about the COVID-19 pandemic?

2. Have you ever met with someone whose cultural background differs from yours? How did you communicate with him or her?

1.1   A Glimpse into TCM Interculturalization

COVID-19 as a Global Threat

Almost five years ago, the sudden outbreak of **COVID-19** (新冠) caused chaos worldwide. Due to the airborne transmission (空气传播) of the virus, there was a high demand for personal protective equipment (PPE) such as face masks. Consequently, PPE rapidly became unavailable in supermarkets and drugstores. To combat COVID-19, numerous countries collaborated and healthcare professionals as well as researchers offered their assistance to China. Aid supplies were sent to China, including contributions from the JYDA, a non-profit organization based in Japan. In January 2020, the JYDA sent aid shipments to Hubei Province and inscribed a line of poem on every box. The poem, composed of eight Chinese characters, conveyed the message: "Mountain, River, Different, Areas / Wind, Moon, Same, Sky", symbolizing that despite living in different places, we all coexist under the same sky. This heartfelt gesture gained widespread attention on the Internet, touching the hearts of many Chinese netizens. More aid from abroad followed suit.

The rapid spread of the virus and its extensive impact on the global economy have greatly emphasized how interconnected the world is. The movement of people and goods around the world demonstrated the significance of these global connections, which were severely disrupted by the pandemic. Consequently, the flow of goods and people was either slowed down or halted completely. This disruption in goods had a significant impact on China, the world's second-largest economy and one of the most extensive producers, and the US, the world's largest economy and a prominent consumer. According to a UN report, while trade in services finally recovered to pre-COVID-19 levels, reaching more than $32 trillion in 2022, there was a continuation of trade stagnation (停滞) seen in the first quarter of 2023 (UNCTAD, 2023).

As the pandemic continued to spread, many nations resorted to traditional border practices by implementing restrictions on cross-border movements. Some countries had even gone as far as completely closing their borders, trying to block the spread of the virus. At the time of writing this book, COVID-19 is already declining. Yet, we still remember vividly that over the past three years, millions of people have been infeeted by the virus, which causes hundreds of thousands of deaths and widespread economic crisis. This global crisis has brought about tremendous changes in life across the entire world.

Global Responses to COVID-19

COVID-19 has already established itself as one of the most devastating pandemics in recent history, which has undoubtedly had an impact on everyone. It has not only resulted in significant advancements in science and medicine, but has also spurred the largest global vaccination campaign ever witnessed. At that time, many universities and colleges had transitioned to online classes; factories were closed; shopping malls were silenced; some people we know may have been robbed of their lives. Right from the start, countries responded to the crisis in varying ways, with some variations being quite significant. Can individualistic cultures expect their citizens to follow rules? Are collectivistic cultures better equipped to handle these public health challenges? Our responses to such crisis situations are influenced by our cultural backgrounds and frameworks. From time to time, we find ourselves thinking of the following questions:

- Should we prioritize our own desires?
- Do we consider the well-being of others?
- Will we witness a trend towards closed borders?
- Will we extend a hand in greater engagement with the world?

It is essential to reflect on these questions before moving forward.

Intercultural Challenges

The field of intercultural communication presents numerous challenges and raises a series of complex questions for those involved in studying, teaching, and conducting research in this area. One significant issue revolves around whether discussions on cultural differences might reinforce stereotypes. Additionally, understanding the wider social, political, and historical contexts becomes crucial when engaging in intercultural communication. We must also explore how our intercultural communication skills can contribute to enhancing our own lives as well as the lives of those around us. Finally, an important question arises: Can scholars of intercultural communication promote a more inclusive and harmonious world for everyone? These thought-provoking questions deserve our attention in response to the rapidly changing dynamics of culture.

From one perspective, natural disasters such as the wildfires in Australia and the US have generated a range of positive reactions, fostering (促进) significant care and compassion across diverse cultural and international boundaries. The global efforts to combat COVID-19 also serve as a compelling illustration of how humans can collaborate by surpassing cultural and ideological differences. Conversely, the reinforcement of national borders amidst global migration, conflicts between law enforcement and communities of color in the US, and the dissemination of racist, hateful, and sometimes false content on social media worsen the situation and contribute to heightened intergroup conflict. These extremes vividly exemplify the dynamic relationship between culture and communication.

The unarmed combat against COVID-19 is an on-going endeavor. Both Western and Eastern medicine can offer feasible solutions to winning this war without gunpowder. However, significant obstacles, both visible and invisible, clearly hinder (阻碍) the complete integration of traditional Chinese medicine (TCM) in addressing this health crisis.

Communicating TCM Across Cultures

Across continents, spanning from East to West, a significant divergence exists in the mindset regarding the perception of the world. The intense embrace of the "America First" policy by American politicians serves as a perfect example of how the US has insensitively disregarded international norms, retreating into unilateralism (单边主义) and isolationism. If China were to follow in America's footsteps, it might be tempted to adopt a similar "China First" approach, simplistically based on a tit-for-tat strategy. However, this is not the case. Instead, China proposes a completely different ideal: building a community of a shared future for humankind (人类命运共同体) through initiatives like the Belt and Road, alongside other intercultural cooperation projects, in response to the backdrop of **deglobalization** (去全球化).

Narrowly speaking, this difference merely pertains to individual pursuits. However, from a broader perspective, it is intertwined with culture. Remarkably, Chinese civilization has thrived for approximately 5,000 years, exceeding the history of the US by a significant margin. By **communicating TCM across cultures**, people outside China can gain a deeper understanding of splendid and diverse Chinese culture, as well as the Chinese approach to healthcare. Western medicine and TCM are similar to a bird flying through the sky and a fish swimming underwater — two distinct species thriving in different environments. It is doomed to failure to force a swimming fish to learn how to fly, as it simply cannot be done. Unfortunately, some individuals perceive TCM solely as complementary and alternative medicine (补充替代医学). This biased perception is a stereotype or preconceived notion (成见) that requires dismantling (消除).

In this textbook, a comprehensive three-step process is outlined to enhance your intercultural competence, with a focus on transmitting TCM across different cultures. Fundamental concepts from intercultural communication studies, including perception, culture, communication, adaptation, stereotypes, ethnocentrism, values, and ethics, will be thoroughly explored. Additionally, theories and principles of TCM such as yin-yang will be discussed to provide you with a strong foundational understanding. Subsequently, both verbal and nonverbal communication behaviors will be emphasized, paving the way for a transformation in your perspectives and actions, enabling you to engage effectively and appropriately in intercultural interactions.

Finally, the most frequently used term of our theme is "communicating TCM across cultures". At times, "across cultures" is interchanged with "interculturally" or "globally". After all, our main goal is to promote TCM on a global scale. This is why "TCM globalization" is also appropriate. "Interculturalization" is derived from "interculturalize", indicating the process of making something intercultural. Therefore, "TCM interculturalization" is both suitable and concise. When referring to participants involved in TCM interculturalization or TCM globalization, expressions like **TCM cultural ambassador**, **TCM culture facilitator**, or publicist for TCM interculturalization are used if necessary.

Activities

Comprehension Questions

1. How did Chinese netizens respond to the generous donation from the JYDA?

2. In what way(s) does the outbreak of COVID-19 demonstrate the interconnectedness among people around the globe?

3. What do you think could prevent TCM from fully participating in the fight against pandemics like COVID-19?

4. What are some possible topics that will be covered in this book?

5. What example(s) can you give to illustrate the possible stereotypical understanding of TCM?

Group Work

1. Think about people around you. How would you describe their level of awareness of domestic and international cultures and identities? How about your own? What are some specific areas in which you would like to develop in terms of your cultural knowledge and skills during this course?

2. In what way(s), if any, do you think the globalization of media, especially social media like Weibo or TikTok, is influencing your culture? Does it influence all cultures equally? Why or why not?

Translation

Translate the following text into English.

"中医药学凝聚着深邃的哲学智慧和中华民族几千年的健康养生理念及其实践经验,是中国古代科学的瑰宝,也是打开中华文明宝库的钥匙。"回顾历史,张骞西行、鉴真东渡、玄奘取经、郑和远航,这些名垂青史的中外文明交往佳话,把中医药传播到了世界各地,体现了和而不同、海纳百川的大同思想,折射出兼济天下、悬壶济世的胸襟气度。

Before reading this section, please consider the following questions:

1.How much do you recommend TCM to foreign friends? Why?

2.Why do we need to promote TCM globalization?

1.2　Rationale for Communicating TCM Across Cultures

Preliminary Definitions of Four Key Concepts

In the previous section, we observed a significant global health crisis that necessitates cooperation among diverse cultures and nations. While this case clearly demonstrates the need for intercultural communication, individuals can also derive personal benefits from such education, even if they never venture beyond their hometown. Presently, many students worldwide are actively engaging in community development, displaying a greater sense of social responsibility compared with their parents' generation. Many of you belong to this particular group. In this section, we emphasize the importance of understanding TCM interculturalization. Subsequently, we direct our focus towards the reasons why it is essential to globally communicate TCM, i.e., enriching the diverse world we inhabit, and bringing that understanding back to our local and regional communities.

Before we begin, it would be beneficial to establish definitions for some key terms. Each of these terms possesses complexity and will be further elaborated on in subsequent chapters. Firstly, let us define **culture** as the collective way of life adopted by a group of people, including symbols, values, behaviors, artifacts, and other shared aspects. Culture undergoes continuous evolution as individuals exchange messages. According to *The Law of the People's Republic of China on Traditional Chinese Medicine* (NPC, 2016), TCM serves as the overarching term for the medical practices of all Chinese ethnic groups, including both the Han ethnic group and ethnic minority groups. It reflects Chinese nation's understanding of life, health, and diseases, representing a system of medicine and pharmacology (药理学) with extensive historical traditions, as well as unique theories and technical methods. For the time being, **communication** is understood as the process of creating and conveying symbolic behavior, and interpreting behavior between individuals. Consequently, **intercultural communication** occurs when culture influences the communication process. If the message is related to TCM, it is considered as one aspect of TCM interculturalization. For instance, if a TCM physician from China takes a medical history (病史记录) of a German patient, that interaction would typify TCM interculturalization. In its summary of the "2019 World Report", UNESCO (2020) emphasized the necessity of dialogue across numerous domains of social and global development. However, as we shall soon discover, addressing global issues represents merely one of the reasons to study intercultural communication.

Three Motivating Factors

What is the importance of understanding intercultural communication? This question is frequently raised and has gained attention from university researchers, journalists, and even vloggers. If it was necessary to provide justification for organizations or individuals studying other cultures in the past, in today's globalized world, the necessity to understand intercultural communication seems to be widely acknowledged without question. The reasons and benefits of studying intercultural communication are extensive, ranging from personal growth to community engagement and even career boost. We will delve into these motives and explore others as well.

• Personal Growth

Let us move to the motive of personal growth. Our initial incentive revolves around the advantages that learning about other cultures can bring to you as an individual. While there are numerous personal benefits associated with this learning experience, we will specifically focus on three: developing a global mindset, increasing self-awareness, and boosting personal capabilities.

To begin with, the process of learning about cultures and engaging in intercultural communication can greatly enhance our understanding of others worldwide. As Hall *et al.* (2018) suggested, one of the obvious benefits of studying intercultural communication is the liberation from ignorance. Acquiring knowledge about different cultures enables us to be more accountable and mindful (考虑周到的) individuals, approaching each interaction with a heightened awareness of others and a greater level of competence, or a global mindset. Furthermore, as we explore deeper other cultures, we simultaneously gain a fuller understanding of our own culture and ourselves. Just as studying other languages expands our understanding of our native language, the same applies to culture learning. This increased self-awareness, in turn, facilitates us to communicate with others with ease. Lastly, possessing intercultural experience greatly cultivates our flexibility. It has long been proposed that immersing ourselves in new cultures provides us with alternative ways of thinking, feeling, and behaving, thus empowering (允许) ourselves to get away from any cultural cage we are in (Hall *et al.*, 2018). Over time, we may even become intercultural individuals, capable of effortlessly navigating between cultures or, at the very least, comprehending different cultural perspectives more readily.

• Community Engagement

We are not isolated individuals; we exist in constant interaction with others and bear the responsibility of coexisting peacefully and ethically. Marshall McLuhan's metaphor of the global village (McLuhan, 1964) aptly demonstrates how our communities have become increasingly interconnected due to advancements in technology, media, and travel convenience. In the face of global environmental changes, there arises a heightened necessity for leaders to engage in global discussions, where policies that are fair to all nations can be formulated with the aim of preserving and enhancing the environment.

Certainly, the environment represents just one among numerous issues that necessitate global collaboration. With the world population progressively growing and encountering challenges related to aging and other health factors, successful coping approaches must consider local cultural perspectives. This principle remains valid when addressing concerns like the quest for remedies for diseases (疾病) such as AIDS, cancer, or heart disease. TCM, renowned for its efficacy in fostering well-being, can present an additional choice for healthcare practitioners worldwide.

• Career Boost

It has become evident thus far that gaining knowledge about another culture and mindset can greatly enhance one's prospects of securing a well-paying job, boosting one's career development. Given the increasing global interconnectedness in various fields, facilitated by the Internet, people around the world are united not physically but virtually. Consequently, businesses aiming to expand globally must consider hiring an intercultural expert or practitioner who can guide their business planners in adapting to local cultures, catering to a global audience, and seizing opportunities in the global market. University students who possess a substantial understanding of transcending (超越) cultural barriers, therefore, have undoubtedly gained a competitive advantage in the challenging job market. For those aspiring to work for multinational corporations, learning about intercultural communication provides them with essential tools, acting as a stepping-stone into a vibrant world where cultural diversity is the norm. Even for those who choose to remain within their home country, such knowledge becomes financially rewarding as they are more likely to be employed by domestic companies serving international customers.

Benefits of Promoting TCM Globalization

Now it is time to address a commonly asked question: Why is it important to promote TCM on a global scale? During the ongoing global impact of COVID-19 in 2022, the Director-General of the World Health Organization, Tedros Ghebreyesus, emphasized at a press conference, "Rather than letting our guard down, now is the time to intensify our efforts to save lives. This entails (有必要) investing in the equitable distribution of COVID-19 resources while concurrently strengthening healthcare systems" (Ghebreyesus, 2022). Numerous countries and international organizations extended assistance and support to China during its challenging period. In turn, China also made significant efforts to aid the global battle against COVID-19, firmly believing that solidarity and cooperation are the only appropriate choices for the international community in response to such a major crisis. Conversely, acting selfishly and scapegoating others would only bring harm to all members involved.

First, it is meaningful to provide an additional, equally effective, and simple method for treating diseases. TCM is comparatively affordable, enabling more individuals worldwide to benefit from this ancient healing practice. Notably, China has become the first major economy to experience a turnaround in the economy amid the COVID-19 pandemic, demonstrating leadership in both epidemic control and economic recovery on a global scale. TCM physicians collaborate closely with Western-trained doctors in tackling one of the most severe pandemics in human history, and the effectiveness of TCM has been proven. For instance, a two-week clinical trial overseen by the renowned Chinese researcher Zhong Nanshan has shown that the consumption of Lianhua Qingwen capsules (连花清瘟胶囊), a botanical TCM product, in conjunction with standard therapy, can speed up the recovery of COVID-19 patients (Li *et al.*, 2020). China is willing to share its knowledge and experience as long as other nations are open to accepting them.

Moreover, the global promotion of TCM is essentially equivalent to the intercultural dissemination of Chinese culture. The fundamental principles of TCM, such as the harmony between humans and nature, the five-phase theory, and the yin-yang theory, are an integral part of Chinese culture. By publicizing elements of TCM, we are essentially introducing the world to a better understanding of China.

Lastly, an equally significant impact of TCM's inter culturalization is to benefit TCM itself. By embracing the global community and assimilating into world medicine, TCM practitioners can gain a clearer understanding of their own shortcomings. Historically, the introduction of Western medicine during the late Qing Dynasty posed an unprecedented challenge to TCM. Many individuals started doubting its theories and effectiveness, and some even completely abandoned TCM in favor of Western medicine. However, this period also presented a valuable opportunity for TCM physicians to initiate (发起) reforms and acquire knowledge from Western medicine. In essence, every challenge serves as an opportunity. Promoting TCM across cultures enables us to confront critics and opponents, ultimately making TCM more coherent, effective, and globally recognized.

Significance of Communicating TCM Across Cultures

Up until now, we have observed that studying culture entails certain risks, such as overgeneralization, oversimplification, and exaggeration of cultural aspects. However, it also offers numerous advantages. Understanding culture and engaging in intercultural communication can enhance our global citizenship, equipping us with the necessary skills to participate in the dialogues advocated by the UN *Annual Report* (UN, 2022), ultimately contributing to a better world tomorrow. Additionally, gaining knowledge of different cultures empowers us as individuals, granting us greater control over our own choices within the context of this globalized world.

Likewise, communicating TCM across cultures holds significant importance in multiple respects. Firstly, TCM provides an alternative approach to disease treatment that is equally effective, simple, and cost-efficient, as evidenced by its successful application in combating COVID-19. Given the vast cultural differences between the East and the West, meaningful cultural dialogues serve as an initial step towards mutual understanding. Secondly, deeply rooted in traditional Chinese culture, TCM acts as a representative of China to the world, showing its vibrant and practical aspects while closely intertwining with human health, thus offering a perfect gateway to understanding Chinese culture. Lastly, the challenges confronted by TCM practitioners both domestically and internationally serve as opportunities for self-improvement, enabling them to enhance their ability to care for global well-being. As President Xi Jinping emphasizes, we are living in a community of a shared future for humankind in which TCM plays an indispensable role in preventing and treating diseases.

Activities

Comprehension Questions

1.What are the three major reasons for studying intercultural communication?
2.How does an individual benefit from learning different cultural patterns?
3.What are the three main reasons for promoting TCM across cultures?
4.What could be some possible negative consequences of studying cultures?
5.In what way is TCM globalization at once an opportunity and a challenge?

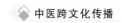

Survey

It is commonly acknowledged that promoting TCM on a global scale is both a personal endeavor and a government priority. To date, the Chinese government has issued several significant documents and policies aimed at fostering the cross-cultural promotion of TCM.

What actions do you believe Chinese college students can take as individuals to contribute to the advancement of TCM interculturalization? Conduct a survey among some Chinese students and report it to the class.

Translation

Translate the following text into Chinese.

China pursues an ideal world where the Great Way rules for the common good, respects the principles of good neighborliness and harmony in relations with all other countries, and advocates cooperation and mutual help. Deep rooted in Chinese culture, these are the firm beliefs that inspire China's development cooperation.

Group Work

1. Have each individual in the group bring an item that represents their culture and request them to share the reasons behind their choice. Have a discussion on the meaning of culture in our everyday lives.

2. In a group of three, take turns discussing a topic about which you have different opinions on parking, a recent movie, or experience in seeing a (TCM) physician. When the first person talks, the others should listen and support him or her. When the second person talks, the others should act uninterested. And when the third person talks, the others should strongly disagree with his or her opinion. Use these experiences to talk about cultural norms and how communication can depend on the situation and the people involved.

3. Read national newspapers or magazines to explore their perspectives on intercultural events. Look for articles about the same incident from other newspapers or magazines that represent communities different from your own, such as the English version of *China Daily, Japan Times*, or *Washington Post*. Compare and contrast their viewpoints.

1.3 Brief Overview of TCM Interculturalization

TCM as Representative of Traditional Chinese Culture

If a foreigner is asked to identify the essence of China and its culture, he or she might mention Chinese Kungfu or Chinese cuisine. However, there is now a third answer: traditional Chinese medicine (Lin, 2019). TCM has emerged as a medical science that has developed and prospered within the daily lives of Chinese people, throughout their enduring battle against diseases spanning thousands of years. It embodies the core value of Chinese civilization by applying principles such as "observing the law of nature and seeking for the unity of heaven and humanity" (顺天行道,天人合一), "maintaining a balanced harmony between yin and yang to achieve the golden mean" (阴阳平衡,调和致中), and ensuring that "practice of medicine should aim to help people" (以人为本,悬壶济世). TCM also advocates "full consideration of the environment, individual constitution, and climatic and seasonal conditions when practicing syndrome differentiation and determining therapies" (三因制宜,辨证论治), and "mastership of medicine lying in proficient medical skills and lofty medical ethics" (大医精诚,仁心仁术). All of these concepts enrich Chinese culture and provide a solid foundation for studying and transforming the world. TCM encompasses a harmonious integration of natural sciences and humanities with philosophical ideas unique to the Chinese nation. As perceptions of well-being and medical paradigms (范式) continue to evolve and progress, TCM increasingly assumes its profound value.

TCM in the World

Having originated in China, TCM has assimilated the essence of other civilizations, evolving and gradually disseminating across the globe. As early as the Qin and Han dynasties (221 B.C.–A.D. 220), TCM gained popularity in neighboring countries and regions, greatly influencing their traditional medical practices. For instance, TCM has had a longstanding impact on the development of Korean medicine. During the Ming and Qing Dynasties (1368–1911), the technique of TCM smallpox vaccination had already extended beyond China's borders (Ma, 2010).

According to the keynote speech at "The 6th Belt and Road Forum for TCM Development" (6th September, 2023), TCM has been disseminated to 196 countries and regions. Additionally, 30 overseas TCM research centers have been established, and TCM has been utilized to treat over one third of the global population. According to statistics from the WHO, among the 179 Member States, 113 have granted approval for the practice of acupuncture and moxibustion, 30 have implemented specific regulations regarding acupuncture, and 20 have incorporated acupuncture into their medical insurance coverage (WHO, 2019a).

Acupuncture is widely practiced in the US and the UK as a popular method for relieving pain and treating various ailments. While the earliest recorded instances of TCM in Europe date back 350 years, acupuncture gained significant prominence in the UK and other Western countries following American President Nixon's visit to China in 1972. In 2007, the first Confucius Institute for TCM was established in London, symbolizing the extensive collaboration between British and Chinese universities in the TCM field (Wu *et al.*, 2013).

Even in the US, where Western medicine is highly prevalent, 48 out of 50 states and one special administrative region have implemented legal regulations regarding acupuncture (Liu and Zhou, 2023). Notably, California, Florida, New Mexico, Texas, and Washington DC have legalized both acupuncture and Chinese herbal medicine. In states that recognize acupuncture, most insurance companies provide coverage for acupuncture treatments, although the extent of coverage may vary. Since the 1990s, many renowned universities like Harvard, Yale, Stanford, and Cornell have incorporated TCM courses into their medical programs. As a result, the study of TCM has become an integral part of medical education in these prestigious institutions.

In Australia, there is a national registration management system for TCM practitioners. Since July 2015, the process of qualification certification for TCM practitioners has become standardized. The efforts of TCM practitioners, including Professor Lin Ziqiang, President of the Federation of Chinese Medicine and Acupuncture Societies (Australia), have played a crucial role in this development. In February 2000, the state of Victoria passed the *Chinese Medicine Registration Act 2000*, making it the first Australian state to enact legislation specifically for TCM. Furthermore, in 2012, the Australian Federal Government passed legislation that incorporated TCM into the national health industry registration management and qualification certification system (Dong *et al.*, 2022).

In Continental Europe, France is among the first European countries to have widely accepted and practiced acupuncture, not only for humans but also for animals in clinics (Zhu *et al.*, 2018). In Germany, only registered doctors and practitioners are permitted to practice TCM. The Hungarian Congress officially passed the *TCM Act* in 2013, making Hungary the first European country to establish legislation regarding TCM (Xia, 2016). Portugal has maintained regular contact with China for approximately 500 years and is a leading contributor to the development of TCM among European countries (Yan *et al.*, 2021). In the 12th century, Portugal witnessed acupuncture for the first time, and in the 16th century, a Portuguese missionary wrote the first article about acupuncture in Portuguese. Nowadays, Portugal has established two centers committed to the research and development of TCM. These centers not only contribute to the spread of TCM within Portugal but also among other EU countries. Portugal's dedication to advancing TCM serves as a valuable resource for the broader European community seeking to explore and benefit from this ancient medical tradition.

TCM is experiencing significant growth among the member countries of BRICS, which encompasses regions across Africa, Asia, and Europe. Initially, BRICS referred to five emerging markets in Asia and Africa. However, at its 15th summit meeting in 2023, BRICS invited other six countries, representing half of the world population. As the Belt and Road Initiative continues to deepen and cooperation among BRICS members strengthens, the popularity of TCM is expected to grow steadily.

TCM and ICD-11

TCM is making its way into clinics worldwide as well. On 25th May 2019, the World Health Assembly approved the eleventh revision of the International Statistical Classification of Diseases and Related Health Problems (**ICD-11**) (WHO, 2019b). In comparison to the previous version, ICD-11 includes a supplementary Chapter 26 dedicated to optional use, which incorporates 150 disorders and 196 patterns originating from TCM and commonly employed in China, Japan, the Republic of Korea, and other parts of the world. This recognition signifies that TCM is now officially acknowledged as an integral part of mainstream medical practice.

It is important to note that patterns included in Chapter 26 of the ICD-11 only represent a small portion of TCM clinical practices. Nevertheless, this inclusion marks a significant milestone for TCM global recognition. Historically, TCM was excluded from the ICD system. The incorporation of TCM in the ICD-11 represents not only a landmark for the classification system but also a crucial moment for TCM itself, for this integration allows statistical data to include information beyond Western medicine, providing a more accurate depiction of healthcare systems among WHO member states.

This initiative aligns with the "WHO Traditional Medicine Strategy (2014–2023)" (WHO, 2013), which highlights the WHO's recognition of TCM's past contribution to global healthcare as well as its response to the current needs of member states. Furthermore, this action will have long-term impacts on TCM as it opens doors for further development, improved service levels, education, research, and regulation among WHO member states. Additionally, it contributes to the progressive reform of the global healthcare system by fostering the integration of TCM with various disciplines rooted in Western medicine. Ultimately, people worldwide will benefit from this initiative.

International Recognition of TCM Classics

TCM classics such as *Huangdi Neijing* (*Huangdi's Internal Classic*) have long been considered as the masterpieces of medical research. Charles Darwin, the British biologist, hailed *Ben Cao Gang Mu* (*Grand Compendium of Materia Medica*) as an "ancient Chinese encyclopedia" (Zhang, R X, 2018). Both *Huangdi Neijing* and *Ben Cao Gang Mu* were listed in the UNESCO's **Memory of the World Register** (世界记忆名录) in May 2011. *The Four Treatises of Tibetan Medicine* (《四部医典》) joined the big family of Memory of the World Register in 2023. *The Four Treatises of Tibetan Medicine*, which was compiled from the 8th to the 12th centuries and is considered the most fundamental classic of traditional Tibetan medicine (TTM), part of TCM, is divided into four parts: tsagyu (root treatise), shegyu (explanatory treatise), managagyu (treatise of oral instruction), and chimagyu (the last treatise). *The Four Treatises* comprehensively showcases the growth and transformation of TTM. Not only does it represent the pinnacle of medical knowledge in ancient Xizang, but it also reflects the exploration of humanities, history, traditions, literature, art, and craftsmanship during earlier periods of Xizang civilization.

China's Foreign Health Aid

Acupuncture and moxibustion have gained popularity worldwide due to their remarkable efficacy. The discovery of qinghaosu (artemisinin) has been responsible for saving millions of lives, particularly in developing countries. With advancements in modern medicine, the value of TCM is becoming increasingly recognized, leading to its growing popularity on a global platform. While pursuing its own development, China has consistently provided aid and assistance to other developing nations to fulfill its international obligations. During the past 60 years, China has sent medical teams, including TCM professionals, to more than 70 countries across Asia, Africa, and Latin America (Yu, 2023). These dedicated teams have played a crucial role in combating the diseases and ensuring the well-being of affected populations. This demonstrates the significant contribution of TCM in safeguarding people's health and promoting its philosophical values globally, making it an essential component in addressing public health challenges.

Chapter Summary

- The field of intercultural communication presents numerous challenges and raises a series of complex questions for those involved in studying, teaching, and conducting research in this area.
- By communicating TCM across cultures, people outside of China can gain a deeper understanding of the splendid and diverse Chinese culture, as well as the Chinese approach to healthcare.
- Names of our themes are as follows: communicating TCM across cultures, TCM interculturalization, TCM globalization.
- The participants of TCM interculturalization are named as TCM cultural ambassador, TCM culture facilitator, or publicist for TCM interculturalization.
- Culture is defined as the collective way of life embraced by a group of people, including symbols, values, behaviors, artifacts, and other shared aspects.
- TCM serves as the overarching term for the medical practices of all Chinese ethnic groups, including both the Han ethnic group and ethnic minority groups, reflecting Chinese nation's understanding of life, health, and diseases, and represents a system

of medicine and pharmacology with extensive historical traditions, as well as unique theories and technical methods.

- Communication is understood as the process of creating and conveying symbolic behavior, as well as interpreting behavior between individuals. Consequently, intercultural communication occurs when culture influences the communication process. If the message is related to TCM, it is considered as one aspect of TCM interculturalization.
- The reasons and benefits of studying intercultural communication are extensive, ranging from personal growth, community engagement to career boosting.
- Communicating TCM across cultures serves to provide an additional, equally effective, and simple method for treating diseases, helps disseminate Chinese culture, and encourages TCM culture facilitators to embark on self-improvement.
- TCM has been disseminated to 196 countries and regions. Additionally, 30 overseas TCM research centers have been established, and TCM has been utilized to treat over one third of the global population. So far, among WHO's 179 Member States, 113 have granted approval for the practice of acupuncture and moxibustion, 30 have implemented specific regulations regarding acupuncture, and 20 have incorporated acupuncture into their medical insurance coverage.
- ICD-11 includes a supplementary Chapter 26 dedicated to optional use, which incorporates 150 disorders and 196 patterns originating from TCM.
- Three TCM classics are listed in the UNESCO's Memory of the World Register.

Checklist	Yes	No
Cognitive: I have mastered the core information		
Behavioral: I have the ability of putting what I've learned into practice		
Affective: I am willing to carry out what I've learned		
Moral: I will take the ethical consideration into account during practice		

Chapter 2

Ethical Considerations in TCM Interculturalization

Chapter Objectives

After reading this chapter, you should be able to:

◆ Define principles of TCM interculturalization.

◆ Describe ethical rules of TCM interculturalization.

◆ Describe medical ethics both in TCM and Western medicine.

◆ Summarize Sun Simiao's contribution to medical ethics.

─[**Key Terms**]────────────────────────────────

bioethics

Confucian ethics

ethical relativism

four principles plus scope (principlism)

humanistic principle

medical ethics

TCM ethics

universalistic guidelines

Quotes

"The mind's feeling of pity and compassion is the sprout of humaneness; the mind's feeling of shame and aversion is the sprout of rightness; the mind's feeling of modesty and compliance is the sprout of propriety; and the mind's sense of right and wrong is the sprout of wisdom." (恻隐之心,仁之端也;羞恶之心,义之端也;辞让之心,礼之端也;是非之心,智之端也。)

——孟子(公元前372—前289年)

"Peace and development: this has have been the aspiration held dear by mankind over the past century. However, the goal to achieve peace and development is far from being met. We need to respond to the people's call, take up the baton of history and forge ahead on the marathon track toward peace and development." (这100多年全人类的共同愿望,就是和平与发展。然而,这项任务至今远远没有完成。我们要顺应人民呼声,接过历史接力棒,继续在和平与发展的马拉松跑道上奋勇向前。)

——2017年1月18日习近平《共同构建人类命运共同体》

"When one wants to enter another country, he has to get familiar with the customs followed by people in that country; when one wants to go to others' family, he must try to know the taboos held in that family; when one wants to enter into a hall, he has to inquire about the etiquettes; when one is going to treat a patient, he must be clear about the preference of the patient." (入国问俗,入家问讳,上堂问礼,临病人问所便。)

——《灵枢·师传》

Before reading this section, please consider the following questions:

1. What is your understanding of Confucian ethics? Share your knowledge with your partners.

2. What ethical factors need to be considered when promoting TCM across cultures?

2.1　Ethical Principles of TCM Interculturalization

Maltreating or Treating

Jack moved to the US eight years ago. He now has a wonderful wife and a five-year-old son named Daniel. Jack's father, Old Jack from China, is visiting him. One day, Daniel returned from nursery school and told his grandpa that he had a bad headache and was having difficulty breathing. Florida in June is very hot during the daytime. After simple examination, Old Jack suspected that Daniel might suffer from heat exhaustion. Because he did not read and write in English and thus was not able to buy medicine from a local drugstore, Old Jack gave Daniel a simple guasha. Guasha is a traditional healing technique originated in ancient China. It involves scraping the skin with a smooth-edged instrument, often made of jade, horn, or other materials, to stimulate blood circulation and promote the healing of various ailments. Guasha is commonly used to treat conditions such as chronic pain, muscle stiffness, respiratory issues, and even the common cold. In traditional Chinese medicine (TCM), it is believed that the practice helps restore balance and harmony within the body. However, one side effect of guasha is that it leaves a long strip of bruising, skin irritation, or even bleeding. Daniel did feel good after guasha. Jack knew nothing about it.

A few days later, Daniel went for a normal check-up at a local hospital. When the doctors saw Daniel's severely injured back, they informed Jack and contacted the police. The local police accused Jack of committing domestic violence. The situation worsened when the court ultimately decided to remove Jack's custody of his son, Daniel.

Some of you might doubt the authenticity of this story, and did not think that it could be real. After all, guasha is a widely practiced and well-accepted therapeutic method in China. For others, however, seeing is believing. The bruised back of Daniel serves as tangible evidence suggesting Jack is mistreating his son. It may seem absurd to believe that scraping one's back can be a cure for heat stroke or a common cold. Jack's yelling at the court did not help him get out of the trouble. The judge simply ignored Jack's "self-claimed" explanation. Is it only about intercultural misunderstanding? Or is it related to ethics? If your answer to the latter question is no, consider the following statements:

- The timing of death should be determined solely by nature.
- Mercy killing should be legalized.
- Women possess the right to govern their reproductive choices.
- Artificial birth control is wrong.

Deciding how you feel about these ideas involves considering what is right or wrong, good or bad. You also need to think about them on a global scale and decide whether what works for your society is suitable for the whole world. That is what intercultural ethics is about.

The doctors, policemen, and court officials in the above scenario (场景) fail to recognize an important fact in dealing with culturally different behavior and conduct. They are not aware that what they consider as illegal behavior could be rationalized from a totally different angle. Their professional and ethical knowledge helps them interpret Daniel's skin bruise as strong evidence of domestic violence. Yet, from a different point of view, the same scar on the back could be interpreted as effectiveness in treating heat stroke. Ethics is shaped by cultural beliefs and serves as a set of principles that influence how you communicate with others. It guides your actions, behaviors, and interactions with people, helping you determine what is right, proper, and how you should engage with others.

Ethics and Morality

Ethics and morality are connected to the concepts of right and wrong. Morality encompasses all behaviors that can be considered right or wrong, and ethics focuses on the application of morality in our interactions with others (Wines and Napier, 1992). While morality can be universal across cultures, ethics may vary from culture to culture.

As we interact with others, it is common for us to adhere to certain guidelines or principles. Let us imagine that you wish to take some goods from abroad without declaration. Different ethical approaches can lead to different decisions (Baldwin *et al.*, 2014). You might think about who benefits from the tax or who might hurt from it. It is called utilitarianism (功利主义), determining the greatest benefit for the greatest number of people. The golden mean (中庸之道), avoiding going to extremes, may tell you that if the total value of the goods is not huge enough, you may try it out but not very often. Ethical altruism (利他主义) refers to making choices based on what seems to be good or beneficial to others rather than yourself—in that case, you refrain from illegally bringing back some goods without paying tax because it hurts others. On the contrary, ethical egoism (利己主义) is about making choices totally based on whether the beneficiary is yourself–you definitely avoid paying the import-tax because you want them.

Engaging TCM interculturalization poses ethical challenges as well. Some scholars (e.g., Martin and Nakayama, 2022) are working for constructing **universalistic guidelines** of ethical behavior toward others that can be applied to everyone, irrespective of their cultural diversity. Some of these principles include humanistic principle (e.g., never do harm to others), dialogic ethic (e. g., encourage free discussion with mutual respect), among others. Other scholars are advocating **ethical relativism** (Baldwin *et al.*, 2014). In other words, in every culture, individuals establish their own accepted standards regarding what is considered right or wrong. Each ethical system holds equal acceptability as any other system. Since the principles of TCM interculturalization are guidelines that help individuals effectively and ethically navigate communication across different cultural backgrounds, we would like to offer some suggestions on how to be an ethical TCM culture facilitators as follows.

Guidelines for TCM Interculturalization

Ethical Rule 1: Respect for cultural differences. Show respect for the cultural practices, beliefs, and values of others, even if they differ from your own. Avoid ridiculing or demeaning (贬低) another culture. Avoid behaving in a way that may be considered disrespectful or offensive in another culture. Embrace cultural diversity and promote cultural autonomy.

Ethical Rule 2: Non-discrimination and non-harm. Treat individuals from different cultural backgrounds with fairness and equality. Avoid discrimination based on race, ethnicity, religion, gender, or any other cultural characteristics. Strive to avoid causing harm, offense, or distress to individuals from different cultures through your verbal and non-verbal cues.

Ethical Rule 3: Informed consent (知情同意). Obtain informed consent before using or sharing information related to individuals or groups from different cultures, especially in research or media representation.

Ethical Rule 4: Privacy and confidentiality (保密). Respect the privacy and confidentiality of individuals, especially when discussing sensitive cultural matters or personal experiences.

Ethical Rule 5: Intercultural sensitivity. Be aware of your own cultural biases and strive to understand how they might impact your communication and perceptions of others.

Ethical Rule 6: Honesty and transparency. Be truthful and transparent in your intercultural interactions. Avoid misre presenting information or intentionally deceiving others.

Ethical Rule 7: Avoidance of cultural appropriation (文化挪用). Refrain from appropriating cultural symbols, practices, or artifacts without proper understanding, acknowledgment, and respect for their cultural significance.

Ethical Rule 8: Ethical use of technology. Use technology responsibly in intercultural communication, considering the potential impact on cultural understanding and relationships.

Intercultural communication in general, and TCM intercul turalization in particular, are not merely cultural activities but a commitment to fostering understanding, respecting, and cooperating across cultural boundaries. By adhering to these principles, individuals can build positive intercultural relationships, reduce misunderstandings, and promote effective communication across cultural boundaries.

──┤ **Activities** ├──────────────────────────────────────

Comprehension Questions

1. Do you agree that morality and ethics differ from each other? Why or why not?
2. How do you translate "morality" and "ethics" into Chinese? How do Chinese "道德" and "伦理" differ from each other? Why or why not?
3. What are some of the merits of a relativistic approach to developing an intercultural ethic? Of a universalistic approach? What are some of the dangers?
4. What are the guidelines or rules of TCM interculturalization and how can they be applied in practice?
5. Can you list other principles or ethical rules of intercultural communication?

Translation

Translate the following text into English.

2014年5月4日青年节,习近平总书记考察北京大学时说:"社会主义核心价值观,其实就是一种德,既是个人的德,也是一种大德,就是国家的德、社会的德"。

今天,我们的国家要有持之以恒的精神力量,就要努力践行社会主义核心价值观,提高整个社会的道德水平。首先要以教育为根基,提高人们的内在修养;其次,法律是道德规范和社会文明的风向标,要以法律和制度作为保障,稳固整个社会的道德基石;最后,每个人都要做社会道德的学习者和践行者,道德大厦的建设需要每个社会成员添砖加瓦。

——2014年5月4日习近平在北京大学师生座谈会上的讲话

Speech

Please prepare a speech on the following topic.

German philosopher Kant once said, "Two things fill the mind with ever new and increasing admiration and awe, the more often and steadily we reflect upon them, the starry heavens above me and the moral law within me." Similarly, the statement "morality makes a prosper country and virtue makes a decent man" can be understood as a new era's pursuit for spiritual strength.

Prepare to deliver a speech in English on the given topic.

My Understanding of Morality in the New Era

Before reading this section, please consider the following questions:

1.Please collect some medical oaths across the globe; compare and contrast them to identify their similarities and differences.

2.What could be some possible issues in bioethical debates? How does culture play a role in those debates?

2.2 Ethics in TCM Practice

Two Scenarios

The following are stories shared by two Clinicians.

Clinician 1

I vividly remember a patient who first visited me in April 2019. I designed a treatment plan for him, and he went back for treatment. It seemed to have had a great effect. When he returned in mid-2020, I noticed that his tumor had worsened significantly. He was from a community severely hit by COVID-19, and I understood the challenges he faced during the pandemic. However, I discovered that he had stopped receiving treatment for a long time.

I was puzzled. Why did he stop the treatment when it was working so well? He explained that his family believed he was already cured, so he thought the treatment was no longer necessary.

But in reality, he was in the late-stage case of the disease and needed ongoing treatment. Unfortunately, his family kept this information from him, so he believed he was "cured" without knowing the truth. This patient was in his forties and was an important contributor to his family. This situation was undoubtedly harmful to both the patient and the family.

Clinician 2

Once, some family members of the patient asked the doctors to keep the patient from knowing his condition, but they did not notice everyone to keep the "secret". The patient got the news when he was informed by the nurses on how to take medicine. Or sometimes, the patient might know about his cancer from inmates (病友) because his family members shared the news with others without informing the latter not to tell. Upon knowing his true condition, the patient became extremely depressed and wanted to leave the hospital, no longer willing to cooperate. At the same time, the family was dissatisfied and filed a complaint to the administration of our hospital, claiming that the doctor did not do a good job of confidentiality; they felt that confidentiality is the doctor's obligation.

If you were the doctor in the above two scenarios, what would you do? Would you choose to tell the patients in person? Or would you persuade the patients' family to tell the truth? Or would you do your best to keep the patients from knowing his condition even if you knew this patient might only have no more than six months to live? If you believe it is wise to keep the condition from the patient, then you would definitely feel guilty or at least sad because your colleagues did not help you keep the information. On the contrary, if you think the patient has the right to know his condition, then you would blame his family members who said nothing about the patient's terminal cancer.

Defining Medical Ethics

There is a protocol (规约) or medical regulation in China informing how doctors should do in face of the similar situation, especially in terms of informed consent. Sometimes out of humanistic care, and sometimes out of reality, especially when the patient is illiterate (不识字的) or is in deep coma, it is the responsibility of the family who makes the decision on behalf of the patient. Doctors, in this situation, still have something to do. And a lot of times, doctors are kept in dilemma. To tell or not to tell; that's the question. It is moral or ethical obligation. That is what morality or ethics can work in the healthcare setting, i.e., medical ethics.

Medical ethics is a branch of ethics which pertains to medical practice. It is sometimes viewed as part of the larger field of **bioethics**, which concerns ethics in the medicine and life science, and is closely related with nursing ethics and other areas of ethics which intersect with medical practice. "*Bio* refers to life, and issues in bioethics are often life-and-death issues. Ethical and bioethical standards can be personal, organizational, institutional, or worldwide" (Lewis and Tamparo, 2007, p. 4). Since bioethical considerations are about critical issues with no clear-cut answers, they are usually tricky and difficult to handle. Complicated by cultural variability, medical ethics in practicing TCM across cultures can be even more troubling. The following part is committed to exploring the depth of medical ethics from both Western and Eastern perspectives.

Biomedical Ethics in the West

Hippocrates, often considered as the father of Western medicine, initiated the first ethical code of medicine, "At least do no harm" (Magner and Kim, 2018, p. 67). The well-known Hippocratic Oath (希波克拉底誓言) is the earliest document of Western medical ethics, which has greatly influenced the development of medicine and medical morality in later generations. The Hippocratic Oath, while not as emphasized in medical schools today, can still be found on the walls of many healthcare settings and clinics in the US and other nations. It is relevant today because this Oath protected, though tentatively, the rights of the patients.

Beauchamp and Childress (2013) are among the first researchers who are trying to theorize biomedical ethics. Their biomedical framework, known as **"principlism"**, includes four moral principles, namely, respect for autonomy, non-maleficence, beneficence, and justice, which are applied in professional-patient relationship.

Since the 1970s, it has been warmly welcomed both by researchers and healthcare practitioners, and later has been promoted by Raanan Gillon as the "four principles plus scope" approach in Europe (Gillon, 1994, p. 184). It has been popularly accepted, especially in Western medical circles, as a set of universal guidelines for bioethics, despite strong criticism. This framework claims that regardless of personal beliefs or values, whether they be philosophical, political, religious, or ethical, people around the world should have no difficulty in embracing four fundamental moral principles and carefully considering their applicability. Furthermore, these four principles, along with a thoughtful examination of their scope, cover the majority of moral dilemmas that arise in healthcare.

The claim of universality (普遍性) may be the most significant merit of this theory, as if these moral principles were culture-general and applicable to everyone, thus helping construct global bioethics that transcends cultural variability. "However, perhaps ironically, it is also the most challenging position." (Tsai, 1999, p. 315) Critics argue that principlism, which claims to be a universal norm for bioethics, cannot be accepted as such because it is rooted in a specific culture. Since the theory is based on American common morality, it may reflect certain aspects of American society and therefore may not be applicable or transferable to other contexts and societies.

Likewise, TCM also has its unique understanding of medical ethics, the best proponent (倡导者) of which is Sun Simiao (孙思邈), honored as King of Medicine, whose contributions to TCM practice and ethics are unparalleled.

TCM Ethics

Huangdi Neijing has already discussed medical ethics in some chapters. For instance, Chapter 48 in *Lingshu* (《灵枢》)

records that in ancient times, physicians were required to engage in specific rituals and take a blood oath before embarking on the study and practice of acupuncture. These traditions are believed to be essential in upholding the integrity of their profession. Other medical monographs (专著) include discussions of bioethical considerations such as Zhu Huiming's *Dou Zhen Chuan Xin Lu* (《痘疹传心录》,[明]朱惠明撰) (*Medical Cures of Smallpox Learnt by Heart*) (1594), or Chen Shigong's five admonitions and ten requirements for physicians in *Waike Zhengzong* (《外科正宗》,[明]陈实功撰) (*An Orthodox Manual of Surgery*) (1617). However, the most representative literature of medical ethics in ancient China appeared in the seventh century during the Tang Dynasty. Sun Simiao wrote *Qianjin Yaofang (Essential Prescriptions Worth a Thousand Pieces of Gold)* (《备急千金要方》), in which he put forward the notion of "the absolute sincerity of great physicians" (大医精诚) for the first time, offering an all-round argumentation on the guiding rules of medical ethics a TCM physician must hold on to. He argued that "human life is of paramount importance, more precious than a thousand pieces of gold; to save it with one prescription is to show your great virtue" (人命至重,有贵千金,一方济之,德逾于此). Su Simiao himself is a perfect example of such a noble moral character.

Sun Simiao emphasized the importance of thorough education, conscientiousness, and self-discipline in medical practice. He believed that "compassion" (恻隐之心) and "benevolence" (仁慈) were the basic values that should guide physicians. The principles of TCM ethics thus can be approached from five interrelated aspects: purpose of medical practice, requirements of a great physician, manner of medical practice, attitudes towards patients, and attitudes towards other physicians.

These principles demonstrate the following characteristics.
• TCM ethics is built upon the principles of **Confucian ethics**. For over 2,500 years, Confucian scriptures such as *The Analects* have

served as vital educational resources for students, and Confucian ethics has remained the prevailing moral philosophy and ideology in Chinese culture (Cui, 2017). The moral expectations for TCM physicians align closely with those tenets, for an ideal Confucian individual, known as "*jun zi*" ("superior man"), was a doctor as well, which is vividly reflected in the Chinese adage (箴言) "*gong tong liang xiang*" (the achievement of a good physician equals that of a good prime minister 功同良相).

- Humaneness lies at the core of its principles. In other words, the practice of medicine is the realization of humaneness. This is why the Chinese employ the saying "*ren xin ren shu*" (a heart of humaneness, the skill of humaneness 仁心仁术) to praise the virtues of exceptional physicians. It is the innate (与生俱来的) quality of humaneness that bestows (赋予) value and respect upon medical practice.

- TCM ethics has a strong emphasis on duty and virtue. Physicians are responsible for caring for and assisting their patients, without seeking personal gain or giving way to selfish desires. Confucian philosophy advocates that the moral development of an individual is crucial for maintaining social harmony and promoting human well-being. As most learned scholars are also quite skilled physicians, scholar-physicians can ensure that their medical practice conforms to ethical principles by cultivating virtue. The Chinese adage "*shu de bing zhong*" (both skill and virtue are admirable 术德并重) is used to praise a TCM physician who is both ethically and medically superb.

Both medical practitioners at home and abroad highlight the importance of bioethics in medical practices. These moral constraints such as lofty medical ethics, friendly interpersonal relationships between doctors and patients, and among doctors themselves, including others, are meant to benefit not only patients but also doctors. TCM ethical principles reveal that Confucianism is the underlying paradigm, with Taoism and Buddhism playing some parts in providing core values. TCM ethics reminds us of a valuable element present in traditional healing practices, i.e., benevolence. Embracing this element in modern times can help alleviate the alienation between doctors and patients and restore significance to the doctor-patient relationship.

Activities

Comprehension Questions

1. What is the four-principle approach to biomedical ethics?
2. What is the essence of Sun Simiao's medical ethics?
3. Search as many as possible Chinese phrases that describe good TCM physicians and/or charlatans and put them into proper English or other foreign languages.
4. How is Confucianism reflected in TCM ethics?
5. Collect as many as possible Chinese idioms or adages on medical ethics and put them into proper English or other foreign languages.

Translation

Translate the following text into Chinese.

凡大医治病,必当安神定志,无欲无求,先发大慈恻隐之心,誓愿普救含灵之苦。若有疾厄来求救者,不得问其贵贱贫富,长幼妍媸,怨亲善友,华夷愚智,普同一等,皆如至亲之想。亦不得瞻前顾后,自虑吉凶,护惜身命。见彼苦恼,若己有之,深心凄怆,勿避险巇、昼夜、寒暑、饥渴、疲劳,一心赴救,无作功夫形迹之心,如此可为苍生大医,反此则是含灵巨贼。

——[唐]孙思邈《大医精诚》

Case Study

Fan Zhongyan, a well-known government official during the Northern Song Dynasty, had big dreams at a young age. Despite being born into a poor family, he believed it was his duty to serve the people. One day, Fan Zhongyan went to a temple seeking divination. He drew a lot and asked, "Will I become a prime minister in the future?" The lot indicated no. He prayed again, asking, "Will I become a good physician instead?" Once again, the answer was no. Fan Zhongyan sighed and said, "Neither of those paths seems possible. How can I fulfill my lifelong aspirations in the future? " Others were taken aback and questioned him, saying, "It's understandable for a person to pursue their dream by becoming a prime minister. However, isn't it a shame to be content with becoming a physician?" Fan Zhongyan replied with determination, "I have a strong desire for knowledge, and naturally, I hope to have the opportunity to serve the country under a wise emperor in the future. Becoming a prime minister is the ultimate way to contribute to the well-being of the people. However, since this path is not available to me, there is nothing more worthwhile than becoming a physician. As a physician, I can utilize my knowledge to benefit others. I can heal the illnesses of my parents and patients, educate people about health management and longevity. Therefore, is there a profession better than being a physician to bring benefits to people and alleviate their suffering?"

Questions

1. What did Fan Zhongyan want to be when he was young?

2. What are the similarities between being a prime minister and a physician according to Fan Zhongyan?

2.3   Bilingual Excerpts about TCM Ethics

Excerpt One: Ethical Discussions from Huangdi Neijing
(Wu and Wu, 1997)

The Yellow Emperor said, "I am told that the preceding masters had many personal understandings which were not recorded in the plate, and I hope to hear about these understandings. I will keep them with good care and will take it as the norm of my behavior to treat the people and myself, so that the people may be exempted from diseases, people in the upper class and the lower class in the society may keep harmonious, to have kind relations and good will between them, as love and kindness are prevailing among the people, their descendants will live peacefully without mental and physical disturbances and the good tradition may pass to the future generations without end."

黄帝曰:"余闻先师,有所心藏,弗著于方,余愿闻而藏之,则而行之,上以治民,下以治身,使百姓无病,上下和亲,德泽下流,子孙无忧,传于后世,无有终时。"

——《灵枢·师传》

Qibo said, "The patient should be left alone in the room, the windows and doors should be shut to eliminate all the misgiving of the patient, and ask him about the condition of disease confidentially in detail..."

岐伯曰:"闭户塞牖,系之病者,数问其情……"

——《素问·移精变气论》

"Those who are keen in palpation of the pulse in diagnosis must investigate carefully to know whether the five viscera are agreeable with the energy and blood, the comprehensive condition of yin and yang, superficial and interior, male and female to the exquisite extent by deep consideration, and at the same time, be familiar with the principles and be skillful in treating. When one is proficient in such a degree, he may select and teach someone and hand down the knowledge. It is only the person with such an achievement is deserved to be the one who has really known the essentials of diagnosis."

"故善为脉者,谨察五脏六腑,一逆一从,阴阳表里,雌雄之纪,藏之心意,合心于精,非其人勿教,非其真勿授,是谓得道。"

——《素问·金匮真言论》

Excerpt Two: Ethical Discussions from *Dayi Jingcheng*
Doctor's Code of Conduct

The code of conduct for doctors should be one of cautions in speech and action, refraining from casual jokes, noise, discussing others' shortcomings, or boasting about their own reputation. They should never slander or attack other doctors to exaggerate their own achievements. When successfully treating a patient, they should not become self-congratulatory or arrogantly satisfied, considering themselves unmatched. These are bad habits that doctors must overcome.

Laozi once said, "When a person openly does good deeds, people will naturally repay him; when a person secretly does good deeds, spirits and gods will repay him. When a person openly does evil, people will naturally seek revenge; when a person secretly does evil, spirits and gods will bring calamity upon him." Regarding these two aspects of a behavior, positive deeds yield positive consequences, while negative deeds yield negative consequences. This is not deceiving people. Therefore, doctors should not solely pursue wealth based on their expertise. As long as they harbor the desire to alleviate the suffering of others, they will surely experience blessings in the underworld.

Furthermore, they should not arbitrarily prescribe expensive medications to individuals who cannot afford them just to showcase their skills, as this goes against the Confucian principles of loyalty and benevolence. I am dedicated to saving and assisting humanity, which is why I have discussed these matters in detail. Those who study medicine should not feel ashamed due to the straightforwardness of my words.

夫为医之法,不得多语调笑,谈谑喧哗,道说是非,议论人物,炫耀声名,訾毁诸医。自矜己德。偶然治瘥一病,则昂头戴面,而有自许之貌,谓天下无双,此医人之膏肓也。

老君曰:人行阳德,人自报之;人行阴德,鬼神报之。人行阳恶,人自报之;人行阴恶,鬼神害之。寻此二途,阴阳报施岂诬也哉。所以医人不得恃己所长,专心经略财物,但作救苦之心,于冥运道中,自感多福者耳。

又不得以彼富贵,处以珍贵之药,令彼难求,自炫功能,谅非忠恕之道。志存救济,故亦曲碎论之,学者不可耻言之鄙俚也。

——《大医精诚·为医之法》

Excerpt Three: Ethical Considerations from *Five Medical Admonitions*

Admonition No. 1: See patients without delay whoever they are, be they rich or poor, suffering from minor or severe illness. Do not procrastinate, pretend to go, or be unapproachable. Try your best to treat your patients no matter how much they can afford to pay you. And do not go against your conscience. If you do go, your medical business will boom day by day.

一戒：凡病家大小贫富人等，请视者便可往之。勿得迟延厌弃，欲往而不往，不为平易。药金毋论轻重有无，当尽力一例施治，自然生意日增，毋伤方寸。

Admonition No. 2: Do not enter the rooms of women, widows, monks, or nuns unless you are accompanied by a second one. Diagnose your patients with care, especially those who suffer from illnesses that are related to private parts. Do not share your patients' histories with your wife because they are quite personal.

二戒：凡视妇人及孀妇、尼僧人等，必候侍者在旁，然后入房诊视，倘傍无伴，不可自看。假有不便之患，更宜真诚窥视，虽对内人不可谈此，因闺阃故也。

Admonition No. 3: Do not take precious medicinal materials like pearls or amber, which would be misunderstood as the possibility of replacing the authentic with the fake. Ask the patients themselves to prepare the precious medicinal materials. Even if the medicine does not work, they will not doubt or slander you. Furthermore, you should not compliment how effective the patients' medicinal materials are, which is not what a superior man should do.

三戒：不得出脱病家珠珀珍贵等送家合药，以虚存假换。如果该用，令彼自制入之。倘服不效，自无疑谤。亦不得称赞彼家物色之好。凡此等非君子也。

Admonition No. 4: You should not entertain yourself by climbing, drinking, or leave your consulting room. You should see the patient who comes to your consulting room in person, and hand out the herbs with care. Your prescription must come from classic formulae. Do not make up new prescriptions, which could incur doubting.

四戒：凡为医者，不可行乐登山，携酒游玩，又不可片时离去店中。凡有抱病至者，必当亲视，用意发药。又要依经写出药帖，必不可杜撰药方，受人驳问。

Admonition No. 5: Do not tease women patients who are whores or who have an affair with men. Treat them as gentlewomen. Return to your home as soon as you finish your diagnosis. Return the medicinal money to those who are in poverty. Even if they come to invite you, do not visit the patients again, and just give them the medicinal. Otherwise, they might try to pay you back in an inappropriate way.

五戒：凡娼妓及私伙家请看，亦当正己，视如良家子女，不可他意儿戏，以取不正。视毕便回。贫窭者药金可璧病回，只可与药，不可再去，以图邪淫之报。

——［明］陈实功《医家五戒》

Chapter Summary

- Different ethical approaches such as utilitarianism, the golden mean, ethical altruism, ethical egoism, can lead to different decisions being made.
- Some scholars are working for constructing universalistic guidelines of ethical behavior toward others that can be applied to everyone, irrespective of their cultural diversity, including humanistic principle, dialogic ethic, among others. Other scholars are advocating ethical relativism.
- Medical ethics is a branch of ethics which pertains to medical practice. It is sometimes viewed as part of the larger field of bioethics.
- Four principles plus scope approach, also known as principlism, includes four moral principles, namely, respect for autonomy, non-maleficence, beneficence, and justice, which are applied in professional-patient relationship.
- Sun Simiao wrote *Qianjin Yaofang (Essential Prescriptions Worth a Thousand Pieces of Gold)*, in which he put forward the notion of the absolute sincerity of great physicians, offering an all-round argumentation on the guiding rules of medical ethics a TCM physician must hold on to.
- The principles of TCM ethics can be approached from five interrelated aspects: purpose of medical practice, requirements of a great physician, manner of medical practice, attitudes towards patients, and attitudes towards other physicians.

Checklist	Yes	No
Cognitive: I have mastered the core information		
Behavioral: I have the ability of putting what I've learned into practice		
Affective: I am willing to carry out what I've learned		
Moral: I will take the ethical consideration into account during practice		

Part Two
Theories

Chapter 3

Culture in General and Culture of TCM in Particular

Chapter Objectives

After reading this chapter, you should be able to:

◆ Define and discuss the nature of culture.

◆ Identify the key features of culture and its main functions.

◆ Summarize the basic features of TCM culture.

◆ Comprehend the basic contents of yin-yang theory.

Key Terms

cheng (honesty)

co-culture or subculture

context

culture or *wenhua*

dynamic

he (harmony)

infinite divisibility

interdependence and reciprocity

inter-transformation

jing (excellency)

learned

opposition and mutual constraint

ren (benevolence)

shared

symbolic

TCM culture

transmittable

waning and waxing

yin-yang theory

Quotes

"We are ready to work together with the international community to open up a new prospect of enhanced exchanges and understanding among different peoples and better interactions and integration of diversified cultures. Together we can make the garden of world civilizations colorful and vibrant." （我们愿同国际社会一道,努力开创世界各国人文交流、文化交融、民心相通新局面,让世界文明百花园姹紫嫣红、生机盎然。）

——2023年3月15日习近平在"中国共产党与世界政党高层对话会"上的主旨讲话

"Culture is one of the two or three most complicated words in the English language." （"文化"位居两到三个含义最为复杂的英文词汇之列。）

——Raymond Williams, 1981, *Culture*

"Culture is roughly anything we do and the monkeys don't." （文化大致可理解为我们所为,而猿猴所不为之事。）

——Lord Raglan

Before reading this section, please consider the following questions:

1.Translate the following Chinese into English:

· 人把自己从野兽中提拔出，可是到现在人还把自己的同类驱逐到野兽里去。祥子还在那文化之城，可是变成了走兽。

· 我的经历告诉你们一个道理：做一个作家只要认识一些字，会写一些字就足够了，有文化的人能成为作家，没文化的人也能成为作家。

2.Do you use the English word "culture" to translate all the instances of "wenhua" mentioned above? If not, what are the reasons behind it?

3.1   Culture: Definitions and Features

Differences and Commonalities

Scientists around the world believe the first humans emerged in Africa around two million years ago. It is the mass migration of these first humans to scatter to other parts of the world that brings about the birth of human society. Biologists contend that the first human woman lived some 200,000 years ago in sub-Saharan Africa (Jandt, 2018). In historical linguistics, some researchers also argue that there is a mother language that "generates later dialects the way plants produce branches or shoots" (Lass, 2015, p. 46). It is universally acknowledged that language and culture are closely intertwined. It follows that there must be a single culture within humanities. Mastering this mother culture would equip us with a magic key that can be used to unlock the secret of human interaction.

Intercultural studies, however, often focus on how cultural groups differ from one another: Jewish differ from Buddhists; Koreans differ from Chinese Americans; the older generation differ from the younger generation. The list can go on and on. It might be tempting to consider the commonality (共性) shared by humans. After all, regardless of cultural backgrounds, people all around the world participate in similar daily activities and share common desires. We all eat, sleep, make friends, and seek respect and love from those who are important to us. Yet, it is also true that how these wants and desires are realized differs from culture to culture. Jewish and Buddhists have different belief systems. Korean Americans and Chinese Americans have different ancestral roots. The old and the young have different goals and lifestyles. In a banquet held by King of Chu in honor of Yanzi (晏子), a famous statesman from the Kingdom of Qi, Yanzi very cleverly refuted (驳斥) King of Chu's claim that people from Qi are habitual thieves by saying that "Oranges grown south of the Huai River are quite delicious; once transplanted to the north, they become uneatable though resembling in shape. Our people become thieves because they now live in Qi". Yanzi's smart retort (反驳) clearly tells us that context or culture plays a key role in determining one's make-up (品格).

Although there are multiple factors that influence our behavior beyond culture, its quality of being everywhere, just like the air that we are breathing, makes culture one of the most powerful. Edward Hall, one of the founding fathers of American intercultural studies, underscores this point when he concludes, "Culture is man's medium. There is not one aspect of human life that is not touched and altered by culture" (Hall, 1976, p. 16). As culture is a core concept in TCM interculturalization, the rest part of this section is devoted to the discussion of the definitions and features of "culture" and its related concepts of context, subculture, and co-culture.

Defining Culture

The human society is as colorful as the sand of the sea, sparkling and shining in its own way to describe, understand, and define the world as well as the behaviors, beliefs, and the identity of an individual. The preceding discussion on the topic of culture should enable you to see that culture is present everywhere and quite complex. It is also difficult to define. Etymologically (从词源角度来看), the English word "**culture**" originated from the Latin nord *cultura*, which denotes (意指) the act of cultivating the land. In the Chinese context, one of the earliest documents containing "文化" is to be found in this statement, "圣人之治天下也,先文德而后武力。凡武之兴为不服也。文化不改,然后加诛。" It can be roughly translated into English as "A wise ruler governs the country with culture and virtue as the first means and then force. Whenever force is used, it is because of the presence of disobedient people. Force is only used when *wenhua* (cultural education) fails". In the traditional Chinese context, *wenhua* is the main method of governing the state advocated by Confucianism, as opposed to *wugong* (the use of force or even violence to achieve social governance (治理) (Editors, 2021). In modern times, *wenhua* is used as the Chinese equivalent of the English word "culture". Over time, the term "culture" has undergone tremendous transformation and evolved to encompass broader meanings related to the cultivation and development of human knowledge, beliefs, customs, arts, and social behaviors.

Turning to the Western academic circle, an early definition was seriously attempted by Edward B. Tylor (Jackson, 2014), an English anthropologist and founder of cultural anthropology, who treated culture as a complex whole of our social traditions. You hear the phrase "popular culture" when people discuss current trends within the culture. In the medical circle, culture can refer to bacteria or cells grown for medical or scientific use. The media also uses the word "culture" to portray aspects of individual taste, such as classical music, fine art, or the appreciation of exceptional food and wine, or even literature. We, as TCM culture facilitators, are concerned with plainer aspects of culture, a definition that can reveal the strong link between culture and communication.

Martin and Nakayama (2018) put forth a definition that

satisfies our criteria. Some modifications have been done to make it in line with TCM interculturalization. Culture can be defined as learned patterns of symbolic systems that guide individuals' perception, values, and behaviors, shared by generations of people, and that are dynamic and heterogeneous. To be concise, culture is a way of life. It guides us in our socialization (适应社会 的过程); it maneuvers us in our interaction; it commands us in our decision-making. We are making culture; meanwhile, culture is making us. Now, let us turn to the features of culture.

Features of Culture

Firstly, culture is **shared**. Whereas our personal experiences and genetic heritage form the unique us, culture unites people with a collective frame of reference. The experience of sharing common reality results in a collective knowledge, a shared sense of identity, common traditions, and unique behaviors that distinguish a particular culture from that of other groups. The idea of culture implies a group of people. An individual's living style can vary from each other; yet the whole pattern in general is a type of living that evolves from the past and shared by a group of people who are experiencing the same environment. For example, in traditional Chinese color symbolism, red represents vitality, celebration, and fertility. In attending wedding ceremonies or observing important festivals like *Chunjie* (Chinese Spring Festival), Chinese people decorate their houses with colorful flowers and couplets. Red is always the main color. Another example of shared perception of culture is evident in how young and old people think of smart phones and other modern technologies. While older people in China usually do not favor smart phones or iPads, younger generations are said to be born with modern technology. This leads to a new concept, **subculture** (次文化), also known as **co-culture** (共文化). In cultures as diversified as Chinese, smaller cultures coexist with each other within the main or dominant culture. They are called subculture. subcultures can be identified in terms of age, dressing style, language, profession, technology, etc. As the term subculture may imply inferiority of some smaller cultural groups, co-culture is preferable.

Secondly, culture is **transmittable**. Closely linked to the first characteristic is the idea that cultural elements are transmitted from one generation to another. For a culture to endure, it must ensure that its essential messages and elements are not only shared but also passed down to future generations. In this way, the past becomes the present and helps create the modern culture and tries to make it last. In his famous poem *My Heart Leaps Up*, William Wordsworth articulates (清楚表明) this cultural transmission clear and loud by singing "The child is the father of the man". This process of transmitting culture serves as cultural inheritance. Since TCM is considered as a jewel in the crown of Chinese culture, it is natural for us to do whatever we can to keep it passed down.

Thirdly, culture is **symbolic**. By examining how culture is passed down from one generation to another, we can smoothly move to the next characteristic, i.e., culture is based on symbols. If we are not able to think symbolically and express those symbols fluently, culture could not be passed on. The symbols of the loong and the five-star red flag are just two typical images of Chinese culture. So important are symbols to the study of TCM interculturalization that we have set aside one complete chapter discussing verbal and non-verbal messages to further develop this connection between symbols and human behavior.

Fourthly, culture is **learned**. Culture is not innate. Humans are not born with culture. Rather, it is acquired. What is shared, transmitted from generation to generation, and symbolized needs to be incorporated into members of each culture through learning. It has direct implications for the study of TCM interculturalization. If you were reared in a home where your family spoke Cantonese, you learned to communicate in that language. If your family engaged in a great deal of touching, you learned about touch as a form of communication. It is important to be aware that not every group responds to the environment equally. In a community where people can meet face to face daily or quite easily, there is probably no need to develop rather sophisticated writing system. However, as China is a vast country with an immense and varied landscape, a coherent written form of Chinese is essential for transcribing and retaining a way of life. For hundreds of years, it has been a tradition for a TCM student to learn after his TCM master by observing, listening, and helping. A learned scholar in ancient China was not only proficient in their prose-making and versed in governance, but also adept (擅长的) in treating patients. This versatility (多才多艺) requires years of learning, training, and practicing.

Finally, culture is **dynamic**. Culture is constantly changing over time. Change may occur during the process of cultural transmission from generation to generation, group to group, and place to place. Five major factors account for the change of cultures (Chen, 2009a): technological innovation such as the invention of new technologies leading to the modernization of TCM, natural and human calamities such as the black death in the Middle Ages, political factors such as Second World War, cultural contact such as globalization bringing out the publicity of TCM, and social considerations such as urbanization. Sometimes, changes can be acute and instantaneous. On numerous occasions, however, change is slow and imperceptible (难以觉察的). It does not occur overnight but requires years of accumulation before reaching a critical moment where there is sharp distinction between the old and new cultures.

Functions of Culture

Perhaps, at this stage of our exploration of culture, it would be easy to answer the following question: What is the basic function of culture? In its simplest form, culture has served the purpose of facilitating human adaptation to their environment for thousands of years and continues to do so today. It guides us in our daily life to deal with familiar and unfamiliar occurrences with appropriate responses (at least we think they are) so we will not feel surprised or unprepared.

As the software of human mind, culture, in addition to allowing our participation in a specific group, serves two major functions. First, culture provides a **context** in which three aspects of human society are constructed and maintained: linguistic, physical, and psychological. Context is commonly shaped by the physical, virtual, or social elements of the situation in which communication takes place. It may have multiple layers such as social, political, and historical. (Consult Chapter Five for more information about the relationship between culture, context, and communication). Second, culture functions to provide structure, stability, and security that are used by the group members to maintain themselves as a healthy system. For example, from a macro perspective, traditional Chinese culture set up a stable and self-contained social system in which Chinese people in Chinese feudal society fared rather well. It is due to the clash with Western culture in the early 19th century that such a fixed pattern began to transform. In the 21st century when globalization has become a reality, such cultural contacts can only become more frequent. How to positively embrace this contact while at the same time without losing the true essence of Chinese culture is a challenge that is worth considering.

Activities

Comprehension Questions

1. Compare and contrast the following definitions of culture. Which (aspects) of the conceptions do you find the most agreeable? Which one is the least agreeable?

- "Culture is defined as an accumulated pattern of values, beliefs, and behaviors shared by an identifiable group of people with a common history and verbal and nonverbal symbol systems" (Neuliep, 2018, p. 16).

- Culture is "an ordered system of meaning and symbols... in terms of which individuals define their world, express their feelings and make their judgments" (Geertz, 1973, p.68), or "culture is the fabric of meaning in terms of which human beings interpret their experience and guide their action" (Geertz, 1973, p. 145).

- "Culture, as I understand it, is essentially a product of leisure. The art of culture is therefore essentially the art of loafing. From the Chinese point of view, the man who is wisely idle is the most cultured man" (Lin, 1998, p. 148).

- 文化的本质就是创造,是人类意识克服自然惰性或摩擦力的那种努力。它的动向始终是发展,是前进,是使更大多数人获得更大的幸福。(郭沫若,1947, p. 1)

- 所谓一家文化不过是一个民族生活的种种方面。总括起来,不外三方面:(一)精神生活方面,如宗教、哲学、科学、艺术等。宗教、文艺是偏于情感的,哲学、科学是偏于理智的。(二)社会生活方面,我们对于周围的人——家庭、朋友、社会、国家、世界——之间的生活方法都属于社会生活一方面,如社会组织,伦理习惯,政治制度及经济关系是。(三)物质生活方面,如饮食、起居种种享用,人类对于自然界求生存的各种事。(梁漱溟,1999,p.19)

2. Define subculture/co-culture in your own words with concrete example(s). What are some typical ways in which members of subcultures/co-cultures function effectively?

3. Among the five features of culture that are discussed in this section, which one impresses you the most and why?

Group Work

The following excerpts are focused on "*wenhua*" and "*wenming*" from Chinese classics.

- It is a law of heaven that the hard and soft interweave; it is a rule of humans that they should observe the rites and conduct restraint. By observing the movement of constellations, we can learn about the change of seasons; by observing development of wenhua, we can enlighten the people and build a civilized society. (刚柔交错,天文也。文明以止,人文也。观乎天文,以察时变;观乎人文,以化成天下。《周易·象传》)

• A wise ruler governs the country with culture and virtue as the first means and then force. Whenever force is used, it is due to the presence of disobedient people. Force is only used when wenhua fails. (圣人之治天下也,先文德而后武力。凡武之兴为不服也。文化不改,然后加诛。《说苑·指武》)

Work with your group members to find more excerpts from Chinese classics about "*wenhua*" or "*wenming*". Compare and contrast between "*wenming*" and "*wenhua*", and report to the class.

Translation

Translate the following text into English.

中华优秀传统文化源远流长、博大精深,是中华文明的智慧结晶,其中蕴含的天下为公、民为邦本、为政以德、革故鼎新、任人唯贤、天人合一、自强不息、厚德载物、讲信修睦、亲仁善邻等,是中国人民在长期生产生活中积累的宇宙观、天下观、社会观、道德观的重要体现,同科学社会主义价值观主张具有高度契合性。

——习近平总书记在中国共产党第二十次全国代表大会上的报告

Writing: My Cultural Stories

As a guiding principle, culture influences every aspect of our life. It guides us in our socialization; it maneuvers us in our interaction; it commands us in our decision-making.

Reflect on your upbringing. What influenced you the most? Who or what helped define you as a college student in the 21st century? What kind of books/ movies/ TV programs motivated you the most?

Then, compose your own cultural story. Share your cultural stories with others if you are willing to do so.

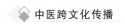

Before reading this section, please consider the following questions:

1. How do you define the cultural aspects of traditional Chinese medicine (TCM)?

2. Do you agree or disagree with the statement that promoting TCM worldwide is a means of communicating traditional Chinese culture globally?

3.2 Essence of TCM

Culture is a complex issue that permeates (渗透) every aspect of our lives. It has a strong impact on individuals within a community, shaping their behavior and thoughts. Cultural influence can even extend beyond the living, as the collective memories of the past are consolidated through present-day cultural practices. To promote the understanding and adoption of TCM across different cultures, it is important to be familiar with both present and past cultural practices. It is equally important to know some highlights of TCM. Otherwise, TCM interculturalization would be out of the question.

Before discussing TCM culture, let us revisit the unveiling (揭幕) ceremony of the TCM Confucius Institute at the Royal Melbourne University of Technology in Australia. During the ceremony, President Xi Jinping has stated that TCM is a valuable asset of ancient Chinese science, a key to unlocking the rich treasure trove of Chinese civilization because it embodies the profound philosophical wisdom and practical knowledge in healthcare that the Chinese nation has accumulated over countless generations. What President Xi Jinping emphasizes here is that TCM is a significant aspect of traditional Chinese culture, serving as one of its prominent carriers. The revival of TCM culture is considered an essential means towards the realization of rejuvenating Chinese culture. To do that, it is of paramount importance to highlight some of the basic features of TCM culture, which is the focus of this section.

Defining TCM Culture

To comprehend TCM culture and its components, it is crucial to devote sufficient time to exploring the relationship between health and culture. After all, TCM aims to manage illnesses and maintain good health. Understanding the role of culture is a prerequisite to comprehending healthcare practices and behaviors since our personal health habits and medical practices are heavily influenced by cultural factors (To learn more about how culture affects our perception of health, please refer to Part 4). In a broad sense, TCM is a branch of natural science that aims to explore human physiology, causes of medical conditions, as well as their treatment and prevention. Therefore, TCM itself can be considered as a component of culture of scientific research. In a narrow sense, TCM embodies the wealth of knowledge that Chinese people have gathered over time to combat diseases. It is intricately intertwined with the Chinese way of life, including philosophy, worldviews, and values. Therefore, one important goal of TCM interculturalization is to foster awareness and appreciation of this specific aspect of TCM culture among diverse societies.

TCM culture consists of both tangible and intangible elements (Zhang Q C, 1999). The intangible part includes Chinese people's attitudes towards life and health, philosophy, values, and worldviews. The tangible part consists of Chinese herbal medicine, medical equipment, medical halls, and diagnostic techniques.

Essential Aspects of TCM Culture

Considering the vast scope of TCM culture, it is more practical to narrow down our focus to its key components. Since TCM is the representative of excellent traditional Chinese culture, which integrates the essence of Confucianism, Taoism and Buddhism, and embodies the core values of Chinese culture, some scholars (e.g., Zheng and Wang, 2012) argue that the core dimensions of TCM culture can be classified into eleven aspects, including the belief in the unity of heaven and humans, the perspective of achieving balance and harmony in life, the emphasis on preventive and timely healthcare, the pursuit of human-centered values, the spiritual quest of respected physicians, the sense of social responsibility in serving patients, people, and the nation, and the adherence to benevolent medical ethics, among others. Professor Zhang Qicheng (2018), a respected scholar from Beijing University of TCM, has condensed the fundamental elements of TCM culture into four Chinese characters, "*ren*", "*he*", "*jing*", and "*cheng*". Each character represents the spiritual, relational, technical, and moral aspects of being a TCM physician.

• Ren (Benevolence)

Simply put, *ren* in Chinese means kindheartedness or benevolence. Professor Zhang Qicheng (2018) argued that this concept serves as the foundation for TCM, reflecting TCM practitioners' belief in demonstrating benevolence through their medical skills and conduct. The renowned philosopher Mencius once stated, "To be a doctor is to display one's benevolent skill," emphasizing the close relationship between doctors and benevolence, which highlights the importance of "*ren*" in TCM physicians' medical practice.

The Chinese character "*ren*" can be written in two ways, each with its own significance. The character consists of a body on top and a heart at the bottom, illustrating that benevolence is expressed through both compassionate intentions and practical actions. Simply claiming to love patients verbally is not enough; it is crucial to demonstrate kindness in one's treatment approach. Additionally, "ren" is written in a way that a body (人) and the Chinese number two (二) stand side by side, symbolizing the equality among individuals. This underscores the importance of doctors treating patients as equals—a key aspect of showing genuine kindness in medical practice.

• He (Harmony)

　　The Chinese culture attaches immense importance to the concept of "*he*", which translates into "harmony" in English. This notion is pervasive (无所不在) and highly valued in various aspects of daily life among Chinese people. During the Spring Festival, greetings such as "*he qi sheng cai*" (和气生财), meaning "harmony brings wealth" are often heard. Chinese people also use the idiom "*jia he wan shi xing*" (家和万事兴) to convey the idea that harmonious relationships lead to prosperity in all endeavors. Confucius specifically acknowledged the significance of harmony, viewing it as a distinguishing factor between individuals of noble character and those of despicable character. He asserted that while gentlemen aim for harmony, mean persons strive for uniformity (君子和而不同, 小人同而不和). This illustrates the paramount importance of harmony in Chinese culture.

　　Harmony, to a certain degree, can be seen as the most essential of the core aspects of TCM culture (Zhang Q C, 2018). From a worldview perspective, the advocacy for harmony between humans and nature is deeply rooted not only in Taoist ideals but also within the practice of TCM. The notion of supreme harmony (太和), which is the ultimate level of harmony described in *The Book of Changes* (《易经》), is also reflected in *Huangdi Neijing*. When asked how one can live a long life, Qibo answered, "Those who knew how to maintain good health in ancient times always aligned their behavior in daily life with nature. They followed the principle of yin and yang and kept in conformity with the art of prophecy based on the interaction between yin and yang." ("上古之人, 其知道者, 法于阴阳, 和于术数") Contrarily, disharmony between yin and yang leads to illness, which underscores the significance of reconciling these opposing forces in the treatment of diseases. Finally, the concept of harmony extends beyond the balance of yin and yang; it is also related to how doctors and patients interact with each other, as well as the harmonious relationships among fellow doctors.

• Jing (Excellency)

"*Jing*", i. e., medical excellency, regarded as one of the essential attributes of exceptional physicians alongside "*cheng*" (honesty), occupies a highly esteemed position. This is primarily because the fundamental purpose of patients visiting a doctor is to seek effective treatment and relief from their sufferings. Therefore, it is imperative for TCM physicians to possess a thorough command of medical skills in order to succeed in their careers. Mastery of these skills serve as a prerequisite (先决条件) for providing optimal care to patients.

In both *Huangdi Neijing* and *Nanjing*, three different levels of "*gong*" (medical practitioners) are outlined: *shanggong* (advanced 上工), *zhonggong* (intermediary 中工), and *xiagong* (elementary 下工). It is the aspiration of every TCM physician to attain the level of "*shanggong*", which represents the highest level of proficiency and expertise in the field.

• Cheng (Honesty)

Sun Simiao, honored as the King of Medicine, places equal emphasis on "*cheng*" (honesty) and "*jing*" (excellency). These values form the cornerstone of ethical conduct and behavioral norms for TCM practitioners. In essence, TCM physicians are expected to be sincere and honest in their dealings with patients while avoiding any form of self-promotion or deceit. The significance of medical ethics, particularly within the context of TCM, is so profound that an entire chapter of Sun Simiao's teachings is dedicated to exploring this ethical framework (For more information, please consult Chapter 2).

TCM culture is deeply intertwined with traditional Chinese culture, making it a distinctive healthcare system that sets it apart from others around the world. To effectively bridge the intercultural gap in TCM interculturalization, it is crucial to understand the core elements of TCM, i. e., "benevolence", "harmony", "medical excellency", and "honesty". Embracing benevolence means displaying compassion and a genuine concern for patients, while harmony emphasizes the balance and synergy (协同作用) between body, mind, and nature. Medical excellence stresses the mastery of TCM skills and knowledge, while honesty underscores the importance of ethical and transparent practices. By recognizing and appreciating these fundamental principles, one can gain deeper insights into the essence of TCM culture and its holistic (整体的) approach to healthcare.

Activities

Comprehension Questions

1. What is the essence of TCM culture?
2. How is the concept of "*ren*" manifested in traditional Chinese medicine?
3. How is the concept of "*he*" manifested in traditional Chinese medicine?
4. How is the concept of "*jing*" manifested in traditional Chinese medicine?
5. How is the concept of "*cheng*" manifested in traditional Chinese medicine?

Debate

Read the following statements.

Culture undergoes constant and subtle yet irreversible changes over time. Traditional Chinese culture, including TCM culture, has a rich history dating back thousands of years. It is widely recognized that culture emerges from human interactions and is influenced by geographical factors and various other elements. Additionally, it is evident that the cultural context of ancient China greatly differs from that of modern China. This leads to an ongoing debate. Some people assert that traditional Chinese culture belongs solely in museums and books, acknowledging its value but considering it impractical in their contemporary life. Others argue that the worth of traditional Chinese culture cannot be solely measured by its practicality; it holds intrinsic value beyond mere functionality.

Discuss with your partners how to appreciate traditional Chinese culture, and then form teams with classmates who share the same side, with 2–4 members on each side. Give alternate speeches for and against the topic.

TCM Stories

Story 1

During the Three Kingdoms Period (220–280 A.D.), there is a story recorded in *The Tales of the Immortals* that explains why TCM and the community of TCM in China are sometimes referred to as the Apricot Grove.

According to the tale, Dong Feng, a Taoist physician, lived in a mountainous region where he selflessly treated patients without accepting any form of payment. Upon curing patients with severe conditions, he requested them to plant five apricot trees, while those with milder ailments were asked to plant just one tree. Over the course of ten years, the whole area was transformed into a magnificent forest with ten thousand apricot trees.

Since then, the term "apricot grove" has become synonymous with TCM. Expressions such as "a warm spring arrives in the apricot grove", "famed in the apricot grove", and "apricot grove master" are used to describe skilled and esteemed practitioners of traditional Chinese medicine.

Questions

1.What implications can be drawn from this story regarding the practice of TCM?

2.What are alternative names for TCM? How do these expressions come to be associated with TCM?

Story 2

Long ago, a child named Zhou came down with a cold and the local doctor advised him to avoid certain types of food that may worsen his condition. The list of prohibited foods was quite extensive, but Zhou strictly followed the advice even as his condition worsened. Later, a renowned TCM physician named Fan Wenfu (1870–1936) was invited to diagnose the child. He found that although most of the pathogens had been eliminated, Zhu's body was still quite weak. Fan then said, "I'm hungry." Quickly, the family cooked a large bowl of noodles with shredded pork and vegetables for him. Fan gave the nourishing dish to the child who enthusiastically ate it. As soon as he received proper nutrition, Zhou's energy was replenished, and he was instantly cured.

Questions

1.What can we learn about TCM syndrome differentiation from this story?

2.Could you tell your class about the stories of other renowned TCM practitioners?

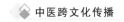

3.3　Yin-Yang Theory and TCM

The philosophical foundation of TCM finds its roots in ancient Chinese philosophy, which emerged from the observations made by early civilizations regarding the existence and transformation of elements, phenomena, and living beings in nature. Through these observations, the Chinese people were able to identify and outline the fundamental principles governing the workings of the world. Yin-yang theory, along with five-phase theory and the theory of qi, constitutes some of the fundamental philosophical components used to comprehend and explain the world and the human body (Chai, 2007). This section primarily focuses on the essence of yin-yang theory since it represents the core of TCM philosophy.

Taichi and the Original Meaning of Yin and Yang

Taichi is a pivotal concept in Chinese cultural legacy, and the Taichi diagram (also known as the Yin-Yang Figure) is revered as "the first diagram in China's nature map" (Editors, 2018, p. 775). It is extensively employed on the pillar of Confucian Temple, the robe of Taoist priests, the emblem of TCM associations, and in book covers centered around TCM culture. In general, the white portion of the diagram implies yang while the black implies yin. The two segments resemble two fish that are head-to-tail, with the corresponding fisheyes (one black and one white) signifying the presence of yang within yin, and vice versa.

Originally, the terms yin and yang were used to describe the shaded or sunny side of a hill — the side facing the sun was considered yang, while the opposite side was referred to as yin (Xie, 2010). Subsequently, these terms were expanded to encompass the contrasting aspects of interconnected entities or phenomena in the natural world. For instance, yang is associated with concepts such as heaven, fire, daytime, qi, anything that embodies light, brightness, warmth, formlessness, and activity. On the other hand, yin is associated with earth, water, night, blood, anything that represents heaviness, darkness, coldness, form, and tranquility. The Chinese ancients perceived that all things or phenomena were both opposites and interconnected. This fundamental understanding forms the basis for the beginning and development of the yin-yang theory.

Basic Features of Yin-Yang Theory

Yin-yang theory represents a Chinese perspective and methodology for comprehending and explaining the world, serving as a prominent philosophy in the history of Chinese thought. It serves as a fundamental theory within TCM, providing insights into the physiological functions and pathological changes of the human body, and guiding clinical diagnosis and treatment. The key characteristics of yin-yang theory encompass the following five aspects, namely, opposition and mutual constraint, interdependence and reciprocity (互惠), waning (衰减) and waxing (增加), inter-transformation, and infinite divisibility (Wang, 2016).

· Opposition and Mutual Constraint of Yin and Yang

Opposing characteristics can be found in all sorts of entities and phenomena in nature, giving rise to what is known as the opposition of yin and yang. The concept of mutual constraint within yin and yang implies that the two opposing forces exhibit a relationship of mutual restraint and control. For instance, spring is associated with warmth, summer with heat, autumn with coolness, and winter with coldness. The warmth and hotness experienced during spring and summer are counterbalanced by the cold and cool qi of autumn and winter. Similarly, the coolness and coldness of autumn and winter are moderated by the warm and hot qi of spring and summer.

· Interdependence and Reciprocity of Yin and Yang

In order for yin and yang to exist, the presence of their respective counterparts is a prerequisite; neither can exist independently. Additionally, the interdependence of yin and yang often signifies a relationship of mutual generation and promotion. For instance, water and fire are regarded as symbols of yin and yang, respectively, enabling people to recognize and experience sensations of coldness and hotness. However, without understanding the concept of cold, it becomes impossible to comprehend heat. This connection is aptly explained by the quote, "Yin cannot be generated without yang, and yang cannot develop without yin" (无阳则阴无以生，无阴则阳无以化).

· Waning and Waxing of Yin and Yang

Waning signifies a decrease in power, vigor, importance, brilliance, size, and so on, while waxing denotes an increase in size, strength, power, and so forth. Therefore, the waning and waxing of yin and yang indicate a state of equilibrium between these interdependent counterparts. Let us consider the yearly climatic change as an example: The transition from winter to spring and then to summer gradually brings warmer weather, representing the process of yin waning and yang waxing. Conversely, the transition from summer to autumn and then to winter progressively brings colder weather, indicating yang waning and yin waxing. Consequently, the climate maintains its balance through such dynamic changes.

· Inter-transformation of Yin and Yang

Nothing remains fixed or unchangeable in the natural world. Yin and yang are no exception. In fact, both yin and yang have the ability to transform into one another under specific conditions, suggesting that yin can transition into yang, and vice versa. This transformation typically takes place during the "extreme phase" in the process of transformation itself. Just as *Su Wen* highlights, "extreme yin gives rise to yang, while extreme yang gives rise to yin", and "extreme cold brings on heat, while extreme heat turns to cold" (阴盛则阳,阳盛则阴;寒极生热,热极生寒).

Fundamentally, in the development of any object or phenomenon, there are two inseparable stages: the waning and waxing of yin and yang, and the inter-transformation of yin and yang. The former can be understood as a process of quantitative change, while the latter represents qualitative change. Put differently, the quality of the waning and waxing serves as a prerequisite for inter-transformation, and inter-transformation is the result of the waning and waxing.

· Infinite Divisibility of Yin and Yang

Yin and yang not only undergo dynamic and constant changes but also possess the ability to be further subdivided. This implies that within each yin and yang category, an infinite number of yin and yang differentiations can be made. This concept is referred to as the infinite divisibility of yin and yang. To illustrate this, let us consider one of the most common and straightforward examples: the division of a day into daytime, representing yang, and nighttime, representing yin. However, the daytime itself can be divided into morning and afternoon, while the nighttime can be divided into the period from nightfall to midnight and the period from midnight to dawn. According to the principles of yin-yang theory, morning is a subset of yang within yang, afternoon is a subset of yin within yang, the period from nightfall to midnight is a subset of yin within yin, and the period from midnight to dawn is a subset of yang within yin.

Application of Yin-Yang Theory in TCM

The relationship between function and substance can be explained through the principles of yin-yang theory. Function is associated with yang, while substance is linked to yin. The physiological activities of the body rely on the metabolism of substances. On one hand, without substances, there would be no support for functional activities. On the other hand, functional activities serve as the driving force for the production of substances in the body. In other words, without functional activities, the metabolism of substances would be impossible to carry out; without necessary substances, functional activities would have no means of being performed. It is no wonder that TCM practitioners adhere to the belief that "yin remains inside to act as a guard for yang, while yang stays outside to act as a servant for yin" (阴在内,阳之守;阳在外,阴之使也).

The origin of yin and yang remains a subject of ongoing debate. Some scholars posit (假定) that the concept of yin and yang emerged no later than the Shang and Zhou Dynasties (1,300 B.C.–256 B.C.), as evidenced by the existence of symbols for both yin and yang documented in the *Book of Changes* (Jiang, 2017). Meanwhile, in the ancient TCM classic *Huangdi Neijing*, yin and yang are widely described and manifested through various opposing elements such as heaven and earth, men and women, fire and water, among other contrasting pairs. In modern times, as TCM culture continues to spread, an increasing number of Westerners have recognized and embraced the concept of yin and yang. Consequently, it has deepened their understanding and acknowledgment of TCM.

Chapter Summary

- The English word "culture" originated from the Latin word *cultura*, which denotes the act of cultivating the land.
- In the Chinese context, one of the earliest documents containing "文化" is to be found in this statement, "圣人之治天下也,先文德而后武力。凡武之兴为不服也。文化不改,然后加诛。".
- Culture can be defined as learned patterns of symbolic systems that guide individuals' perception, values, and behavior, shared by generations of people, that are dynamic

and heterogeneous. To be concise, culture is a way of life. It guides us in our socialization; it maneuvers us in our interaction; it commands us in our decision-making. We are making culture; meanwhile, culture is making us.

- Culture is shared, transmittable, symbolic, learned, and dynamic.
- In a broad sense, TCM can be considered as a component of culture of scientific research. In a narrow sense, TCM embodies the wealth of knowledge that the Chinese people have gathered over time to combat diseases, encompassing philosophy, worldviews, and values.
- The fundamental elements of TCM culture are summarized into four Chinese characters: "ren", "he", "jing", and "cheng". Each character represents the spiritual, relational, technical, and moral aspects of being a TCM physician.
- Yin-yang theory, along with five-phase theory and the theory of qi, constitutes some of the fundamental philosophical components used by Chinese people to comprehend and explain the world and the human body.
- The key characteristics of yin-yang theory encompass five aspects, namely, opposition and mutual constraint, interdependence and reciprocity, waning and waxing, inter-transformation, and infinite divisibility.

Checklist	Yes	No
Cognitive: I have mastered the core information		
Behavioral: I have the ability of putting what I've learned into practice		
Affective: I am willing to carry out what I've learned		
Moral: I will take the ethical consideration into account during practice		

Chapter 4

Human Communication: Concepts, Models and Features

Chapter Objectives

After reading this chapter, you should be able to:

◆ Define and discuss the nature of communication.

◆ Understand two models of human communication.

◆ Explain the relationship between communication and culture.

◆ Offer an insightful analysis of features of TCM interculturalization.

◆ Become aware of the greatness of TCM interculturalization as part of a larger national policy.

Key Terms

communication

constancy

creative

encoding and decoding

flexible

harmony

hierarchy

holistic

I Ching model

imbalanced

interconnected

noise

official

process

reciprocal

symbol

systematic

transactional model

Quotes

"Tolerance, coexistence, exchanges and mutual learning among different civilizations play an irreplaceable role in advancing humanity's modernization process and making the garden of world civilization flourish, as the future of all countries is closely connected nowadays." (在各国前途命运紧密相连的今天，不同文明包容共存、交流互鉴，在推动人类社会现代化进程、繁荣世界文明百花园中具有不可替代的作用。)

———2023年3月15日习近平在"中国共产党与世界政党高层对话会"上的主旨讲话

"Qibo answered, 'Generally, everyone is afraid of death and prefers living, if the physician tells the patient what is beneficial and what is harmful to his body, shows him the proper way of treating which will benefit him and relieve his misgiving that causes him miserable, he will not neglect your advice even if he is a somewhat unreasonable man.'" (岐伯曰：人之情，莫不恶死而乐生，告之以其败，语之以其善，导之以其所便，开之以其所苦，虽有无道之人，恶有不听者乎。)

———《灵枢·师传》

"Confucius said, 'The superior man has nine things which are subjects with him of thoughtful consideration. In regard to the use of his eyes, he is anxious to see clearly. In regard to the use of his ears, he is anxious to hear distinctly. In regard to his countenance, he is anxious that it should be benign. In regard to his demeanor, he is anxious that it should be respectful. In regard to his speech, he is anxious that it should be sincere. In regard to his doing of business, he is anxious that it should be reverently careful. In regard to what he doubts about, he is anxious to question others. When he is angry, he thinks of the difficulties his anger may involve him in. When he sees gain to be got, he thinks of righteousness.'" (子曰："君子有九思：视思明，听思聪，色思温，貌思恭，言思忠，事思敬，疑思问，忿思难，见得思义。")

———《论语·季氏》

Before reading this section, please consider the following questions:

1. The English word "communication" can be translated into several different Chinese phrases such as " 传播、沟通、交流、交际 ". Discuss with your partner(s) this terminological diversity in Chinese community.

2. Have you ever encountered or read about any communicative barrier due to the influence of power? Share the story with your partner(s).

4.1   Defining Human Communication: Western Perspective

Several years ago, in a class discussion on definitions of communication, a student once offered a very clever response when asked, "What is communication? " She answered, "Communication is when my mom says something to my dad or my dad shows something to her, that's it. But I don't get it why there is so much going on to describe it." Perhaps this is the reason sometimes we hate definitions. Where there is a definition, there is a test.

However, definition is useful because it offers us a clear understanding of the topic under consideration. Through analyzing and discussing the essence of communication, we are better equipped with its power in our social life. Unfortunately, like culture, another key concept in TCM interculturalization, it is difficult to find a single definition for the word "communication". If you search for "definition of communication" on the Internet, you will find countless attempts to define this word. Since, to be a competent TCM culture facilitator, it is essential to understand the process of human communication, we would like to spend some time on a detailed exploration of the true essence of communication before proceeding.

Understanding Communication

Because of the difficulty in defining "communication" and its ubiquity in a variety of disciplines such as speech communication studies, linguistics, second language acquisition, and even telecommunications, scholars have put forward a wide variety of definitions. The table below shows common communication elements and their definitions, with some overlap (重叠) in between (adapted from Jackson, 2014).

Elements	Definitions	Disciplines
Symbolic	the symbolic nature of communication means that the words we speak or the gestures we make have no inherent meaning. Rather, they gain their significance from an agreed-upon meaning. When we use symbols to communicate, we assume that the other person shares our symbol system. (Martin and Nakayama, 2022, p. 87)	Intercultural Communication
Process	Communication is a symbolic process whereby reality is produced, maintained, repaired, and transformed (Jackson, 2014, p. 74)	Applied Linguistics
Intentional or Unintentional	Humans are capable of producing sounds and syllables in a stream of speech that appears to have no communicative purpose. These outpourings sound like language, but with no speaker control it is not intentional communication (Yule, 2020, p. 14)	General linguistics
	Communication does not have to be intentional. Some of the most important (and sometimes disastrous) communication occurs without the sender knowing a particular message has been sent (Martin and Nakayama, 2018, p. 41)	Intercultural Communication
Interactive	Communication in face-to-face encounters can be seen as constituted by interactive exchanges of moves and countermoves involving speakers and listeners who actively co-operate in the joint production of meaningful interaction (Gumperz and Cook-Gumperz, 2012, p. 66)	Sociolinguistics
Culture	Culture is communication and communication is culture (Hall, 1976, p. 191)	Intercultural Communication

Infante *et al.* (1990, p. 6) provided a great explanation for the challenge of establishing a single definition:

"Definitions differ on such matters as whether communication has occurred if a source did not intend to send a message, whether communication is a linear process (a source sending a message in a channel to a receiver who then reacts), or whether a transactional (交互的) perspective is more accurate (emphasizing the relationships between people as they constantly influence one another)."

To make things more complicated, when attempting to translate the word "communication" into Chinese, we can end up with at least seven different phrases. It appears that we find ourselves in a rather challenging situation. Thankfully, Hall (1959, p. 191) provided us with a clear and concise definition by claiming "culture is communication, and communication is culture". Does this imply that these two are identical? Certainly not. Hall did not consider the sameness between the two, but rather underscored the intimate interconnectedness between communication and culture. In fact, when examining communication and culture, it is hard to decide which is the voice and which is the echo.

The fundamental reason behind this duality (二元性) stems from the fact that our culture is acquired through the process of communication, while simultaneously, communication serves as a representation of our cultural values and norms. To put it in a slightly different way, culture is both a teacher and a textbook. If you are studying communicating TCM across cultures as part of a degree in some area of humanities such as English, you may already have met some sort of definition of communication, like communication is the transfer of meaning between a sender and a receiver. Infante and his colleagues (1990) overlooked the complexities that arise from the inclusion of digital-mediated (以数字为媒介的) communication. In our daily lives, we are constantly surrounded by digital media like televisions, mobile phones, tablets, and computers. Inevitably, a variety of communicative activities take place under new media and social media.

Miller (2005) summarized the debate surrounding the

notion of communication in a thorough way. She argued that most scholars agree we should refer to communication as a **process**, rather than simply as a single message. The concept of process refers not just to the message itself, but how it is intended, sent, received, and interpreted. We can think of a message as a set of **symbols** like words, sounds, or images, placed together to represent some ideas. While a message might transfer an idea from one person to another, that transfer exists in an ongoing set of messages and ongoing relationships.

For the sake of further study, we consider Samovar and his colleague's definition of **communication** appropriate, "Human communication is a dynamic process in which people attempt to share their thoughts with other people through the use of symbols in particular settings" (Samovar *et al.*, 2017, p. 28). Intercultural communication, therefore, occurs when culture plays a significant role in communication. And TCM interculturalization involves the transmission of TCM-related elements across cultures.

Samovar and his colleagues' understanding of communication encompasses several features that are to be discussed in detail in the next part.

Features of Communication

One model of communication devised by Shannon and Weaver (Baldwin *et al.*, 2014) describes communication as a message produced intentionally by a source and encoded by a transmitter. The encoded message, now a signal, travels through a channel, be it airwave or electric wave, and is decoded by a receiver so that a message can arrive at a destination. **Encoding** (编码) refers to the process of using symbols (e.g., words, gestures, pictures, objects, etc.) to represent ideas or messages, and **decoding** (解码) is the opposite of encoding. Noise (干扰信号) or interference can be physical, as the real, extra, and unpleasant or disturbing sound that can interfere with the passing of the message through the channel.

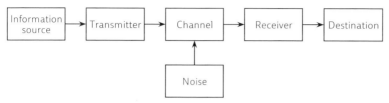

Shannon and Weaver's Mathematical Theory of Communication

This model applies, for example, to a video-chat discussion between Ying Ying, a PhD student of TCM, and her classmates who are international students from several different countries. Her friends do not hear her voice directly, but sound waves coming through cyberspace, and "noise" can be interference in the transmission, a poor Internet connection, or laughter in the office where she is typing. In face-to-face communication, Ying Ying's voice and gestures become the transmitter, as she translates her ideas into a message. The channel is airwaves and the receiver, her friends' ears and eyes. In modern context, noise can be physical, such as whether the room is too cold, or it can be psychological. In this case, cultural and language differences are a type of noise.

This model emphasizes the process aspect of communication, which is almost universally agreed upon. Yet, some argue that this model is too simplistic because, especially in face-to-face communication, both parties exchange messages simultaneously. The inclusion of feedback to the model somewhat addresses this criticism. It means that the person receiving the message can respond verbally or nonverbally to the sender, either immediately or later. In other words, scholars agree that communication is transactional or dynamic. It involves giving and taking, not just message exchange, but mutual influence. Hence, the addition of feedback to the process leads to a new model called the **transactional model** of communication.

A third area of agreement is that communication is

symbolic — participants use verbal and nonverbal messages to represent something else. The fact that communication is symbolic is important for the study of TCM interculturalization, as it deals with the meaning of words. It shows that communication breakdowns can happen not just due to psychological or physical distractions, but also because of misunderstandings in the meaning conveyed. According to the semantic (语义的) triangle theory (Ogden and Richards, 1923, p. 11), we establish a connection between words and our lived experiences through concepts or thoughts. This is important in intercultural communication because same symbols can be associated with different cultural realities. For example, for TCM physicians, "邪气", literally meaning "evil air", is a certain kind of pathogenic (致病的) factors, but among the majority of Caucasian (白种人) doctors trained in Western medicine, "evil" usually is associated with devil. Transmission can break down unless cultural barrier is dismantled. For more information, please refer to Chapter 7 on verbal communication.

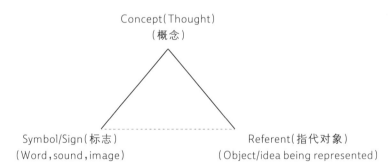

The relationship between symbol/sign and referent is unstable

Semantic Triangle Theory

However, scholars disagree on other aspects of communication. For example, they sometimes have different opinions on whether it is possible to communicate with oneself. As you wonder what kind of doctors you should visit, are you communicating? Some call this thought. Others call it intrapersonal communication (自我沟通), when one creates messages for oneself, within the mind. There is another debate about whether communication always requires intention. While some scholars insist on the senders' intentionality as the prerequisite for communication (Baldwin *et al.*, 2014), Watzlawick *et el.* (1967, p. 51) argued that "one cannot not communicate", emphasizing the persuasiveness of communication. Suppose someone is nearby, when any intentional and unintentional behavior such as dozing off in class or ignoring an inquiry from a patient is observed. As long as this person gives meaning to the behavior/message, it is communication (Baldwin *et al.*, 2014). Martin and Nakayama (2022, p. 41) shared the same view by arguing that "some of the most important communication occurs without the sender knowing a particular message has been sent".

Ongoing Debate

The debate on whether intention is a prerequisite for communication or not is relevant to the study of TCM interculturalization, especially in terms of nonverbal communication. While it is meaningful to examine how individuals from diverse cultural backgrounds intentionally construct messages, it is equally important to acknowledge the unintended consequences of our TCM intercultural activities. Sometimes, non-intentional message could leave a deeper impression, which may even serve to negate the intentional one.

—— **Activities** ————————————————————————

Comprehension Questions

1.Summarize the debates on the understanding of communication.

2.In what way are culture and communication intertwined? Use examples if necessary.

3.What is semantic triangle theory? In what way do cultural elements influence the communicative process from the perspective of semantic triangle theory?

4. Explain the transactional model of communication with concrete TCM intercultural activities.

5. Neuliep (2018, p. 14) argued that "Communication is dependent on the context in which it occurs". Explain what is meant by the claim that "communication is contextual". Can you think of examples of how context has influenced your behavior?

Group Work

1. Do bibliographical research to locate at least four models of communication put forward by overseas scholars. List their features and key components. Apply each model to analyze one TCM intercultural activity to find out their advantages and drawbacks respectively. Report to the class orally.

2. The following dialogue comes from *Mo Zi* (《墨子》), one of the most important books in the history of Chinese philosophy. Master Mo Zi was angry with Geng Zhu Zi. Geng Zhu Zi asked, "Do I not surpass other men?" Master Mo Zi in turn asked, "If I were about to ascend Taihang Mountain and I yoked a thoroughbred horse and an ox to my cart, which one would I urge on?" Geng Zhu Zi replied, "You would urge on the thoroughbred horse. " Master Mo Zi asked, "And why would I urge on the thoroughbred horse?" Geng Zhu Zi replied, "Because the thoroughbred horse is up to the task." Master Mo Zi said, "I also take you to be up to the task." Geng Zhu Zi was enlightened. (子墨子怒耕柱子。耕柱子曰:"我无俞于人乎?"墨子曰:"我将上太行,以骥与牛驾,将谁策?"耕柱子曰:"将策骥也。"墨子曰:"何故策骥而非策牛也?"耕柱子曰:"骥足以策。"墨子曰:"我亦以子为足以策,故怒之。"耕柱子悟。)

What do you learn from this anecdote about the importance of effective communication?

Translation

Translate the following text into English.

加强国际传播能力建设,全面提升国际传播效能,形成同我国综合国力和国际地位相匹配的国际话语权。深化文明交流互鉴,推动中华文化更好走向世界。

——习近平总书记在中国共产党第二十次全国代表大会上的报告

Debate

Read the following statements.

Professor Watzlawick claims that we cannot avoid communicating, while Professor Martin argues that messages can be captured by the receiver with the sender's unawareness. Does eavesdropping constitute a communicative behavior or not?

Form teams with classmates who share the same side, with 2–4 members on each side. Give alternate speeches for and against the topic.

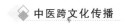
Before reading this section, please consider the following questions:

1. It is said that Chinese style of communication is indirect and implicit. Do you agree or disagree with it? Choose your side and defend your position with examples.

2. "Reading between lines" is an advanced human cognition that can also be culturally conditioned. Discuss with your partner(s) to find out how culture plays a role in uncovering the hidden meaning.

4.2 Defining Human Communication: Chinese Perspective

Chinese Style of Communication

Communication is a universal activity that exists in all societies. Every day, we are sending and receiving messages to others, and even to ourselves, with or without our awareness. Hence, the development of a universal model or theory of human communication is possible, especially when applied to the explanation of the existence, nature, and components of communication. Yet, as what has been discussed in the first section of this chapter, there is still no consensus about a unified model of communication. One important reason is that the way to perceive the concept and to exercise communication activities is subject to the influence of the culture a person lives in. This is also the key element centered on our book about TCM interculturalization.

To illustrate the involvement of culture in communication, let us revisit the classic model of human communication formulated by Shannon and Weaver (Baldwin *et al.*, 2014). Encoding, a necessary internal process of creating messages out of ideas, is thought to be the first step in communicative process. It is well acknowledged that people from different cultural backgrounds tend to rely on different symbols to represent the same idea. Chinese people, therefore, may have different symbolic systems from the British. Besides, research (Fang and

Faureb, 2011) shows that Chinese communication style has at least five distinctive characteristics, namely, implicit communication (含蓄式沟通), listening-centered communication (倾听式沟通), polite communication (客气式沟通), insider-communication (内外有别式沟通), and face-directed communication (重面子沟通). For Chinese people, communication serves to strengthen or weaken each other's face or self-esteem. To reduce the negative impact of communicative behavior, strategies such as being economical with the fact (不把话说满) are employed to allow some room for others to fill in, just like working out a jigsaw puzzle.

Traditionally, the way in which Chinese philosophers and artists expressed themselves can be rather vague. Feng Youlan (1966, p. 12), a famous modern Chinese philosopher, argued that "Suggestiveness, not articulateness, is the ideal of all Chinese art, whether it being poetry, painting, or anything else". Chinese style of communication is no exception. According to Chinese literary tradition, in good poetry, "the number of words is limited, but the ideas it suggests are limitless" (Feng, 1966, p. 12). An intelligent reader of poetry, therefore, seeks to read what is outside the poem. Widely known proverbs such as "Silence is gold" and "Who talks much, errs much" (言多必失) warn people against unnecessary speech. From a cultural standpoint, it becomes evident that people from Chinese cultural communities have distinct communication styles.

A New Model of Human Communication with Chinese Characteristics

Working in the domain of intercultural communication for years and as a Chinese American, Professor Chen Guoming (2009b) has developed a model of communication from the Chinese perspective, specifically based on *The Book of Changes*. It is assumed that this model can be used to better understand Chinese communication behavior from a micro perspective.

In order to understand his model, it is useful to take a look at *The Book of Changes*, an ancient collection of Chinese wisdom that appeared more than two thousand years ago. "Bian" or change is a key concept of *I Ching*, and this is why *I Ching* is translated into English as *The Book of Changes*. *I Ching*, which serves as a guide for decision-making and understanding of the dynamic changes in the world, is based on the principle of the interconnectedness of all things and the notion that change is constant. The dialectical (辩证的) interaction between the two opposite but complementary forces, i.e., yin and yang, is the origin of change. While yin represents the friendly, yielding (顺从的), or submissive force, yang is unyielding and dominating. They are interchangeable and interpenetrating (相互渗透). Three assumptions are found in *I Ching* as follows, which are meant to regulate the alternate and continuous change of yin and yang (Chen, 2009b, p. 73):

• The universe, including human interaction, is a great whole, in which all is but a transitional process.

• The transformation of the universe is moving in a cyclic manner.

• This cyclic transformation of the universe is an on-going, endless process. Thus, all the contradictions in human society will be resolved in this continuously transforming process of the universe.

The interaction between yin and yang has become a fundamental Chinese philosophy to explain the rise and fall of life. It is also used to explain the changes and outcomes in human activities aiming to reach harmonious balance. (For more information about yin and yang and their relationship, please refer to the further reading section in Chapter 3.) In a sense, it can be used to explain human communication with Chinese characteristics. Professor Chen Guoming thus put forward an *I Ching* model which is diagrammed in the following figure.

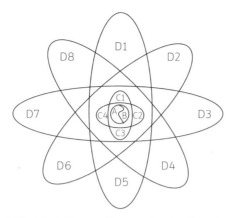

Dialectical Model of Human Communication Based on *I Ching*

Characteristics of Human Commination

This model highlights five features of human communications, holistic, creative, hierarchical, interconnected, and harmonious.

Firstly, human communication is **holistic** in nature. Right in the middle of the diagram are located participants represented by A and B as the two or more interdependent forces. Every force can change itself and go through an internal process of transformation, occupying the lowest level of communication. It is the interaction and connection of these forces that come together to create a whole and integrated system. Contradictions and conflicts can arise during the interaction, but effective communication relies on the interactions maintaining a dynamic balance.

Secondly, human communication is creative. The cyclic interaction between A and B results in C1, C2, C3, and C4, forming larger subsystems than those created by the communicators themselves. The interaction of A and B keeps happening at an upper level, which is represented by D1 to D8. Of course, the highest level is human communication.

Thirdly, the creative feature is accompanied by a third characteristic, i. e., **hierarchy** （层 次 体 系） which is further determined by two elements: time and space. The time factor requires the communicators to know when it is appropriate to begin, keep, and end an interaction verbally and nonverbally. The space factor refers to the fixed markers such as position, status, in addition to physical environment (Consult Chapter 5 for information about how context plays a role in human communication).

Fourthly, human communication is **interconnected**. Each layer is closely linked to the one below and the one above. All subsystems contain the elements of yin and yang. In other words, they are interconnected, interpenetrated, and interdetermined. Familiar Chinese sayings like "Things go into reverse when pushed to the extreme" (物极必反) and "Out of extreme joy comes extreme sorrow" (乐极生悲) reflect this philosophical idea which runs in the blood of Chinese people.

Finally, human communication is harmonious, or **harmony** is the goal of human communication rather than its means. It is conditioned by the dynamic balance between yin and yang, and it is also the driving force for the two elements to penetrate each other. The loss of balanced forces leads to breakdown in communication, which is unnatural, thus must be corrected.

Chinese model of human communication emphasizes holistic, creative, interconnected, hierarchical, and harmonious nature of communication. Instead of resorting to a universal communicative model, a Chinese model as developed by Professor Chen Guoming is useful in describing and analyzing Chinese communicative behavior. As this model incorporates some key features of Chinese culture, it is also applicable to TCM interculturalization, reminding TCM culture facilitators to be aware of differences of value orientations towards communication.

─── Activities ──

Comprehension Questions

1. Summarize the Chinese style of communication as discussed in this section with concrete examples.

2. In what way does Chinese style of communication facilitate TCM interculturalization? In what way does it impede communicating TCM across cultures?

3. What are some of the Chinese value orientations incorporated in the *I Ching* model of human communication?

4. Compare and contrast the *I Ching* model of human communication and the transactional model to discover their similarities and differences.

5. Shao *et al.* (2014) put forward another Chinese mode of communication based on Confucianism. They argue that four communication modes can be summarized, namely internalization mode of value communication, emotion mode of morality communication, extrapolation mode of interpersonal communication, and situation mode of knowledge communication. Compare and contrast this model with Chen (2009b)'s to discover their similarities and differences.

Group Work

The following excerpt comes from "Autumn Floods" in *Zhuang Zi* (《庄子·秋水》), one of the foundational texts of Taoism.

The Spirit of the Ocean replied, "You cannot speak of ocean to a well-frog, who is limited by his abode. You cannot speak of ice to a summer insect, who is limited by his short life. You cannot speak of Tao to a pedagogue, who is limited in his knowledge. But now that you have emerged from your narrow sphere and have seen the great ocean, you know your own insignificance, and I can speak to you of great principles." ([北海若答]"井蛙不可以语于海者,拘于虚也;夏虫不可以语于冰者,笃于时也;曲士不可以语于道者,束于教也。今尔出于崖涘,观于大海,乃知尔丑,尔将可与语大理矣。")

What is the basis for communication, according to the Spirit of the Ocean? Idioms like "对牛弹琴" are concerned about the impossibility of conveying messages under specific circumstances. Find more similar idioms and/or sayings, and then discuss with your partners their causes and offer some possible strategies if possible.

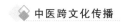
Case Study

Case 1

Paige Yang grew up with Chinese family members in Kailua, Hawai'i. As the oldest granddaughter, she's very close to her grandmother from Zhongshan, China. Yang says her grandmother taught her Chinese traditions.

Yang's entire family lives in the same neighborhood, and her mom is one of five children. "I was at my grandmother's house every day and would stay the night a lot," Yang says. Growing up in a Chinese family, she says that she always wanted to be a doctor. Western biomedicine never resonated with her because she felt it didn't address the spirit and emotions adequately.

Yang studied abroad in Hangzhou, China, during her junior year and took a one-on-one TCM course from Dr. Zhang, a professor at Zhejiang Chinese Medical University. "That course completely changed my aspirations and career path," she says. After graduating from college, she spent a gap year abroad in China, taking more elective classes in TCM theory before returning to the US and studying at the American College of TCM in San Francisco, receiving both her master's and doctorate degrees.

"I do the work because of the profound changes that take place in my treatment room and on the treatment table," she says. "I often feel like in the 'sick care' system of us, people are not heard, seen, or provided with thorough enough healthcare." Yang laments how little time most patients get with their doctors. "I often find my patients have a lot of the answers to their own health questions, but nobody sat with them to flesh it out," she says. "My patients feel so empowered when they're heard and their ideas about their own bodies are validated."

Questions

1.What factors have prompted Paige Yang to embark on a TCM career?

2.What role does communication play in healthcare management?

Case 2

In recent years, elements of TCM have become suddenly trendy. Cupping, which uses suction on the skin to improve the flow of energy known as qi, surged in popularity after the world saw Michael Phelps' cupping marks at the 2016 Olympics. "I think it's great that TCM is trending because it's such a wonderful medicine, "says Paige Yang, a Chinese American TCM physician.

Still, she does have concerns. "If the people spreading the information don't have the proper training, credentials, or expertise and are positioning themselves that way and teaching about a TCM modality without being a TCM practitioner, then I do think it's harmful," she says.

To avoid cultural appropriation—adoption of certain language, behavior, clothing, or tradition belonging to a minority culture or social group by a dominant culture or group in a way that is exploitative, disrespectful, or stereotypical, Yang suggests investing time studying the roots and origins of the practice, remaining humble, and not assuming that you are an expert. Thinking of TCM merely as a new spa treatment to try or a trendy addition to a beauty routine leaves out the tradition's rich history and breadth of knowledge, as well as a valuable lens through which to see and experience health. Yang hopes that people realize TCM is a full medical system, developed over thousands of years with a rich cultural heritage.

Questions

1.In what way may the popularity of cupping and guasha on the social media do harm to TCM? How do you understand Yang's warning in paragraph two.

2.What is cultural appropriation? In what way could TCM be culturally appropriated? Can you find some examples? How can we prevent it from happening?

Survey

As social media has had a huge impact on human life, the way how TCM can be transmitted across cultures is also changing drastically. Before the widespread use of internet, it is often necessary to get a face-to-face contact with cultural strangers in order to engage in TCM interculturalization, which can be time- and money-consuming. Now, social media such as TikTok offers an easy-to-access and quick-to-reach approach. Conduct a survey on how social media has impacted TCM interculturalization. Weigh the pros and cons of each platform.

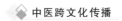
4.3 Features of TCM Interculturalization

The Rise of China

While Westerners treat the theory behind TCM with curiosity or even skepticism, its most important attribute is effectiveness. Much like Chinese medicine, China is adaptable and flexible. In 2021, China Global Television Network launched a series of programs aiming to uncover the secrets to China's success, as part of a larger program to mark the centenary (一百周年纪念) of Communist Party of China. In an interview between the host Tian Wei and the guest Hiria Ottino, President of the Council on Pacific Affairs and a TCM practitioner, they are trying to find out how Chinese people can look back at the 100th anniversary of the Communist Party of China with pride without becoming complacent. When asked about his impression of TCM, Dr. Ottino recounted an unforgettable experience of several years ago. A group of smiling yet doubtful Western doctors finally were convinced by the effectiveness of TCM though miles of barriers exist between them about the comprehensibility of Chinese theories such as qi, acupoint (穴位), etc. In other words, it is possible to communicate TCM across cultures if some commonalities are found; in this case, efficacy is the golden rule.

Under the guidance of Global Civilization Initiative (全球文明倡议) proposed by President Xi Jinping, TCM culture facilitators have assumed a new responsibility, i.e., to advocate the respect for the diversity of civilizations, the common values of humanity, the importance of inheritance and innovation of civilizations, and robust international people-to-people exchanges and cooperation. Because TCM does have its own features and cultural particularities (特殊性) that require constant interpretation and adjustment, some of the essential characters of TCM interculturalization are summarized in this section.

Hybrid of Dynamics and Constants

It is well-known that TCM has its roots in traditional Chinese philosophy, especially that of Taoism and Confucianism. Among three dominant ideas of TCM, that is, yin-yang theory, five-phase theory, and theory of visceral manifestation(藏

象理论), the former two are part of greater Chinese canons. The basic principles and rationales remain a constant, unlikely to change and evolve in their own nature. This **constancy**, however, does not equal theoretical and practical stagnation. Quite the opposite. Their realization requires constant adaptation to the current conditions. Another example goes to TCM diagnostics (诊断学). The four basic diagnostic methods, i.e., inspection, auscultation and olfaction (闻诊), inquiry, and palpation or pulse-taking (切诊), remain unchanged for thousands of years. Yet, their implementation has undergone improvement. All contribute to the dynamic communication conditioned by firmly believed theories and ideas.

This hybrid of dynamics and constants reminds TCM culture facilitators to remain at once flexible and autonomous. Flexible TCM interculturalization is about managing cultural differences creatively and adaptively across a wide variety of situations. It emphasizes the importance of integrating knowledge and an open-minded attitude and putting them into adaptive and creative practice in communicating TCM across cultures. Different perceptions toward health, body, and nature must be taken into consideration. For instance, some people around the world might consider five-phase theory as primitive and backward. Flexible and creative ways of transmitting this and similar concepts must be worked out to create a mutual space of communication which is both dynamic and amicable so the stereotypical and shallow perception of TCM can be dismantled. At the same time, however, TCM culture facilitators must remain autonomous. It means the participants must stand firm and no concessions can be made regarding some core issues that are likely to do harm to individual integrity and/or national image.

Systematic and Official Agenda

Since the launch of the Belt and Road Initiative, the promotion of TCM globalization always occupies an essential part of the overall agenda. In other words, the whole project has been endorsed by the Chinese government, embraced by Chinese people, and welcomed by friends all over the world. It is **systematic** in nature. Governments at different levels have issued documents and guiding policies to support "TCM Going Global" project. Chinese universities and research institutes (like Zhejiang Chinese Medical University, Beijing University of Chinese Medicine, to name just two) have cooperated with organizations / institutions of higher education abroad to establish TCM Confucius Institute, TCM Overseas Research Center where courses on all aspects of TCM such as traditional Chinese culture, Chinese reading and writing, elements of TCM, philosophical foundations of TCM, tai-chi are offered to local people. These programs have received warm welcome for their easy-to-access and learner-friendly nature.

The scientific formulation and implementation of development plans have become an important way for China to govern the country. *Outline of the 14th Five-Year Plan (2021–2025)*, the newest national plan, has identified six key areas for the development of TCM, one of which is the emphasis on the immediacy (紧迫性) of its globalization. With this outline as the general guiding principle, each province and municipality has released their own *14th Five-Year Plan*, all of which include the official requirements and goals of TCM globalization. Thus, platforms and opportunities for communicating TCM across culture abound.

Mixture of Tangible and Intangible Cultural Transmission

TCM culture and theories have a part to play in TCM interculturalization. What is of equal importance is Chinese materia medica (中药材), including Chinese patented medicine (中成药) and various dosage forms. What makes TCM even more charming lies in its flexible employment of local resources in choosing medicinal herbs. Finally, because of the emphasis on moral quality as well as superb medical skills, anecdotes of great TCM physicians have become wonderful inspiration for young pupils of TCM, which are also engaging to cultural strangers. All the above-mentioned tangible and intangible cultural elements have become key components of TCM interculturalization.

TCM culture facilitators are required to master some basic understanding of cultural stories, philosophical and diagnostic theories, principles related to TCM. Preferably, additional mastery of some practicalities like how to do household massaging, taichi, and even Chinese paper-cutting, calligraphy (书法), etc., is also desirable.

Imbalanced as well as Reciprocal Intercultural Activity

Unlike other instances of intercultural communication whose meaning is negotiated and shared, TCM interculturalization, to a great extent, is **imbalanced**, if not unilateral, requiring constant interpretation, clarification, and adjustment. It is undeniable that TCM classics are difficult to crack, not just because they are written in classic Chinese two or three thousand years ago, but also because scholars and practitioners of TCM of later generations have projected their personal understandings into these classics, something like biblical exegesis (诠释). This reflects a dynamic and flexible translation of theories into practice. It is out of Chinese culture that TCM is derived; and it is natural to look to Chinese scholars for help in terms of textual and/or explanatory confusion. It follows that the scales of binary communication among cultures about TCM would tilt toward the originators or masters of the host culture.

This imbalance of communication requires TCM culture facilitators to be aware that power is not a simple one-way proposition but is dynamic. Other participants in TCM interculturalization are not powerless; they may assert and negotiate their power. After all, as the *I Ching* model of human communication clearly indicates, communicators are constantly changing. We, dominant cultural groups of TCM, of course, want to safeguard our positions of privileges. However, too firm grasp of this power would only serve to frighten others away. Sometimes, a little surrender of power to the weaker would result in unexpected yet wonderful outcomes. It requires years of practice and learning to strike a balance.

TCM interculturalization is also **reciprocal** in that it benefits TCM to embrace modernization, thus initiating a new round of renovation. It is noteworthy that by promoting TCM across cultures, we are actually offering Chinese wisdom in combating diseases, contributing to a global community of health for all (人类健康命运共同体). At the same time, it pushes TCM practitioners to actively embrace new methods, applying internationally recognized ways to keep up with the trend.

Part of Chinese Dream

Transmission of TCM across cultures is part of a larger cultural transmission project which is incorporated into the great rejuvenation of the Chinese Nation. The pursuit of Chinese dream has become a highly discussed goal since the 18th National Congress of the Communist Party of China. The concept of Chinese dream was put forward by Xi Jinping, after he was sworn in as the General Secretary of the Communist Party of China. When he visited "The Road Toward Renewal Exhibition" in Beijing along with the other members of the Political Bureau Standing

Committee, Xi Jinping emphasized that realizing the nation's great rejuvenation "is the greatest dream in the country's modern history".

Chinese dream, a wonderful and realistic ambition, features national prosperity, rejuvenation, and people's welfare. Conceptually, the last one has a lot to do with healthcare, in which TCM plays a pivotal role. Chinese dream is neither a closed nor an exclusive dream. Inclusiveness, mutual-benefit, and common development are innate characters of the Chinese dream. Communicating TCM across cultures is an indispensable component of Chinese dream whose realization also contributes to the fruition (取得成果) of TCM interculturalization.

Communicating TCM across cultures is a project that is characterized as being dynamic as well as constant, systematic and official, intangible as well as tangible, imbalanced as well as reciprocal, and great. It has its own characteristics besides sharing commonalities with other types of intercultural activities. A more comprehensive exploration will be offered in the subsequent chapters about the cultural influences on healthcare and TCM interculturalization.

Chapter Summary

• A variety of definitions of "communication" as well as half a dozen Chinese equivalents indicate the complexity of this common human activity.
• When examining communication and culture, it is hard to decide which is the voice and which is the echo.
• Human communication is a dynamic process in which people attempt to share their thoughts with other people through the use of symbols in particular settings.
• Human communication is dynamic, symbolic, transactional, and (un)intentional from the perspective of Western culture.
• From the perspective of *I Ching*, human communication is meant to achieve harmony. It is holistic, creative, interconnected, hierarchical, and harmonious.
• Being adaptable and flexible is a secret to China's success.
• Global Civilization Initiative advocates the respect for the diversity of civilizations, the common values of humanity, the importance of inheritance and innovation of civilizations, and robust international people-to-people exchanges and cooperation.
• Communicating TCM across cultures is a project that is characterized as being dynamic

as well as constant, systematic and official, intangible as well as tangible, imbalanced as well as reciprocal, and great.

Checklist	Yes	No
Cognitive: I have mastered the core information		
Behavioral: I have the ability of putting what I've learned into practice		
Affective: I am willing to carry out what I've learned		
Moral: I will take the ethical consideration into account during practice		

Chapter 5

Culture Values and TCM Interculturalization

Chapter Objectives

After reading this chapter, you should be able to:

◆ Learn about cultural values and their functions.

◆ Identify and describe two cultural value orientations.

◆ Gain a deeper understanding of TCM values.

◆ List strengths and limitations to each framework for understanding culture.

◆ Offer suggestions about how to communicate TCM across cultures effectively.

Key Terms

activity orientation

explanatory function

human nature orientation

human-nature orientation

identity meaning function

individualism vs. collectivism

long-term vs. short-term orientation

masculinity vs. femininity

motivational function

power distance

relational orientation

time orientation

uncertainty avoidance

value

─ Quotes ─────────────────────────────────

"I hope all Chinese will continue to carry forward Chinese culture and draw strength from it, while promoting exchanges between Chinese civilization and other civilizations. Let us tell the stories of China   well, and make our voices heard; let us promote mutual understanding between the people of our own country and those of other lands and create a better environment for achieving the Chinese Dream." (希望大家继续弘扬中华文化,不仅自己要从中汲取精神力量,而且要积极推动中外文明交流互鉴,讲述好中国故事、传播好中国声音,促进中外民众相互了解和理解,为实现中国梦营造良好环境。)

——2014年6月6日习近平在会见第七届世界华侨华人社团联谊大会代表
时的讲话

"Man correlates with heaven and earth and corresponds with the shifting of the sun and the moon." (人与天地相参也,与日月相应也。)

——《灵枢·岁露论》

Consider the past and you will know the present. (鉴古知今)

——Chinese saying

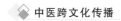

Before reading this section, please consider the following questions:

1. What factors may influence your decisions on what to think about, what to disregard and how to act?

2. At the cultural, ethnic, gender, professional and relational level, why do people have different value systems?

5.1 Basics of Cultural Values

Defining Values

In the previous chapter when culture was explored, we temporarily provided a very limited definition of the term "values": Cultural values are a set of statements that a group of people believe to be beneficial, correct, or valuable. Cultural values, which vary from culture to culture, can be understood as the cultural commonalities that a nation presents in dealing with issues like self-perception, interpersonal relationships, among other things (Xue, 2015). Different cultural values bring out different attitudes and lifestyles, thus constituting different cultural characteristics and determining the development trajectory of the nation (Harrison and Kagan, 2006). It is considered as the national spirit of a country, the ideals, beliefs, and consensus that are held in common. A nation's culture usually has systematic values. Although there are countless exceptions in any one culture, we can still make relatively accurate or broad statements about a particular culture.

For the sake of practicality, **values** are defined in this textbook as shared ideas about what counts as important or unimportant, right or wrong, fair or unfair, ethical or unethical. To put it in another way, values are "the worldview of a cultural group and its set of deeply held beliefs" (Yan *et al.*, 2020, p. 97). Although each of us has developed our unique set of values based on our socialization and life experience, there are also larger values at work on a cultural level. Values are considered as the spiritual aspect of a specific culture, which is observed unconsciously in one's daily life. Therefore, it is of high importance to explore the function of cultural values in order to practice TCM interculturalization effectively.

Functions of Cultural Value Patterns

Cultural value patterns serve many functions, including the **identity meaning function, explanatory function,** and **motivational function**, to name just three.

The first important function of cultural values is to offer identity meaning. As you can see, cultural values provide the points of reference to answer the most fundamental question of each human being: Who am I? For example, in the larger US middle class, American values often emphasize individual initiative and achievements. A person is considered "qualified" or "successful" when he takes the personal initiative to realize his American dream of becoming rich. However, in China, financial success is only a minor scale. What matters in deciding whether a person is successful or not is to see how much he has done to the prosperity of the community. In his first volume of *Essential Prescriptions Worth a Thousand Pieces of Gold,* Sun Simiao, King of Medicine, clearly states that "the object of medical practice is to help, not to gain material goods" (所以医人不得恃己所长，专心经略财物).

Still, some universal values of the world can be deduced from human history. Peace, freedom, social progress, equal rights, and human dignity are highly praised in the *Charter of the United Nations.* These are values that can transcend cultural differences. At the Communist Party of China in Dialogue with World Political Parties High-Level Meeting (中国共产党与世界政党高层对话会) which was held in March 2023, General Secretary Xi Jinping delivered a keynote address in which he proposed the Global Civilization Initiative. As part of the Initiative, Xi Jinping advocated that the common values of humanity, claiming peace, development, equity (公平), justice, democracy, and freedom are the common aspirations of all peoples.

Secondly, cultural values also function as explanation for our actions. Within our own group, we experience acceptance and sense of belonging; we do not have to constantly explain our actions or rationale. Our commonly shared values are understood without explanation. With people of different groups, however, we may need to explain or even defend our culture-based behavior with a lot of effort. For example, it is only too natural for a Chinese patient to feel OK when his TCM physician tells him that he may suffer from liver heat (肝火). However, a person from another culture who has no clue as to what liver heat is might naturally associate it with the dysfunction of liver. Intercultural misunderstandings may pile up if we do not attach the appropriate cultural values to explain the expressions.

Still another very important function of values lies in the ability to motivate us, serving as the internal drives because they determine, though implicitly, what rewards or punishments can result from our obeying or disobeying the basic norms. For example, in the US, proverbs like "Time is money" "There is no time like the present", and "He who hesitates is lost", underscore the idea that people who do not waste time and make quick decisions are highly valued. In Chinese culture, respect for the wisdom of the elderly is embodied in those proverbs like "You'll suffer loss if you don't take advice from the old" (不听老人言, 吃亏在眼前). No wonder, the experience accumulated by great TCM physicians are worth studying.

Confucian ideas such as "by nature men are similar to one another; but learning and practice make them different" (性相近也, 习相远也。) or the Confucian mediocrity(平庸) of harmony and inclusiveness provide complementarity among the diverse cultures of the world. Each culture is unique. Amid such a diversity of human culture, cultural value frameworks help us better understand the cultural complexity, thus facilitating TCM interculturalization. The next three sections, therefore, are devoted to the discussion of three most prevalent cultural value frameworks uncovered by intercultural researchers.

Activities

Comprehension Questions

1.What is your understanding of cultural values?

2.What are functions of cultural value patterns?

3.What do you think of the Chinese proverb "You'll suffer loss if you don't take advice from the old"?

4.What are the core values of socialism with Chinese characteristics in the new era?

5.How can we inherit our traditional values?

Case Study

Case 1

The famous inscription of "Abstaining from Deception" on the plaque that is hung high at the front gate was written by Hu Xueyan, the founder of Huqingyu Tang (胡庆余堂), a historically significant Chinese pharmaceutical company in Hangzhou, Zhejiang Province. As the motto of the drugstore, he admonished his followers to do business in good faith with no adulteration in the slightest. With a reputation as the "King of Medicine in Southeastern China" for more than 140 years, Huqingyu Tang has always been adhering to the spirit of "Abstaining from Deception" to make good medicines and provide a guarantee for the clinical efficacy of traditional Chinese medicine. It has continuously launched various kinds of prescriptions that meet the needs of the times and insisted on innovation to publicize the culture of traditional Chinese medicine through live broadcasting.

——Adapted from Chen and Zhang (2020)

Questions

1.What inspiration can we draw from Huqingyu Tang for the development of TCM as it connects to the past and future and guards its integrity and innovation?

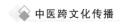

2.How is the spirit of "Abstaining from Deception" reflected in TCM history?

Case 2

Vinca Chu, a Chinese American, was given a promotion to supervise the health management department in her company. In her new role, she oversees a diverse group of eight clerks who were previously her friends. As a caring supervisor, Vinca regularly gathered with her employees and their families twice a month outside of work. Her division perceives her more as a friendly ally rather than just a supervisor.

Vinca has been feeling really anxious lately because her employees are not cooperating. They ignore her requests, gossip behind her back, and act disrespectfully. It makes Vinca dread going to work. She thinks, "Where did I go wrong? Was I too friendly? Am I an incompetent supervisor?"

Their team is planning to organize an annual Chinese cultural event which is meant to exhibit the colorful life of Chinese people and their health management system. Vinca intends to hold this event on a weekend in a large shopping mall to attract a wide variety of participants. While some of her employees show enthusiasm and cooperation, others are reluctant to work on the weekend.

The next week, Vinca has to undertake her annual year-end performance reviews, and it is a tough situation for her. She does not want to write anything negative about her employees because it goes against her values and how she sees herself as a caring person. But she feels like she has no choice but to address these issues honestly. She could expect the worse in the next year, working with her employees.

Questions

1.What can account for Vinca's frustration?

2.What advice can you give Vinca?

Translation

Translate the following text into Chinese.

The use of multimedia platforms to disseminate TCM culture is an important approach to enhancing the image, recognition, and influence of overseas dissemination of TCM culture, which is also a realistic demand for TCM culture to go global. We can utilize the advantages of traditional and new media platforms to expand the dissemination channels and coverage of the story of traditional Chinese medicine.

Before reading this section, please consider the following questions:

1. How much do you know about Value Orientations Theory?

2. In what way may values be related to economic status or rural-urban distinctions?

5.2　Value Orientations and TCM Culture

In order to understand intercultural communication, it is necessary to have a way of discussing how cultures differ. However, here lies a question: How can we compare one culture with another to find out their similarities and differences when there are so many dimensions in which cultures may differ? American anthropologists, Kluckhohn and Strodtbeck (1961), have provided us with a useful tool for cultural comparison. Their theory is based on the idea that every individual, regardless of culture, must deal with five universal questions, which are:

- What is the character of human nature?
- What is the relation of humankind to nature?
- What is the orientation toward time?
- What is the value placed on activity?
- What is the relationship of people to each other?

They posited a list of answers to these five questions, claiming that all cultures can be summarized into a cultural value framework according to their positions in answering each of the above questions. For the sake of discussion, we tend to consider each answer as a definitive mark, creating five continua(连续体) along which each culture is positioned.

Although the value orientation theory has been frequently used to discuss different cultural patterns around the world (Baldwin *et al.*, 2014), it is more appropriate to claim that the focus of this list is on a key component of culture — world view, our personal views and attitudes towards how humans are connected to different elements like nature and time. It also

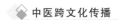

touches upon our overall attitudes towards activities and ourselves.

Kluckhohn and Strodtbeck's Value Orientations (1961)

Orientation	Variations		
Human Nature	Evil	Neutral/Good + Evil	Good
Human - Nature	Subjugation to nature	Harmony with nature	Mastery over nature
Time	Past	Present	Future
Activity	Being	Being-in-becoming	Doing
Relational	Hierarchy	Collaterality	Individualism

Human Nature Orientation

Discussions of human nature often deal with divisions of evil, good and something in between. The traditional Western belief is that human beings are basically evil because Christianity argues humans have original sin. However, one can perfect human nature if one keeps doing good things. People with a Taoist worldview believe that two opposing forces, good and evil, co-exist in the world because the universe is best seen from the perspective of dynamic yin and yang. Yang increases while yin decreases, and vice versa. This view of the good and evil nature of humanity proposes that evil cannot be eliminated because it is an integral part of the universe. The third answer to human nature is good. "*San Zi Jing*" (*Three Character Classic*), a household primer for young children in China, begins with the familiar line, "man at birth is fundamentally good in nature" (人之初,性本善). This indicates at least many Chinese people believe in the benevolence of human nature. This is also in line with Confucian thoughts.

Yet, there is a variation. Some scholars add an additional factor, claiming human nature is corruptible. In other words, human nature is not fixed but changeable. Chinese readers are all familiar with the story of Mencius' mother moving three times in order to live close to good neighbors. Why did she do this? She believes one can be environmentally influenced. You may be virtuous when you are born. However, if you do not choose your friends wisely, you might end up being an evil-doer. Similar ideas are found in *The Analects*, which goes like this, "It is virtuous behavior that constitutes the excellence of a neighborhood. If a man in selecting a residence does not fix on one where such prevail, how can he be wise?" (里仁为美, 择不处仁, 焉得知).

TCM believes in good nature (Hong and Chen, 2016). It respects patients and never takes them as passive objects waiting to be handled. They are with soul and human nature. In prescription and treatment, TCM physicians are expected to negotiate with their patients to make sure patients have understood the pathogenesis (发病机制) and cooperated willingly in the treatment.

Human-Nature Orientation

In human-nature orientation, three types of relationships characterize how different cultures relate to and interact with nature. The first answer is subjugation (臣服) to nature. Human beings are powerless and at the mercy of nature. For cultures that are frequently attacked by natural disasters, it is understandable to foster such an attitude toward the world. "This perspective is found in India and parts of South America" (Samovar *et al.*, 2017, p. 216). At the other end of this continuum lies mastery of nature, which is the opposite to the first answer. People from Western countries, including the US Americans, are said to historically believe that nature is something that is approachable and employable to their advantage. Somewhere in-between lies the cooperative view toward nature, i.e., harmonious co-existence with the universe. This worldview is often observed in greater Chinese cultural community, including Chinese, Korean, Japanese and their expatriates in other parts of the world. The theory that man is an integral part of nature is a good example to show how Taoists do not perceive nature either hostile or profitable, but friendly and welcoming. The practice of feng shui builds on this view.

Harmony with nature has profound influences on TCM (Hong and Chen, 2016). To fully understand health and disease, one has to study not only the inherent characteristics of diseases, but also the environmental factors. For example, TCM treatment to the common cold varies in different seasons. Cold occurring in summer very often goes with summer-heat and dampness. Therefore, the treatment should be meant to eliminate summer-heat and dampness. Cold in winter is mostly caused by winter cold, so the solution would be to expel wind and cold (Tian, 2023).

Time Orientation

As per orientation toward time, the greatest differences are in the respective importance placed on the past, present, and future and on how each influences interaction. At one end of the continuum lies the past orientation, which honors history and tradition. In most Asian nations and South America, respect for the past is prevalent because of their long and eventful histories. Chinese people boast a long history of over five thousand years. President Xi Jinping asserted in his *Foreword to the Revitalization Library* (《复兴文库》序言) that "for thousands of years, the Chinese nation has the tradition of documenting historical records and compiling classic works, so as to draw on the lessons of history and civilize the people through cultural development" (Xi, 2022b, p. 1). Moving from the past arrives at the present. Present-orientation argues that the current time scale assumes the most significant. The past is over that one can do nothing about; the future is unpredictable that is beyond one's reach. Only the moment is worth noting. The famous Latin adage, "carpe diem" (及时行乐), perfectly summarizes this time orientation, enjoying the pleasures of the moment without concern for the future.

Latin American cultures are "notoriously" known to have a casual, relaxed lifestyle. They might be perceived by people valuing the future as being idle and inactive. At the far side of the scale lies the emphasis on the future. For cultures embracing future orientation, the future is expected to carry more significance than the present or past. Most US Americans, who are constantly thinking about what is lying ahead, hold this view toward the future (Samovar *et al.*, 2017). Lingering on the past is definitely not quite favorable.

This time orientation, which is significantly different from past-oriented culture, deserves the attention of TCM culture facilitators. Generally speaking, Chinese people tend to be proud of having a long history. The history of TCM clearly shows its past orientation. The emergence of TCM can be traced back to the Shang Dynasty (ca. 1600–1046 B.C.) when people already had some understanding of diseases. The TCM theoretical system was established during the Warring States Period (475–221 B.C.) and the Han Dynasty (206 B. C. – 220 A. D.) after millennia of explorations and practice. From then on to the Ming (1368–1644) and Qing (1644–1911) Dynasties, many aspects of TCM were significantly expanded, both theoretically and practically. After the Opium War broke out in 1840, TCM was greatly impacted by the import of Western medicine, and it was forced to convert from the past to the future, but its essence is unchangeably past-oriented. This past preference might influence TCM culture facilitators in their communicative behavior, including agenda setting (议程设置) and content delivery. Too much emphasis on the long history of TCM might leave a negative impression on the future-oriented culture. This does not imply that Americans completely disregard the past or ignore the present. However, it is indeed the case that a considerable number of US Americans, whether in their thoughts or actions, often adopt a short-term, future-oriented outlook. One more interesting thing deserves noting, i. e., the essence of TCM is actually future-oriented because TCM aims to prevent rather than cure.

Activity Orientation

There are three common attitudes toward activity: being, being-in-becoming, and doing. Let us begin with "being-in-becoming". Being-in-becoming stresses the idea of personal development and spiritual growth. It focuses on engaging in activities that contribute to the overall improvement and well-being of oneself as a whole. "This orientation seems to be less prevalent than the other two, perhaps practiced only in Buddhism and as a cultural motif in the US in the 1960s" (Martin and Nakayama, 2022, p. 96). The opposite of being-in-becoming orientation is doing, which characterizes most US Americans. The doing orientation describes activity in which accomplishments are measured by external standards. The key to this orientation is a value system that stresses action. It seems the US Americans tend to do or move all the time. Getting ahead is a motto in their life. Academic achievements and career promotion are two very important life activities. They seldom sit and meditate (冥思). A pause of two or three seconds in conversation might be sensed as uncomfortable. Being able to make quick decisions is considered as a virtue in the US. Yet, in a culture that emphasizes less on activity, say China, thinking twice before leaping is preferable, as the Chinese idiom goes, "Hasty men don't get to eat hot tofu" (心急吃不了热豆腐). Finally, a being orientation means accepting people, events, and ideas as they naturally unfold. In Mexico, for example, building strong relationships is valued more than accomplishments, and Mexican people find happiness in simply talking and spending time with family and friends (Samovar et al., 2017). In other words, being orientation tends to combine personal growth with experience. There is no need to separate what you are doing and what you are meant to achieve.

Being-in-becoming is the mode of activity orientation in TCM. TCM philosophy is greatly influenced by Confucianism, Taoism and Buddhism. Taoism's inactivity, Confucianism's morality cultivation and Buddhism's emptiness are all trying to reach an ideal status of tranquility which TCM takes as a goal to maintain health. Specifically, TCM puts character cultivation ahead of physical treatment (Hong and Chen, 2016). Character cultivation is important for both the doctor and the patient. If there is no good character, it is hard to maintain health. Sun Simiao, the King of medicine, advocated such a noble character this way, "A doctor should treat all patients like his own family, whether be they rich or poor, old or young, pretty or ugly, friend or foe, domestic or foreign" (若有疾厄来求救者,不得问其贵贱贫富,长幼妍蚩,怨亲善友,华夷愚智,普同一等,皆如至亲之想). This noble thought has become part of TCM culture.

Relational Orientation

There are three variants in this dimension of value variation: hierarchy, collaterality (群体合作制), and individualism. Individualism, as the term indicates, means members of the culture are independent, separate, autonomous, and unique entities. Individualism, "often cited as a value held by European Americans, places importance on individuals rather than on families, work teams, or other groups" (Martin and Nakayama, 2022, p. 94). The direct opposite to this orientation is hierarchy, in which people are segments of a chain formed by time and interdependent to one another. Also known as collectivist culture, hierarchical society emphasizes the importance of a big extended family and group loyalty. Authority figures such as parents in the family or bosses in the company play a key role in maintaining the healthy functioning of the group.

The last one is called collaterality, which assumes people are members of their collateral group and interdependent even after death. Ancestral worship is an important ritual in a collateral culture. Examples include some Chinese families where there is a table in the house to honor the deceased ancestors who are often consulted in terms of important decision making. Collaterality is also reflected in TCM practice. TCM practitioners view the body as an integrated whole, rather than an assortment of parts which must be treated individually. Since people are complex beings, the philosophy of treating the whole being not just the symptoms is upheld by Chinese medicine. Some of the concepts integrated into TCM practice include theory of visceral manifestation, five-phase theory, and the concept of meridians (经络) (Hong and Chen, 2016).

Though value orientation model is based on the study of five small but culturally rich communities in a region of northwestern New Mexico, US, it is widely acknowledged as a useful tool for interculturalists to understand actions and thoughts of people from different cultural backgrounds. It follows that this value framework can also inform effective TCM interculturalization. It can be concluded that TCM culture is determined by good human nature, harmony with nature, past orientation, being-in-becoming and collaterality. Mastering the five variants is conducive (有助于) to understanding TCM culture and facilitating intercultural communication and globalization of TCM.

─────────────── **Activities** ───────────────

Comprehension Questions

1.What are the five value orientations proposed by Kluckhohn and Strodtbeck?

2.In terms of time orientation, Hall (1983) established a classic framework for examining the link between time and communication. He proposed that cultures organize time in one of two ways—either monochronic (M-time) or polychronic (P-time), which represents two approaches to perceiving and utilizing time. Find more information and explain how it is related to TCM interculturalization.

3. Why is character cultivation important for both doctors and patients from the perspective of TCM?

4. How does the human-nature orientation exert a profound influence on TCM?

5. Please provide examples to show that TCM theory and practice are both past and future-oriented.

Survey

Kluckhohn and Strodtbeck (1961) were pioneers in the study of cultural value orientations. They singled out five universal problems faced by all human societies. The passage above has analyzed the value orientation of TCM, which is worth further exploration. Conduct survey among some TCM physicians and find out more TCM values from the perspective of this value framework.

Translation

Translate the following text into Chinese.

TCM has created unique views on life, on fitness, on diseases and on the prevention and treatment of diseases during its long history of absorption and innovation. It represents a combination of natural sciences and humanities, embracing profound philosophical ideas of the Chinese nation. As ideas on fitness and medical models change and evolve, traditional Chinese medicine has come to underline a more and more profound value.

Case Study

Case 1

The following anecdote illustrates how complicated intercultural communication can be. It concerns a well-intentioned individual trying to be sensitive to one group (Native Americans) but unintentionally ignoring the feelings and sensibilities of another (Japanese).

I organized a week-long intercultural workshop last summer in which the participants were from a mix of domestic and international cultural groups. The purpose of this seminar was to have a first touch of TCM with an emphasis on recognizing some basic Chinese characters such as "阴" and "阳". On the first day, as an icebreaker, we organized a self-introduction session where everyone was asked to introduce the one sitting next to their right. An older Japanese woman named Natsuko had a little trouble with English. She said that her partner (a white American woman) was "Native American".

Immediately, Emma, an American white, raised her hand. She said that it bothered her that this woman had been called a Native American when she was not. She emphasized how important it was that people be labeled accurately. She meant well. But Natsuko was really embarrassed at being singled out as being incorrect in her language. She did not say anything at the time, but as the session was over, she went to me and asked to be transferred out of the group.

Questions

1. What seems to bother Emma and Natsuko?

2. What would you do to cope with the situation?

Case 2

It is known that the human pox inoculation method was invented during the Song Dynasty, which was later introduced to Europe at the beginning of the 18th century. Inspired by human pox inoculation, Edward Jenner, an Englishman living in the late 18th century, invented a less lethal cowpox inoculation by experimenting on a boy so that smallpox, which had killed millions of people, finally became extinct. Ironically, Jenner's method was initially rejected by the Royal Society of England and his papers were either supported or doubted by scholars in related fields or even opposed and stigmatized. However, doubts and objections were finally crushed by facts. The cowpox inoculation was popularized worldwide.

Questions

1. There have been many treatments for infectious diseases in Chinese history. What implications can we get from them?

2. Nowadays, inoculation has become a very important method to contain infectious diseases, and Edward Jenner is considered as the father of immunology. Yet, the fact that he was inspired by Chinese human pox inoculation is not widely known. What is your interpretation of this awkward situation? What implication does this have on TCM interculturalization?

5.3   Cultural Dimensions and Its Influence on Healthcare

Culture is one of the core concepts in the study of intercultural communication, let alone in practicing TCM interculturalization. How and what people talk with each other is greatly influenced by their cultures. Kroeber and Kluckhohn (1952), from the perspective of anthropology, put forward the following conception of culture, which is still widely quoted today.

"Culture consists of patterns, explicit and implicit, of and for behavior acquired and transmitted by symbols, constituting the distinctive achievements of human groups, including their embodiments in artifacts; the essential core of culture consists of traditional (i.e. historically derived and selected) ideas and especially their attached values; culture systems may, on the one hand, be considered as products of action, and on the other as conditioning elements of further action" (Kroeber and Kluckhohn, 1952, p. 181).

Geert Hofstede, a Dutch scholar, who viewed culture from a psychological perspective, worked out cultural dimensions to identify different cultural forms and patterns, which are based on the surveys done by him and his colleagues of over 100, 000 IBM employees in 71 countries. Through theoretical reasoning and statistical analysis, Hofstede (1984) identified four cultural dimensions: individualism vs. collectivism, power distance, uncertainty avoidance, and masculinity (男性特征) vs. femininity (女性特征). Bond (1991) isolated the fifth cultural dimension which is incorporated into Hofstede's, i.e., long-term vs. short-term orientation to time. In their latest research, a new dimension, indulgence versus restraint, is added to the framework (Hofstede *et al.*, 2010). Each country is given a score on each dimension, which is published online (https://geerthofstede. com / culture-geert-hofstede-gert-jan-hofstede / 6d-model-of-national-culture/). While Kluckhohn and Strodtbeck (1961) highlighted the study of cultural variation within one natural boundary, Hofstede and other specialists tried to explore value orientations by studying organizational behavior at various locations of the world with the underlying assumption of culture as "the software of the mind", explaining the function of culture as a determinant factor of human behavior. Though Hofstede's framework is heavily criticized as too rigid, ignoring regional, personal, or gender variability (Chen, 2009a), his work offers a good starting point for engaging in intercultural activities related to TCM.

Individualism vs. Collectivism

The first dimension, individualism-collectivism, is about interpersonal relationships, or how an individual perceives his role in a cultural group. According to Hofstede (1984), in an individualistic culture, people are supposed to take care of themselves and their immediate family. Individual autonomy is over anything else. There is more emphasis on "I" than on "We". The dominant culture in the US is widely known as a typical example of individualistic culture. Famous sayings and adages like "God help those who help themselves", or "To be yourself in a world that is constantly trying to make you something else is the greatest accomplishment" are vivid examples of praising the individualistic or independent spirit. People in an individualistic culture tend to stress self and personal achievement. Competition, therefore, is encouraged in this culture.

On the other end of this continuum is collectivism. In a collectivist culture, people make a very clear distinction between in-groups and out-groups. In-groups include the nuclear family, the extended family, relatives, friends, and acquaintances. Out-groups are those who are basically strangers. People from a collectivist culture keep the out-groups out and only take care of their in-groups. Similarly, their in-groups are supposed to care for them. A child of an extended family is seldom alone, whether during the day or at night. Besides, in the majority of collectivist cultures, it is seen as impolite and undesirable to directly confront another person. In many cases, people avoid using the word "no" directly as it can be seen as confrontational. Instead, they opt for polite phrases like "you may be right" or "we will think about it" to decline requests. Similarly, "yes" may not necessarily mean "accepted" or "understood" or "approved". In Japanese culture, for instance, the listener constantly replies to the speaker with "*Hai* (yes)", only indicating "yes, I heard you", so the conversation may keep going.

This different attitude toward interpersonal relationship is linked to health issue. For example, individualist and collectivist cultures deal differently with disability. A survey (Hofstede *et al.*, 2010) done in Australia showed different reactions to being disabled. In individualist communities (Anglo and German), disabled people tend to remain cheerful and optimistic, to favor independency and self-reliance, and to plan a life as normal as possible. In collectivist communities (Greek, Chinese, Arabic), the disabled person has more expressions of grief and shame than their individualist counterpart, pessimistic rather than optimistic. Family members of the disabled would be asked for advice and support more frequently. Another survey done across the globe also indicates a difference in perception toward disability held by individualist and collectivist cultures (Meyer, 2010). A disabled person in an individualist culture tends to be integrated into the society. In contrast, in a collectivist culture, a disabled person is more likely to be separated from the larger group. It may sound strange for a person from an individualist culture because one is expected to look after himself in an individualist culture, and care is provided for disabled people to lead an independent life as much as possible. In a collectivistic culture, however, the community is supposed to take care of all its members. It is reasonable, therefore, for those disabled people to be gathered in a special house in order to provide medical or other facilities conveniently.

Power Distance

Equality is considered a universal aspect of value system shared by all humanities. Yet, each culture has developed different ways to realize equality. In other words, cultures differ in people's attitude toward status inequalities. Hofstede (1984) created a power distance index (PDI) to assess the extent to which people accept or question the inequality of power distribution and the decisions made by the authority. He defined power distance as "the extent to which the less powerful members of institutions and organizations within a country expect and accept that power is distributed unequally" (Hofstede *et al.*, 2010, p. 61). The PDI scores can tell us about the dependency rate in a culture. In a low-PDI community where people expect short distance of power among members of that culture, boss and subordinates seem to be more equal. Bosses encourage subordinates to use their first name. There is an interdependence between boss and subordinate. On the contrary, in a high-PDI community, the opposite is to be found. Interestingly, students in cultures with low PDI value adaptability and carefulness, while students in cultures with high PDI prioritize few desires, moderation, and disinterestedness

(Bond, 1991).

The difference in power distance between cultures also affects the relationship between doctors and patients (Herzberg *et al.*, 2017). In high-PDI cultures, consultations tend to be shorter, and unexpected information exchanges are less done. The difference can be observed in the use of medication as well.

The following tool helps you evaluate your personal power distance scale (Neuliep, 2018, p. 79).

Power Distance Scale

Directions: The following are 10 statements regarding issues we face at work, in the classroom, and at home. Indicate in the blank to the left of each statement the degree to which you (1) strongly agree, (2) agree, (3) are unsure, (4) disagree, or (5) strongly disagree with the statement. For example, if you strongly agree with the first statement, place a 1 in the blank. Work quickly and record your initial response.

_____ 1. Within an organization, employees should feel comfortable expressing disagreements to their managers.

_____ 2. Within a classroom, students should be allowed to express their points of view toward a subject without being punished by the teacher/professor.

_____ 3. At home, children should be allowed to openly disagree with their parents.

_____ 4. The primary purpose of a manager is to monitor the work of the employees to make sure they are doing their jobs appropriately.

_____ 5. Authority is essential for the efficient running of an organization, classroom, or home.

_____ 6. At work, people are more productive when they are closely supervised by those in charge.

_____ 7. In problem-solving situations within organizations, input from employees is important.

_____ 8. Generally, employees, students, and children should be seen and not heard.

_____ 9. Obedience to managers, teachers, and parents is good.

_____ 10. Managers, teachers, and parents should be considered equal to their workers, students, and children.

Scoring: For items 4, 5, 6, 8, and 9, reverse your responses. That is, if your original response was a 1, reverse it to a 5. If your original response was a 2, reverse it to a 4, and so on. Once you have reversed your responses for these items, sum up your 10 responses. This sum is your power distance score. Lower scores equal smaller power distance.

Uncertainty Avoidance

The third cultural dimension, uncertainty avoidance, relates to how a society deals with ambiguity and attempts to minimize it through the establishment of rules and intolerance toward deviance (异常). In cultures with high uncertainty avoidance orientation like Greece, Portugal and Japan, people tend to make a lot of rules and seek consensus in order to lower the risk of uncertainty. They stress uniformity and dislike deviance. People with low uncertainty avoidance orientation (the UK, Sweden, and the US), by contrast, are more willing to tolerate uncertainty, choosing less rules and accepting dissent.

The difference in uncertainty avoidance between cultures can be seen in healthcare practice. Although medical standards for being healthy do not vary much across cultures, personal perception of health is correlated with cultural variability in the scale of uncertainty avoidance. For instance, Payer (1989) described her personal experiences as a patient in several European countries. that in cultures with low uncertainty avoidance orientation like the UK, low blood pressure is seen as a symbol of longevity, but it is considered a disorder in cultures with high uncertainty avoidance orientation, say Germany, where several drugs are on the market to cure it. One possible explanation for this discrepancy (差异) might lie in the fact that people in a low avoidance orientation culture tend to tolerate the deviation from normal blood pressure as acceptable and thus quite normal. Because older people tend to have higher blood pressure and they are also perceived not as energetic as the youth, low blood pressure is optimistically associated with long and healthy life. By contrast, people from a very high uncertainty avoidance culture feel uneasy when the so-called standard or norm tilts to either side. They rush to correct it to prevent it from becoming worse.

Uncertain avoidance index (UAI) is also associated with patient-doctor communication. One study (Meeuwesen *et al.*, 2009) shows that doctors in low UAI countries more often send the patient away with a comforting talk, rather than giving any prescription. They use more eye contact and spend more time with each patient in the clinic. The opposite is found in some high-UAI cultures where doctors are expected to prescribe several drugs, and they often do so. This research findings are informative for TCM physicians to practice medicine in low-UAI cultures. Chinese medicine formulae usually consist of ten or more herbs, which might frighten away the patient whose main purpose of visiting a doctor is to get comfort.

Masculinity vs. Femininity

In a traditional sense, human world consists of men and women. While men are generally perceived or expected to be aggressive, ambitious, and tough, women are often associated with being cooperative, caring, and soft. A country can be more inclined to manly behavior or womanly conduct in terms of three aspects — directness, task-focus, and role assignment. Hofstede (1984) used a masculinity index (MAS) to assess the extent to which people prefer achievement and competition or cooperation and social support. These variations are referred to as masculinity versus femininity dimension. Masculinity implies aggressiveness and assertiveness, while femininity indicates nurturing, modesty and compassion.

In a society with high MAS, men or manly people dominate the society and gender differences are clear cut; one lives to work; money is important. Japan is ranked first in this dimension where female managers are seldom seen (Hofstede et al., 2010) because women's role in Japanese society is traditionally associated with house cleaning and child-rearing rather than career pursuits. In a cultural region with low MAS like Scandinavia, gender roles are not so rigid; men's and women's occupations are not so different; competition is not idealized; work is not the only thing in one's life; recreation is more important than work.

People from high MAS cultures tend to associate more with people of the same gender, which is enlightening in TCM interculturalization. Gender difference should be taken into consideration in planning cultural events. Otherwise, unexpected communicative barrier might appear, leading to a failure of cultural transmission.

Long-Term vs. Short-Term Orientation to Time

The fifth concern of all cultures relates to the orientation to time. Hofstede's original framework has long been criticized for its Western bias. Bond (1991), a Canadian scholar, conducted a Chinese Value Survey of University Students around the World to address the Western bias problem. He isolated the time orientation dimension which was later incorporated into Hofstede's four cultural dimensions. It was named long-term vs. short-term orientation (LTO) to reflect how strongly a person believes in the long-term perspective. In a high LTO culture, people admire persistence, thriftiness, humility (谦逊) and accept status differences within interpersonal relationships, whereas in cultures with a low LTO, people have an expectation of quick results following one's actions and immediate gratification (满足) of one's needs. Humility is considered a lack of confidence and weakness (Hofstede *et al.*, 2010).

The high LTO is well reflected in TCM, which emphasizes physical fitness and overall health. The concept of preventive treatment of disease in *Huangdi Neijing* is the elaboration of health preservation of TCM. On the contrary, Western medical practice highlights the treatment of the disease itself. It may take a longer time for a TCM physician to treat a disease than a Western doctor to do it. In engaging in TCM intercultural activities, the fifth cultural dimension should also be taken into consideration. As is mentioned in passages about the conceptions of culture, a very important aspect of TCM that can be accepted by people with Western medicine training lies in its efficacy. Now, one more factor, i.e., time, also matters.

Limitations and Applications

Some scholars classified cultures from other perspectives, like Trompenaars and Hampden-Turner (1998). According to their research results, the solutions different cultures have chosen to universal problems can help people identify fundamental dimensions of cultures. A comparison between theirs and Hofstede's cultural framework is given in the following table. Both theories share the same underlying rationale: National cultural index can be averaged to predict individuals' behavior and cultural orientation. This, however, is the biggest weakness. Hofstede himself pointed out the possible misplacement of countries into two conflicting groups like collectivism and individualism, ignoring two facts. Firstly, within one culture or country, sometimes different groups exist with varied cultural traits. For instance, "many Pakistanis will score more individualistic than some Australians, and many Australians will be more collectivistic than most Pakistanis" (Baldwin *et al.*, 2014, pp. 79-80) though Australia and Pakistan occupy two extreme ends of the individualism-collectivism continuum. Secondly, it is tempting to broaden the application of Hofstede's framework to other areas though all the data Hofstede collected is based on IBM. In order to address this issue, it is advisable to avoid overgeneralization by absolutely claiming that "China is collectivistic". Instead, context, or co-culture is a better choice. We should bear it in mind that Hofstede's cultural dimension framework is not meant to describe individuals but only cultures.

Trompenaars and Hampden Turner's and Hofstede and Hofstede's Cultural Frameworks

Trompenaars and Hampden-Turner's Cultural Differences	Hofstede's Cultural Dimensions
Universalism vs. Particularism	Individualism vs. Collectivism
Individualism vs. Communitarianism	Power Distance Index
Neutral vs. Emotional	Uncertainty Avoidance Index
Specific vs. Diffuse	Masculinity vs. Femininity
Achievement vs. Ascription	Long Term Orientation

Hofstede's cultural framework is the dominant cultural paradigm in business studies for its statistical strength and simplicity in application. Many Chinese values can be elaborated from the point of cultural dimensions. TCM with a history of thousands of years, typical of traditional Chinese culture, plays a very important role in Chinese healthcare system. The major difference between TCM and Western medicine may be that the former treats the illness or sickness as a component of the entire body's system, while the latter treats the disease as a single isolated component. The study of cultural dimensions can help people of different backgrounds better understand TCM culture and promote communication and exchange among countries.

Chapter Summary

· Cultural value patterns help establish identity, facilitate interpretation, and boost motivation.
· Kluckhohn and Strodtbeck's five basic questions get at the root of any culture's value system.
· Geert Hofstede's cultural framework positions different cultures along five dimensions: individualism vs. collectivism, power distance, uncertainty avoidance,

masculinity vs. femininity, long-term vs. short-term orientation to time.

•Limitations of cultural value patterns include overgeneralization, ignorance of social, regional, and individual variability.

Checklist	Yes	No
Cognitive: I have mastered the core information		
Behavioral: I have the ability of putting what I've learned into practice		
Affective: I am willing to carry out what I've learned		
Moral: I will take the ethical consideration into account during practice		

Part Three
Messages

Chapter 6

Language, TCM Culture, and Thought: Verbal Communication Across Cultures

Chapter Objectives

After reading this chapter, you should be able to:

◆ Foster a general understanding of linguistics, perception, and thinking patterns.

◆ Describe the process of human perception.

◆ Provide some suggestions on how to develop a good perception of TCM culture.

◆ Describe the relationship between language, culture, and thought.

◆ Perceive image thinking in TCM.

Key Terms

categorization

interpretation

language and linguistics

linear pattern

linguistic determinism

linguistic relativism

Qu Xiang Bi Lei or image thinking

Sapir-Whorf Hypothesis

selection

sensation and perception

thinking pattern

Quotes

Those who know it do not say it;	知者不言,
Those who say it do not know it.	言者不知。
Those who know bar interaction,	塞其兑,
Shut and seal the gates and doors;	闭其门;
They dull their keen edge and	挫其锐,
Resolve their differences,	解其纷;
Reconcile the points of view	和其光,
And blend with the lowly dust.	同其尘,
This we call sublime at-oneness.	是谓玄同。

——《道德经》第五十六章

"Hence those scholars who understand the principles [of life] will take all circumstances into account and conduct a thorough investigation of the cause of a particular [illness]. Only then can they eliminate all doubt and have evidence [at hand]. To those who fail [to conduct such thorough investigations], and who stick to a one-sided perspective, the reality of the facts and principles involved will remain obscure. Their [efforts] will end in confusion in every respect." (故明理之士, 必事事穷其故, 乃能无所惑而有据。否则执一端之见, 而昧事理之实, 均属愦愦矣。)

——《医学源流论·病有鬼神论》

Before reading this section, please consider the following questions:

1.Language undergoes gradual changes that often go unnoticed, but when observed from a historical perspective, these changes become apparent. Explore the semantic change of "Xiaojie" in Chinese.

2.What role does language play in your life?

6.1   Essence of Language and Linguistics

Literacy Test

Hello, Patient X. Time for a test. Please take a look at this card and follow these directions.

Je vais vous montrer des cartes avec trois mots dessus. Tout d'abord, j'aimerais que vous lisiez le mot du haut à haute voix. Ensuite, je vais lire les deux mots ci-dessous, et j'aimerais que vous me disiez lequel des deux mots est le plus similaire ou à une association plus étroite avec le mot du haut. Si vous ne savez pas, veuillez dire : « Je ne sais pas. » Ne devinez pas.

Oh, wait. The instructions are in French, and you don't speak French. (Lucky you, if you do.) OK, here they are in English.

I'm going to show you cards with three words on them. First, I'd like you to read the top word out loud. Next, I'll read the two words underneath, and I'd like you to tell me which of the two words is more similar to or has a closer association with the top word. If you don't know, please say, "I don't know." Don't guess.

So, here are the words on the first card:

sain

gestion

robuste

Which word, gestion or robuste, is most like sain?

Oh, damn it. They're still in French. But that one was pretty easy; you should be able to figure it out. OK, how about this:

صحي

أدار

متين

I am sorry if there was any confusion or difficulty in understanding the information. It seems that you may have some challenges with reading comprehension, and we will make a note of this in your patient record. The doctor will be available to meet with you soon.

This example is obviously exaggerated to make you feel like you have a poor grasp of language while being asked to do a regular health literacy test at your doctor's office. As a TCM culture facilitator, you have the option to choose which language is used in your workplace. You would think English is a best candidate. After all, English has become a de facto (事实上的) lingua franca in many parts of the world. Yet, the world of language is as varied as human culture. The newest 26th edition of Ethnologue(www.ethnologue.com) lists a total of 7,168 living languages worldwide. In Los Angeles city alone, over 80 languages are spoken (Fromkin *et al.*, 2014). It is also possible that your participants attending traditional Chinese medicine (TCM) intercultural activities speak French, Spanish, Arabic, Tagalog, Malay, Japanese, rather than English. They know some English, but not much. Do you still feel confident in effectively and appropriately conveying information about TCM in such a situation? Since language and culture are linked (which will be explored further in the latter part of this chapter), students studying TCM interculturalization would greatly benefit from recognizing the valuable insights that can be gained by exploring the linguistic aspects of cultures beyond their own, which are the focus of this section.

Defining Language and Linguistics

It is said that what makes humans different from animals is

language. While some animals can communicate by sounds and gestures, and a few can even learn bits of human language, humans are unparalleled in their ability to express thoughts due to the creativity and complexity of our communication systems. This system is called **language**, which is usually vocal, but also written or signed.

Humans began to develop interests in exploring language almost 2500 years ago. In ancient China, for instance, Xunzi (ca.313–238 B.C.), a renowned Confucian scholar, proposed the idea of arbitrary connection between objects and names to describe how things are named. His idea of arbitrariness happens to be a key principle in modern language research. **Linguistics**, "the scientific study of human language" (Genetti, 2019, p. 19), generally examines how human beings use language as symbols in communication. It is scientific because the data used by a linguist is empirical and objective, though armchair linguists are still quite active.

Fields of Linguistics at a Glance

We use language every day, but we seldom pause to think about what it means when someone says he knows a language, say, Chinese. One thing is for sure: When you know a language, you can talk to others who know the same language and understand each other. This means you can use speech to convey meanings and understand what others are saying. In other words, our linguistic knowledge includes knowledge of sound system (how certain speech sounds are combined to become meaningful streams), knowledge of words (how letters are combined to become meaningful words), knowledge of sentences and nonsentences (how words are combined to become meaningful phrases, which are combined together to become meaningful sentences), knowledge of meaning (how words and sentences are used to express meaning with or without context). These are the core fields of linguistic research, namely, phonetics, phonology, morphology, syntax, semantics, and pragmatics, the last two assuming special importance for TCM interculturalization.

Some linguists are interested in exploring how humans produce speech sounds that are meaningful, i.e., phonetics. Not every sound articulated by humans is employed in language system. Not every sound is equally used in every human language. To put it in another way, each language develops unique speech patterns, which brings about another field of study called phonology. Finally, not every individual in a particular linguistic community uses the same speech sound to signify the same "idea". This personal variety in language is called idiolect, "the language of an individual speaker with its unique characteristics" (Fromkin *et al.*, 2014, p. 279), not just confined to pronunciation and intonation.

Understanding the pattern of sound is not enough for humans to express ideas. To know a language, one should also know how to put together the independent streams of sounds to form words, i.e., how the unit of meaning is combined to become words. This is called morphology, a linguistic field focusing on the study of words and word building. According to *Shuowen Jiezi* (literally, *Explaining Graphs and Analyzing Characters* 《说文解字》), an early 2nd-century Chinese dictionary from the Han Dynasty, which is focused on the analysis of structures of Chinese characters and to give the rationale behind them, Chinese characters can be classified into six types based on how they are created.

- *Xiangxing* (象形) (pictographs, literally "form imitation"): stylized drawings of the objects they represent. These are generally among the oldest characters. For example, "日" ("sun") is a direct drawing of the sun in the sky.
- *Zhishi* (指示) (ideographs, literally "indication"): expressing an abstract idea through an iconic form, including iconic modification

of pictographic characters.

- *Huiyi* (会意) (compound ideographs, literally "joined meaning"): compounds of two or more pictographic or ideographic characters to suggest the meaning of the word to be represented. For example, "林" ("grove"), is composed of two trees, indicating the cluster of many tress.

- *Jiajie* (假借) (borrowings, literally, "fake and borrow"): characters that are "borrowed" to write another character with the same or similar pronunciation.

- *Xingsheng* (形声) (phonetic compounds, literally "form and sound"): characters that are composed of one part representing the meaning, and the other part indicating its pronunciation.

- *Zhuanzhu* (转注) (mutually explanatory characters, literally "reciprocal meaning"): characters that are mutually explanatory.

   With the help of morphological rules, vocabulary is born. The larger unit of human language is made possible by using words to form phrases and sentences based on rules. The study of these rules is called syntax. While a majority of modern languages rely on word order to decide the relationship between the agent (i.e., the person or thing that does an action) and the patient (i.e., the person or thing that is affected by the action of the verb, not a sick person), word order plays no role in deciding the sentence meaning in some languages such as Latin.

   Finally, in order to rule out meaningless sentences, semantics, or the study of meaning , comes into play. It is necessary, so far, to make a distinction between two types of meaning: linguistic meaning and the user's meaning. While the former usually falls within the domain of semantics, the latter is focused on how language is used in context, which is the main concern of pragmatics. Since language influences thought to a great extent, how language is used to reflect our thoughts also differs. It follows that intercultural pragmatics is a key component of TCM interculturalization because it deals with how language use differs across cultures, which definitely sheds light on communicating TCM across cultures.

Language and Culture

In this textbook, we use culture to refer to our way of life, or all the ideas, customs, and assumptions about the nature of things and the world we are living in, which guides us during our socialization, or helps us become members of the social group (For more information about the discussion of culture, please consult Chapter 3). This kind of knowledge, together with our native tongue, is acquired by us unconsciously, until finally language and culture become cross-influential in shaping us. Just like culture, language is used to describe the world we are living in. For many infants in China, as they are more often than not raised by mothers, the first Chinese character uttered by an infant is usually "*ma*". Then, this "*ma*" can be attributed to anyone or anything nearby, whoever or whatever they may be, including mother, father, grandma, or even a bottle of milk. As they develop a more elaborated linguistic system of Chinese, toddlers learn to categorize different types of entities with "correct" labels. It is understandable that certain vocabulary does not exist in a specific language to signify a certain entity because there is no such entity in their world. In the native culture of the UK, for example, since there is no *doufu*, no native English word is needed for this food. In order to use words such as yin and yang, *shushu* (father's younger brother) or *bobo* (father's elder brother), *shangxun* (the first ten-day period of a month) or *xiaxun* (the last ten-day period of a month), *donggua* (white gourd) or *nangua* (pumpkin), "we must have a conceptual system that includes these people, things and ideas as distinct and identifiable categories" (Yule, 2020, p. 312). If certain people, things, ideas are important in one culture, there is a necessity to use single words to signify those entities or ideas in that culture. As a typical example of collectivist culture where interpersonal relationship is highly valued, Chinese have developed a rather sophisticated system for describing kinship terms. We make a distinction between *waigong* (mother's father) and *yeye* (father's father). However, in English, one word "grandfather" is used for both. This conceptual distinction leads to lexical vacancy (词汇空缺) where certain languages lack an independent expression to signify some concepts which are lexicalized (expressed as a single word) in other languages. We will deal with how language influences our perception of the world in the next section.

•Sapir-Whorf Hypothesis

The above examples vividly demonstrate that people around the world use different linguistic systems to describe the world or talk about external realities. Does that mean the world conceptualized in our mind differs across culture? Though there is a huge distinction between culture and language, language is still a primary medium for humans to express their culture . Anthropologist Sapir and his pupil Whorf were among the pioneers who tried to explore the relationship between language and culture. They posited that the structure of a language influences how its speakers perceive the world around them and therefore, the relationship between language and culture or thought is called the **Sapir-Whorf Hypothesis**. The strong version, **linguistic determinism**, holds that language determines how we think about the external reality. In other words, what we conceptualize about the world is partially true based on our own native tongue. There would be no possibility for another culture to have a connection with what we have conceptualized because of lexical vacancy. This strong form of this hypothesis is of course false. If the speakers of another language could not think about the external reality of a foreigner because their language lacks an independent word for that reality, then translation would be impossible, and engaging in TCM interculturalization would be in vain. It is said that in Navaho, a language used by members of American Indian people of northern New Mexico and Arizona, blue and green are one word. However, that does not mean the Navaho cannot make a distinction between blue sky and green leaves. Maybe it is only because it is unnecessary to tell the difference between these two realities in the eyes of the Navaho people.

However, the weaker version, **linguistic relativism**, might be true. Linguistic relativists hold that the structure of a language we speak helps us know the world around us, thus reflects our thinking, beliefs, and attitudes. In other words, language is a guide to culture. At the same time, culture also influences language, as evidenced by the fact that each year Chinese language has welcomed new coinages because of cultural exchange and/or language contact.

Language, a primary medium for people to get connected, plays a key role in our lives. To know the essence of language, linguists try to explore sound system, structure system, and semantic system, and even the relationship between language and culture in order to figure out how language exerts powerful influence on human as a whole or as an individual.

Activities

Comprehension Questions

1. Can you define human language in your own words?

2. Apart from communication, what other purposes do you think language serves? Give specific examples to explain your point.

3. What are some features of human language? What does human language differ from animal language (if there is such a thing called animal language)?

4. What is the relationship between language and culture?

5. In what way(s) does linguistic relativism shed light on TCM interculturalization?

Survey

What is commonly called shou-ji (hand machine) in China is called a mobile in the UK, a cell phone in the US, cellular in Latin America, keitai (portable) in Japan, nalle (teddy bear) in Sweden, pelephone (wonder phone) in Israel, and handy in Germany. By whatever name, so far, over 95% of the world population owns at least one mobile phone. Every second, there is a call between two or more people. Conduct a survey to find out how people around the globe begin and end their telephone call. Some is done for you.

How People around the Globe Begin and End Their Phone Call

Country/region/culture	Answering the Phone	Ending the Conversation
China	"喂？/您好。您哪位。"(Hello, who is it?)	"再见"(See you)
France	"Allo." The French often add their name and phrase "Qui est à l'appareil?" (Who is on the phone?)	
the UK		
Japan		
Germany		
Spain		
Brazil		

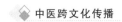
Before reading this section, please consider the following questions:

1. Gatekeeping theory of mass communication was pioneered by German psychologist Kurt Lewin to discuss the possibility of selecting information by an authority to be consumed within the time or space that an individual happens to have. This means gatekeeping falls into a role of surveilling and monitoring data. The gatekeeper decides what information should move past them (through the information "gate") to the group or individuals beyond, and what information should not. They allow certain information to pass through the audience according to personal preference, professional experience, social influences, or even bias. Do you think that gatekeepers exist in the we-media age (自媒体时代) when everyone is a reporter, posting almost anything on the internet? Is it necessary to have a gatekeeper help us avoid being drowned by so much information?

2. Here are two images. What do you see at first glance? A vase or two faces? An old lady or a young woman? Compare your responses with those of your partners. If your answers differ, discuss the possible reasons for the differences.

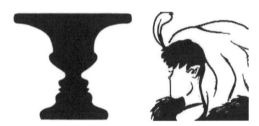

6.2 Understanding Perception of TCM Culture

Defining Sensation and Perception

TCM interculturalization is committed to communicating and promoting the culture of TCM worldwide, so that more people can understand and appreciate the charm and value of Chinese culture. When we try to discuss the possibility of intercultural understanding of TCM, it is necessary for us to probe into the nature of perception itself, the process of perceiving things, and the various factors that can influence perception, which helps us facilitate a better transmission of TCM culture among people.

Every day when we open up our eyes in the early morning, we begin to see, touch, feel, smell, and taste the world. In other words, we rely on our sense organs to connect the physical world with our brain. This process is called sensation. Technically speaking, **sensation** is "the process by which receptor cells are stimulated and transmit their information to various brain centers" (Shiraev and Levy, 2017, p. 105). However, mere feeling is not enough. Humans have the ability to understand the world and the curiosity to explore what is going on by "organizing various sensations into meaningful parts" (Shiraev and Levy, 2017, p. 105), which is called **perception**. To put it another way, it is out of perception that we are connected to the external world. Therefore, perception is a way for us to understand TCM culture.

Process of Perception

Though cognitive psychologists have explored different modes of perception, visual perception is of enormous importance in our daily life. No matter what it is, be it static or dynamic, 2D or 3D, the process of perception is composed of three stages: selection, categorization, and interpretation, each of which is influenced by culture (Jandt, 2018).

Selection, as the first stage, is the process of converting the contextual signals or stimuli, like what we see, smell, feel, etc., into meaningful experience. Too few stimuli fail to excite the nervous system. Too many stimuli increase the burden of neural processing, straining our brain, leading to sensory overload (感觉超载). Thus, as we face a large variety of stimuli every day, we are only capable of perceiving parts of them through a selective process. For example, when you are asked what you see the moment you walk into the consulting room of a TCM physician, you may say that you have seen a doctor dressed in white, or a mini-acupuncture model on the desk. But do you see something else, say, the dresses of other patients, the hair style of your doctor, or those clips on the desk? Obviously, we can only perceive parts of the realities around us. The partiality of our perception is the major cause of misunderstanding in interactions, especially when we come from diverse cultural backgrounds with different perception systems.

After the selection, psychologists inform us that we engage in the deliberate or sometimes unintentional organization of the chosen elements into coherent and meaningful arrangements. This cognitive operation is commonly known as **categorization**. We tend to find a certain logical connection among things by arranging similar things together based on such factors as shape, color, texture, size and intensity. Let us proceed with a brief exercise of organization. Presented to you are seven items: a cow, a rabbit, a TCM physician, some pills, Chinese herbs, a tiger, and a car. You are required to group these items into three distinct and non-overlapping groups or boxes. How are you going to do with it?

One of our students did it this way: Box A contains a cow, a rabbit, and a tiger; a TCM physician, pills, and Chinese herbs stay in Box B; the car goes to Box C. Another student from Germany stood up and commented, "Tigers cannot live peacefully with cows and rabbits because they are meat-eating animals. On the contrary, cows and rabbits can be grouped with herbs because both of them take herbs as their food. Pills and cars can be used by doctors. Naturally, they can be grouped together. Hence, Box A contains the tiger; Box B contains a cow, a rabbit, and herbs; Box C contains a TCM physician, pills, and a car."

As you can see, our German student's perspective appears to be entirely valid as well. This exercise effectively illustrates the subjective nature of perception, influenced by individual and cultural factors. The rationale behind this German student's viewpoint, from which he does not associate herbs, pills, and doctors together, likely stems from his personal belief that grass is not synonymous with medicine.

In general, when we try to organize our perceptions into patterns, we also try to make sense of those patterns by giving them meanings simultaneously. And this is the last stage, **interpretation**, which plays a very important role in TCM interculturalization. For example, a group of international students have just finished nursing skills competition. Winners are smiling broadly. Some Japanese girls are also smiling though they have lost the competition. An American student may interpret the smiles on the faces of Japanese students after being defeated as indicating that Japanese students do not care about it. From the Japanese perspective, however, the same smile, which should be read as a painful expression, is used to hide the embarrassment of being defeated.

Factors Influencing Perception

Perception is how our brains make sense of the world. It is our personal way of interpreting what we experience, blending our thoughts with the reality around us. However, perception is not fixed; it can change and be shaped by factors like language, culture, and our own experiences.

Language plays a significant role in people's perception of the world (Vulchanova *et al.*, 2019). There are about seven thousand languages around the world with different sounds, vocabularies, and structures. The grammatical and verbal structure of people's language influences how they perceive the world. Different words mean various things in other languages and not every word in one language has an exact one-to-one correspondence in another language. More often than not, there is no lexical correspondence between two language systems.

TCM is a medicine explained in classic Chinese, while Western medicine is interpreted in modern English or other

European languages. The language of TCM describes "a metaphorical world about human physiology, pathology and treatment of diseases" (Jia Chunhua, 2014, p. 293). For example, yin-yang, as a theory of TCM, has to do with opposing yet complementary energies, which represents harmony and unity. However, it is difficult to find the English equivalent of yin and yang. The same goes to "*jin*", "*mu*", "*shui*", "*huo*", and "*tu*" in five-phase theory. They are by no means "metal", "wood", "water", "fire", and "soil" in English. Therefore, how to explain TCM terms and philosophical ideas in modern English or other foreign languages so they are transmissible across cultures presents itself one of the toughest problems in TCM interculturalization.

"Just as language shapes our thoughts and perceptions of the world, so does one's culture" (Altarriba, 2022, p.861). We view ourselves, others, and the world around us through specific cultural perspectives. Culture not only includes our backgrounds, upbringing, religious beliefs, and political affiliations, but also involves personal factors like gender, race, ethnicity, and nationality. Our perception and understanding of different cultures, people, historical events, and social issues are all influenced by our own culture.

To illustrate this point, we can examine how people from different cultures perceive age. Western cultures often lay strong emphasis on youthfulness, which can result in negative attitudes towards aging and the elderly. Some common stereotypes associated with aging in Western societies include slowness, loneliness, forgetfulness, fragility, financial difficulties, dullness, irritability, and vulnerability (Seeberg, 1984). However, this negative view of the elderly is not found in all cultures. It is generally believed that Asian societies, influenced by Confucian values of *xiaoshun* (filial piety) and the practice of ancestral worship, are thought to promote positive views of aging and high esteem for senior citizens. In China, an old person is a treasure to the family. Chinese people show respect to seniors and seniors try to act as models to their offspring. Therefore, elderly people help keep a family in order. During our younger years, we were often taught the value of showing respect towards older individuals. Filial piety is an indispensable part of Chinese culture, an important trait of being Chinese. Since respect for the old is not encouraged in the US, filial piety is seldom heard in people's daily conversation.

Similarly, the globalization of TCM is influenced by culture as well. For example, Taichi, a Chinese martial art that is both defensive and beneficial to health, is quite popular at TCM universities around the world. In China, it has attracted people young and old. For those who lack the knowledge of Taichi, a group of people practicing Taichi could be perceived as dancing. However, it is an effective way to strengthen the heart and lung besides overall improvement of health. Therefore, unless the patients seeking the help of TCM physicians are informed the efficacy of practicing Taichi while taking Chinese medicines, they would be confused by the doctors' advice to do Taichi daily and even ignore it.

Finally, personal experience also influences our perception. Typically, when we have a specific need or desire, our attention tends to be drawn towards stimuli that are associated with fulfilling that need. For instance, when hungry, we pay more attention to the delicious smell outside a restaurant. However, we do not notice it as much if we are full.

It can also be used to explain our understanding of TCM culture. For example, when an elderly person has suffered from asthma for many years and his condition has not been improved after extensive medical treatment, he is more likely to receive *sanfu* herbal patch (三伏贴), a TCM treatment technique applied during hot summer days to treat diseases that usually recur or worsen in the winter.

Features of Perception

Language, culture, personal experience, and other factors affect the perception of TCM and may even lead to misunderstandings or perception biases. Adler and Gunderson (2008) argued that perception has the following five features:

- Perception is selective; among so many competing stimuli that all try to get the attention of your senses, only a few can successfully become perceived.
- Perception is learned; socialization is also a process of learning how to perceive the world according to the norms and customs of the group you belong to.
- Perception is culturally determined; our culture serves as a textbook guiding us how to understand the world we are living in.
- Perception is consistent; once a certain reality is perceived in a particular manner, it usually stays there, not easy to change.
- Perception is inaccurate; our perceptions of the world are often influenced by our subjective lens, which is shaped by our cultural background, personal values, and individual experiences. This can lead us to see things in accordance with our expectations or desires.

However, communicating TCM across culture is feasible and achievable because humans share common perception of things all over the world. We have similar understandings of health, diseases, medicines, etc., which makes it possible to spread TCM across the globe. A close examination of medical practitioners' oaths both from China and the US turns out that the basic essence of medical practice remains the same: the dedication to medical research and patients, and respect for the rights of patients and colleagues. It is this common perception of responsibilities, duties and rights of medical practitioners that makes it possible to promote TCM across cultures. Moreover, TCM interculturalization is conducive to enriching human language and culture and improving people's perception of excellent traditional Chinese culture, which therefore deserves great attention.

── **Activities** ──────────────────────────────

Comprehension Questions

1.How do sensation and perception differ?

2.Please provide a definition of sensory overload and illustrate it with specific examples.

3.How does the process of human perception work, and how does culture influence each stage? Please provide specific examples to illustrate.

4.What are some key factors that shape people's perception of TCM culture?

5.What are some features of human perception and how do they shed light on TCM interculturalization?

Translation

Translate the following into Chinese.

　　This study aimed to examine the perceptions of healthcare professionals regarding the current use of TCM for prevention and treatment in TCM hospitals and TCM departments within general hospitals...These results indicate a certain degree of inadequate understanding of TCM for chronic disease care and prevention among healthcare professionals. However, it is worth noting that healthcare providers with better knowledge of TCM preventive and healthcare services are more likely to incorporate it into their daily practice.

Survey

　　Please conduct a survey on people's perception of specific TCM techniques such as acupuncture and moxibustion, *sanfu* herbal patches, or tuina. And then provide answers to the following questions.

　　　　• Does one's language or cultural background impact their perception of TCM?

　　　　• To what extent do factors such as gender, age, place of residence, educational levels, and family background influence people's understanding of TCM?

　　　　Lastly, present your findings to the class.

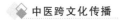
6.3 Thinking Patterns and TCM Culture

Deciphering Thinking Patterns

The strong connection between culture and language brings up intriguing inquiries about the correlation between language and thought. Just as our senses help us perceive the world, our means of communication, both through words and non-verbal cues, allow us to convey our perceptions. Sensory perception depends on physiological input and logical processing, as they help us decide what to pay attention to, how to categorize what is perceived, and what it means to us. As culture influences perception, it also impacts thinking patterns.

Thinking patterns are forms of reasoning and approaches to problem solving. In other words, it is about the way of working out problems. Thinking patterns differ from culture to culture. A logical, reasonable argument in one culture may be considered as illogical in another culture.

Thinking patterns affect not only the way we communicate in our culture but also the way we interact with people from different cultures. One of the pioneers in intercultural research, Kaplan (1966) explained the differences in thinking patterns that are reflected in five language systems, including English and Oriental. He observed that the cultural thinking pattern of English speakers is "dominantly linear in its development" (Kaplan, 1966, p. 4). The **linear pattern** can take either inductive (from specific to general) or deductive (from general to specific) reasoning.

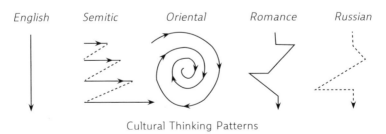

Cultural Thinking Patterns

Comparing Linear and Non-linear Patterns

The following paragraph written by Hsu (1999, pp. 1-2) showcases the deductive development commonly seen in English paragraphs.

Central to this study are the ways in which Chinese medical knowledge and practice are transmitted and learnt in three different social settings. These different modes of transmission may be called "secret", "personal", and "standardized", terms which refer primarily to the observed relationships between the medical practitioners and their acolytes, while simultaneously accounting for overall features of the settings in which the transmission of medical knowledge and practice took place. The "secret", "personal", and "standardized" modes do not describe idealized types; they were not starting assumptions nor hypotheses I set out to test, but have arisen from an interpretation of ethnographic data and correspond, in that sense, to the conclusion of the study.

The above paragraph follows a clear structure: It starts with a thesis statement describing three ways of TCM learning and transmission, and then moves to provide specific examples to support that statement. It remains focused on the central idea without going off on a tangent. Every sentence in the paragraph contributes meaningfully to the overall flow of ideas, leading from the opening sentence to the final sentence in a straight line.

Oriental thinking patterns (Chinese and Korean, excluding Japanese) are marked by an approach of indirection. The writing style of oriental languages is characterized by creating the subject with a variety of "digressive" viewpoints and creating a non-linear movement in which the subject is never mentioned directly. Simply put, the writing focuses on explaining ideas by highlighting what they are not, rather than explicitly stating what they are. In modern English writing, developing ideas by not focusing on what they are supposed to be would seem awkward and unnecessarily indirect to English readers (Kaplan, 1970).

The following paragraph comes from the preface to *TCM for Beginners in English* written by a Chinese scholar (Yin, 1992, preface).

Last year, the Chinese Ministry of Public Health started a two-year project to teach traditional Chinese doctors English in a specialized course. The aim of the course is to bridge the gap between foreign acupuncture students and their Chinese teachers, and to improve future international courses and scientific exchanges. By teaching in English loss of teaching time because of translation is eliminated, and the content is clearer. I was invited to give a four-month course on the fundamentals of traditional Chinese medicine (TCM) in English. When I finished my courses, some of my students encouraged me to publish my lecture notes, for the benefit of readers at home and abroad. Immediately after returning from Beijing, I started to compile and supplement my lecture notes with the help of the comments I received from many hours spent discussing acupuncture with doctors from all over China. This enabled me to improve my writing with new facts and to develop a holistic and systematic structure similar to the TCM concept.

The way this paragraph is structured is completely different from what we typically see in an English passage. The first three sentences provide background information to explain why it is important to train TCM physicians in their English skills. The fourth sentence switches the topic to the author as an English teacher. The fifth seems to emphasize the primary benefit of creating a TCM book in English, which is supported by the last two sentences. The last sentence is worth exploring further because it not only provides an explanation for the importance of classroom discussions with students but also connects to the fourth sentence and the previous one.

The main point of this paragraph is to explain the purpose of compiling a TCM book in English for the benefit of readers at home and abroad. However, this idea is introduced in the middle of the paragraph after the author provides some background context, which could be mistakenly considered as the main focus. Additionally, the author revisits the context towards the end of the paragraph, further adding to the potential confusion. As a result, native speakers of English might have difficulty in understanding the primary objective.

Comparing these two paragraphs provides valuable insights into TCM interculturalization. Paragraphs are constructed concepts used by writers to establish specific structures that are not present in spoken language. Hence, when TCM culture facilitators create written materials for intercultural activities, it becomes crucial for them to invest time and effort in comprehending cross-cultural patterns of thought. This is because they will not have the opportunity to explain or clarify any potential misunderstandings directly to the readers they are targeting.

Thinking Patterns in TCM

In terms of thinking patterns in TCM, *Qu Xiang Bi Lei* (取象比类), literally translated as "taking images to compare and categorize", i.e., using imagery and analogizing to govern changes, or simply known as **image thinking**, is deeply rooted in traditional Chinese culture, which is also a core methodology of Chinese medicine (Lan, 2015). Unlike abstract thinking, image thinking draws on the association of concrete images to uncover the underlying logic through comparison and contrast. To understand the essence of phenomena is to know the regularity. However, the relationship between an phenomenon and an essence is not easy to detect because usually there is no complete one-to-one correspondence. The power of image thinking lies in the fact that the recognition of images out of seemingly chaotic phenomena enables us to seek the essence.

Professor Lan (2015, p. 84) posited that *Qu Xiang Bi Lei* can be summarized into the following four steps:

- Observing the object (观物): directly observing the object or phenomenon.
- Taking image (取象): summarizing and refining the image of the object after repeatedly observing and feeling it.
- Comparing and analogizing (比 类): comparing the things which need to understand or know with the "image" just taken.
- Understanding Tao or the Way, the Rule (道体): finding the rules through the above comparing and analogizing activities.

Image-thinking is complementary to the holistic thinking pattern, another key concept in TCM. While holistic thinking pattern emphasizes wholeness or oneness, image thinking focuses on the separateness and interconnectedness among seemingly separate phenomena. "Imagery is categorized into original or basic image thinking, concrete image thinking, superficial image thinking, and visual thinking at different levels" (Wang, 2019, p. 197). The process of recognizing the original image in Chinese thinking involves experience, observation, and intuition. This pattern of thinking has been the mainstream approach in China for thousands of years.

Language, culture, and thought are intertwined with each other. As we focus on verbal communication in this chapter, language, a carrier of culture, influences and is influenced by thought at the same time. Different thinking patterns across cultures inform TCM culture facilitators to transmit the unique pattern of thinking, image thinking in TCM with care.

Chapter Summary

- Linguistics, the scientific study of human language, generally examines how human beings use language as symbols in the communication process.
- Chinese characters can be classified into six types based on how they are created: pictographs, ideographs, compound ideographs, borrowings, phonetic compounds, and mutually explanatory characters.
- The structure of a language influences how its speakers perceive the world around them and the relationship between language and culture or thought is called the Sapir-Whorf Hypothesis.
- Linguistic determinism holds that language determines how we think about the external reality.
- Linguistic relativism holds that the structure of a language we speak helps us know the world around us, thus reflects our thinking, beliefs, and attitudes.
- Sensation is the process by which receptor cells are stimulated and transmit their information to various brain centers.
- The process of organizing various sensations into meaningful parts, which is called perception, is, composed of three stages: selection, categorization, and interpretation, each of which is influenced by culture.
- Thinking patterns are forms of reasoning and approaches to problem solving.
- The cultural thinking pattern of English speakers is dominantly linear in its development. Oriental thinking patterns are marked by an approach of indirection.
- *Qu Xiang Bi Lei*, i.e., using imagery and analogizing to govern changes, or simply known as image thinking, is deeply rooted in traditional Chinese culture, which is also a core methodology of traditional Chinese medicine.

Checklist	Yes	No
Cognitive: I have mastered the core information		
Behavioral: I have the ability of putting what I've learned into practice		
Affective: I am willing to carry out what I've learned		
Moral: I will take the ethical consideration into account during practice		

Chapter 7

Moving Between Languages: Cultural Translation

Chapter Objectives

After reading this chapter, you should be able to:

◆ Identify two main features of TCM language: literariness and vagueness.

◆ Analyze different translations of titles of four TCM classics.

◆ Define cultural default and describe its value and underlying reasons in translation of TCM classics.

◆ Understand compensatory strategies for cultural default in translation of TCM classics.

◆ Develop a strong sense of pride in being Chinese for having such a profound TCM.

Key Terms

compiled translation	PMPH
cultural default	simile and metaphor
culture-loaded phrases	TCM classics
in-text annotation	vagueness
literary	WFCMS
metonymy	WHO
out-of-text annotation	Wiseman
parallelism	

Quotes

"Translation consists in reproducing in the receptor language the closest natural equivalent of the source language message, first in terms of meaning and secondly in terms of style."（所谓翻译,是指从语义到文体在译语中用最切近而又最自然的对等语再现原语的信息。）

——Eugene A. Nida

"A gentleman has three precepts: When he is young, his blood is uncertain, and his precepts are based on his appearance; when he is strong, his blood is strong, and his precepts are based on fighting; when he is old, his blood is weak, and his precepts are based on obtaining."（君子有三戒:少之时,血气未定,戒之在色;及其壮也,血气方刚,戒之在斗;及其老也,血气既衰,戒之在得。）

——《论语·季氏》

"For us to appreciate the basic differences and parallels between the more than two millennia of Western and Chinese medical traditions, access to English translations of the seminal life science texts of Chinese antiquity, unadulterated by modern biomedical concepts, is essential."（为了更好地理解中西医近两千多年来的发展异同,有必要阅读中国古代有关生命科学重要文献的英文译本。这些译文需要忠实呈现原文内容,且不受现代生物医学概念的影响。）

——Unschuld and Tessenow

Before reading this section, please consider the following questions:

1. What are the key characteristics that distinguish TCM terms from biomedical terminology?

2. What are some instances of TCM terms or expressions that exemplify the holistic approach and philosophical foundations of TCM?

7.1   Features of TCM Language

TCM Language

Traditional Chinese medicine (TCM) is developed in ancient China through observation and experience. In Asia, TCM stands as the oldest medical system. Over thousands of years, TCM has been formulated through extensive empirical testing and continual improvement. Theories, practices, and historical accounts of TCM have been documented and passed down through education and training of practitioners. Prior to the arrival of missionaries in the early 19th century, it served as the sole medical practice in China. These missionaries introduced drugs, devices, and practices of Western medicine, marking the emergence of alternative medical approaches alongside TCM. In countries like Japan, the Republic of Korea, Malaysia, and Vietnam, traditional medicine has its own unique culture. While each country may have different prescriptions and diagnostic methods, the underlying philosophy and principles are similar because they all started in China.

The earliest TCM classic, *Huangdi Neijing*, is one of the most important classical texts in TCM. It is believed to have been written during the Warring States Period (475–221 B.C.) and attributed to the legendary Yellow Emperor, *Huangdi*. Along with other TCM classics, this ancient text serves as the foundation of TCM theory, providing invaluable insights into the diagnosis, treatment, and maintenance of health.

TCM is more than just the product of medical science and technology. It also includes philosophy and way of life, making it a holistic approach to healthcare. TCM emphasizes the connection between the human body, nature, and the universe, perceiving health as a harmonious state, not just the absence of disease. The language used in TCM often includes imagery from nature and ancient mythology, reflecting its rich cultural heritage. This cultural dimension adds depth to TCM, allowing for a more comprehensive representation of its holistic nature. Under standing the cultural aspects of language used in TCM helps us grasp its principles and practices.

Literariness in TCM Language

Overall, TCM language is characterized by two distinctive features: literariness and vagueness. The most prominent feature of TCM language lies in its being **literary** for TCM classics are full of various rhetorical devices such as simile, metaphor, metonymy (转喻), and parallelism. Chinese medical texts are not only the exposition of medical theories and recording of classic prescriptions, but also the practitioners' insights into nature, mankind, and society. Numerous medical stories and cases are highly literary and enlightening.

Simile and **metaphor** are among the most frequently used figures of speech in TCM classics, both trying to extend the meaning of the original by associating two (closely linked) entities or ideas together with or without the use of "like", "as", etc. The employment of simile and metaphor helps readers have a concrete, vivid, and extended understanding of the original concept. Kenneth Burke, an American literary theorist, argued that "it is precisely through metaphor that our perspectives, or analogical extensions, are made — a world without metaphor would be a world without purpose" (Burke, 1984, p. 194).

Now, here comes an example from *Huangdi Neijing*. When the Yellow Emperor asked Qibo about the mutual relations between the twelve zang-organs in human body, Qibo answered, "What an exhaustive question you have asked. Now, let me tell you: The heart is the supreme commander or the monarch of the human body, which dominates the spirit, ideology, and thought of man." (悉乎哉问也！请遂言之。心者,君主之官也,神明出焉。) In this excerpt, heart is likened to a monarch among the five zang-organs. To fully comprehend this metaphor, one would require a rudimentary understanding of the Chinese feudal monarchical system. As the supreme leader of the state, the monarch has not only great power but also supreme status in ancient China. He represents the dignity and image of the country and is the supreme advocate of national interests. The status of the king determines that he must assume the important responsibility of maintaining the security and prosperity of the country. At the same time, he also needs to demonstrate his majesty and authority at all levels. With this information in mind, it is easy for us to understand how important the heart is among the five zang-organs.

When the original concept does not stand together with the concept or the entity that the original is likened to, a new form of figures of speech is employed, i.e., **metonymy**. In other words, the new entity is used to stand for the original one. For instance, in the phrase "*ge huang zhi shang, zhong you fu mu*" (膏肓之上, 中有父母), "*fumu*" ("parents") metonymically refers to the heart and lungs, highlighting their vital roles in sustaining life. As this example shows, metonymy is referential in nature. In addition to providing a familial concept/entity, this entity is used to substitute the original one, increasing the difficulty of meaning perception.

For TCM culture facilitators, it is advisable to use metonymy with care. Though some cognitive linguists argue that some metonymies are unlikely to cause difficulty in intercultural understanding, others do have greater potential to present comprehension difficulties between speakers of different cultures (Littlemore, 2015). Hilpert (2007), for example, investigated the metonymical use of body parts across 77 languages. In 18 languages (including English), the "ear" metonymy is used to imply "paying attention", and in other languages (e.g., Kyaka Enga, a language used in Papua New Guinea), "ears" are used to refer to "obedience". In TCM classics, ear is referred to as "*chuanglong*" (windows of cage), which contains a chain of metonymy. Human head is compared to "*long*" (cage) because both are round; *chuang* (window) is meant to provide an opening to the outside world, just like ears that offer head an opening to the outside. Therefore, the combination of these two entities gives rise to ear. The meaning of this and other metonymies may be less transparent for speakers of other languages, causing difficulties in TCM interculturalization.

TCM classics, especially those produced during the Warring States Period, are also full of poetic elements. For instance, *Huangdi Neijing* is written in a dialogic form. It is both colloquial and poetical, thus containing a lot of verses with rhymes (押韵) (Sun, 2012). **Parallelism** manifests itself in TCM language at multiple levels: lexical, phrasal, sentential, and even textual. Phrasal parallelism is exemplified by the following excerpt:

心欲苦，

肺欲辛，

肝欲酸，

脾欲甘，

肾欲咸。

The heart prefers bitter taste,

The lung prefers acid taste,

The liver prefers sour taste,

The spleen prefers sweet taste,

The kidney prefers salty taste.

In this example, the structure of "A prefers B" is repeated five times to create a smooth flow of the meaning intended to convey. It also helps leave a deep impression among the readers.

Sometimes, complex sentential parallelism is observed as follows:

逆春气,则少阳不生,肝气内变。

逆夏气,则太阳不长,心气内洞。

逆秋气,则太阴不收,肺气焦满。

逆冬气,则少阴不藏,肾气独沉。

If the principle of preserving health in spring being violated, one's *Shaoyang* energy will not be able to bring the function of generation into full play. Thus, the kidney energy will become worse internally.

If the principle of preserving health being violated in summer, one's *Taiyang* energy will not be able to bring the function of growth into full play. Thus, the heart energy will be stirring inside.

If the principle of preserving health being violated in autumn, one's *Shaoyin* energy will not be able to bring the function of harvesting into full play. Thus, the distention of lung energy will occur.

If the principle of preserving health being violated in winter, one's *Taiyin* energy will not be able to bring the function of storing into full play. As the *Taiyin* energy connects with the kidney internally, so when *Taiyin* fails to store, the kidney energy will degenerate, and its functions will become weak.

(Wu and Wu, 2012, p. 16).

In this excerpt, the structure of "A leads to B and C" is employed four times to strengthen the relationship between four seasons and four zang-organs. Interestingly, the middle of the second and four lines is rhymed with "ang", creating a sense of sound beauty.

Vagueness in TCM Language

The employment of so many rhetorical devices helps create a medical text that is quite literary and imaginative. It is also closely related to another feature, i.e., **vagueness**. That TCM language is vague or ambiguous arises from its implicit and sometimes obscure expressions, in addition to being literary or figurative. Examples abound in terms of how the meaning of TCM texts can be hard to understand rather than straightforward. It may sound unbelievable at first glance. After all, diagnosis and the corresponding treatment should be expressed as straight forwardly as possible to help the patient recover as much as possible. How can such an end be achieved if there exists opaque information which definitely impedes health communication? Before doubting the validity of TCM texts, let us examine an expression. The term "*yin qu*" (隐 曲) (literally, "hidden and crooked") denotes two specific parts of the human body: the urethral orifice (尿道口) and the anus (肛门). This indirect mode of expression is rooted in cultural norms of ancient China. In other words, euphemistic expressions are used in order to avoid directly mentioning concepts related to reproduction and private parts of human body. Sometimes, vagueness is caused by polysemy, the coexistence of many possible meanings for a word or phrase. An example is the term "*mingmen*" (命门), which has been translated in two ways: as a literal translation "life gate", and as the name of an acupoint "*mingmen* (GV4)" according to World Federation of Chinese Medicine Societies. This multiplicity of meanings can cause confusion, particularly in TCM inter culturalization. One proposed solution to this issue is to standardize TCM terms by assigning a single meaning to each term.

The vagueness of TCM language can be attributed to two key factors. Chinese is a high-context language, where interpretation relies heavily on contextual cues. Besides, traditional Chinese mode of thinking often employs analogical reasoning, contrasting with the Western approach which prioritizes logical reasoning over intuition. It is important for TCM culture facilitators to provide additional information to facilitate understanding, particularly for speakers of low-context languages like English.

Despite the challenges these linguistic features pose to intercultural communication, they are an integral part of the cultural identity reflected in the TCM language. These features not only add vividness to the language, but also fill it with a unique essence of Chinese culture. The goal of TCM interculturalization should not be to subjugate one culture to another, but rather to bridge the gap between high-context and low-context cultures, preserving the richness and diversity of human communication.

Activities

Comprehension Questions

1. What are the two main linguistic features that characterize TCM classics according to the passage?
2. What causes the literariness in TCM language? Illustrate your points with concrete examples.
3. What are other factors that could contribute to the literariness of TCM classics in addition to the ones discussed in this passage? Illustrate your points with concrete examples.
4. What causes the vagueness in TCM language? Illustrate your points with concrete examples.
5. What are some other linguistic features of TCM classics other than what is discussed in this section?

Debate

Debate topic: The Unique Language of TCM: Strengths and Limitations

Debate statement: TCM language, with its unique features, is a valuable asset in promoting holistic healthcare.

Debate guidelines

- Divide students into two teams: Team A and Team B. Team A will argue in favor of the statement, defending the notion that TCM language is a valuable asset in promoting holistic healthcare. Team B will argue against the statement, highlighting the limitations and challenges associated with TCM language.
- Each team should assign speakers who will present their arguments and provide supporting evidence.
- The debate should consist of an opening statement, rebuttals, and a closing statement.
- Encourage respectful and constructive dialogue, allowing students to present their viewpoints and challenge opposing arguments.
- After the debate, students can engage in a class discussion to further explore the theme and share their personal reflections.

Before reading this section, please consider the following questions:

1.What are the four classics of TCM in Chinese and English?

2.What are obstacles to translating TCM classics into English or other foreign languages?

7.2 Translating TCM Classics into English

Introducing Four TCM Classics

Colorful human civilization is not just about different ways of life; it is also about how different ways of life are conceptualized in languages. Some languages are quite robust; the number of users can exceed over 100 million, or even 1 billion (say, Chinese). Most of these languages reflect how the speakers of that language perceive the world. As TCM is deeply rooted in Chinese language and culture, one issue related to TCM interculturalization is how to render **TCM classics** into the target language properly and accurately. That is what translation should do.

As techniques that help bridge interlingual gaps, translation and interpretation are as old as intercultural activities. No one knows for sure when humans began to engage in translation activities in history. In ancient China, translators, known as *xiangxu* (象胥) in Chinese, are considered as officials who were responsible for entertaining guests from nearby countries in the Zhou Dynasty (1046–256 B. C.), serving as their liaison interpreters. As those guests could fall into sickness, an interpreter was required in their visit to TCM physicians. Unfortunately, no written documents exist about these earliest intercultural activities. Thus far, the first translation of TCM classics to European readers on record is attributed to Michel Boym (1612–1659), a Polish missionary, who must have read some books on TCM, and commented on what he read in Latin

(Ma and Zhang, 2023).

However, systematic translation of TCM classics into English and other modern European languages began in the early 20th century when a six-page English version of *Huangdi Neijing* was published in *Annuals of Medical History* (Wang Y Q, 2023). As is known to all, there are four TCM classics, *Huangdi Neijing*, *Nanjing* (《难经》), *Shanghan Zabing Lun* (《伤寒杂病论》) and *Shen Nong Bencao Jing* (《神农本草经》). The translation of these four classics and other TCM academic literature helps promote TCM across cultures. Due to the immense scope of translation involved, the main focus of this section is twofold: One is on the study of how to translate titles of TCM classics by comparing four major versions, namely, World Federation of Chinese Medicine Societies (hereafter WFCMS) (Li, 2007), WHO West-Pacific Region (hereafter WHO) (WHO, 2022), Nigel Wiseman's version (hereafter Wiseman) (Wiseman, 1998), and Terminology of People's Medical Publishing House (hereafter PMPH); Another is to offer a mini history of translating the earliest and most significant TCM monograph, *Huangdi Neijing*.

Translating Book Titles of Four TCM Classics

The following table summarizes the four English versions of TCM classics. Let us begin with *Huangdi Neijing*, which is viewed universally as the most important classic book on TCM.

Titles of Four TCM Classics in English

| | Huangdi Neijing | Nanjing | Shanghan Zabing Lun | | Shennong |
			shang han lun	jin gui yao lue	
WFCMS	Huangdi's Internal Classic (huáng dì nèi jīng, 黄帝内经)	/	Treatise on Cold Damage Diseases (shāng hán lùn)	Synopsis of the Golden Chamber (jīn kuì yào lüè)	/

Continued

| | Huangdi Neijing | Nanjing | Shanghan Zabing Lun | | Shennong |
			shang han lun	jin gui yao lue	
WHO	Huangdi's Internal Classic (Huangdi Neijing, 黄帝内经)	Classic of Difficult Issues (Nanjing, 难经)	Treatise on Cold Damage and Miscellaneous Diseases (Shanghanzabinglun)		Shen Nong's Classic of Materia Medica (Shenong bencaojing)
Wiseman	huang2 di4 nei4 jing1, 书名 The Yellow Emperor's Inner Canon (1st Century)	nan4 jing1, 书名 The Classic of Difficult Issues (1st Century, Eastern Han4)	shang1 han2 za2 bing4 lun4, 书名 On Cold Damage and Miscellaneous Diseases (Eastern Han4, Zhang1 Ji1 张机[Zhong4-Jing3 仲景]		/
PMPH	The Yellow Emperor's Inner Classic (Huáng Dì Nèi Jīng, 黄帝内经)	The Classic of Difficult Issues (Nàn Jīng, 难经)	Treatise on Cold Damage and Miscellaneous Diseases (Shāng Hán Zá Bìng Lùn, 伤寒杂病论)		Shen Nong's Classic of the Materia Medica (Shén Nóng Běn Cǎo Jīng, 神农本草经)

• Huangdi Neijing

According to WFCMS, *this book* is translated as *Huangdi's Internal Classic* (huáng dì nèi jīng, 黄帝内经), using **transliteration** (音译) (Huangdi), **literal translation** (直译) (Internal Classic) together with Chinese characters. WHO's version is *Huangdi's Internal Classic* (Huangdi Neijing, 黄帝内经). As can be seen, it is quite similar to that of WFCMS. The version by Nigel Wiseman, a well-known TCM translator, is huang2 di4 nei4 jing1, 书名 *The Yellow Emperor's Inner Canon* (1st Century). Wiseman's version is very friendly to common readers, especially suitable for beginners because it includes pinyin, the standard system of Roman spelling in Chinese, with tones, followed by literal translation of the title and even the date when the book was written. This additional information is a good way of transmitting Chinese elements as pinyin is unique and very Chinese in addition to literal translation which is meant to get meaning across.

PMPH, stipulated by one of the leading publishing houses in China with a focus on medicine, translates it as *The Yellow Emperor's Inner Classic* (*Huáng Dì Nèi Jīng*, 黄帝内经), combining literal translation, transliteration and Chinese characters.

The major differences among the four versions lie in how to translate *Huangdi* and *Neijing*. PMPH and Wiseman translate *Huangdi* into Yellow Emperor, an example of literal translation, while WFCMS and WHO choose Huangdi, a typical example of transliteration. Li and Kuang (2021) argued that the adoption of Yellow Emperor only looks at the superficial meaning of the book, ignoring the historical implication associated with the English word "emperor". Since *Huangdi Neijing* was written in the Warring States Period (475–221 B. C.), quite earlier than the establishment of feudalist system in China, the term "di" in Chinese does not necessarily denote an "emperor". In fact, it holds a much greater significance, as during the Shang Dynasty (c. 1600–1046 B.C.), "di" referred to the supreme deity who governed all aspects of the world. It is said that Huangdi originally had the surname Gongsun and the given name Xuanyuan. However, he was given the title Huangdi, thus becoming the ancestor of the Chinese people and worshipped by Chinese offspring. Therefore, it is reasonable to assume that the use of "di" was intended to elevate the mortal to the immortal realm. Additionally, the English term "emperor" typically denotes the ruler of an empire, like Augustus (63 B.C.–A.D. 14), the first Roman Emperor. As the word suggests, an empire encompasses a vast collection of states or countries under a single supreme authority. It is widely believed that Huangdi did not govern an empire but rather acted as a leader of a small tribe. Hence, the English term "emperor" may not be the most accurate choice for *Huangdi* in *Huangdi Neijing*. Otherwise, it could lead to cultural default which is the topic of next section of this chapter.

• *Nanjing*

The discussion around the origin of *Nanjing* remains highly contentious (Xu *et al.*, 2023): One popular belief is that *Nanjing* is an extended exegesis of *Huangdi Neijing* while others argue that *Nanjing* is an independent TCM book written by Bianque (扁鹊) (407–310 B. C.), the earliest known Chinese physician. Mythical stories about how Bianque miraculously cured many seemingly incurable diseases might contribute to the claim that it was Bianque who composed *Nanjing* which is a collection of eighty-one difficult medical issues. Unlike *Huangdi Neijing* which has attracted so many researchers and translators around the world, it was not until in 1986 that the first English version of *Nanjing* was published (Zhao, 2008). *Nanjing* is not included in WFCMS, so there is no English title of this book. WHO translates it as *Classic of Difficult Issues* (Nanjing, 难经), combining literal translation, transliteration and Chinese characters. Wiseman renders it as *nan4 jing1*, 书名 *The Classic of Difficult Issues* (1st Century, Eastern Han4), using pinyin with tones, together with Chinese characters indicating this is a book, followed by the literal translation of the title and the date when it was written. And PMPH translates it as *The Classic of Difficult Issues* (*Nàn Jīng*, 难经), in a way that is quite similar to WHO. In essence, these three versions are quite similar. This is mainly because the meaning of "*Nanjing*" itself is straightforward: "Nan" means difficult, "jing" classic.

• *Shanghan Zabing Lun*

Shanghan Zabing Lun, authored by Zhang Zhongjing (张仲景) (A.D. 150–219), Sage of Medicine, has established the basic framework for the identification and treatment of diseases and norms for the application of TCM in clinical practice, and thus is known as the "Book of Formulas" in TCM practice. To date, this book is still the main guide for the practice of TCM. As a TCM classic, *Shanghan Zabing Lun* has been translated into English and other foreign languages partially or completely. One of the very noteworthy translations is the first full translation of the original texts done by Luo Xiwen, a researcher at the Institute of Philosophy of the Chinese Academy of Social Sciences in 1986 (Chen J *et al.*, 2019). In addition to being poetic and ambiguous, there are other linguistic characteristics that make translation of this TCM classic challenging. These include use of diverse terminology, need for syndrome differentiation, precision in prescribing treatments, flexibility in clinical practice, and conciseness in expression (Chen J *et al.*, 2019, p. 1401).

Since this book is composed of two volumes, *shang han lun and jin gui yao lue*, WFCMS renders two parts instead of one, namely *Treatise on Cold Damage Diseases* (shāng hán lùn) and *Synopsis of the Golden Chamber* (jīn kuì yào lüè). WHO's version is *Treatise on Cold Damage and Miscellaneous Diseases* (Shanghan zabing lun), using both literal translation and transliteration. Wiseman's version is shang1 han2 za2 bing4 lun4, 书名 *On Cold Damage and Miscellaneous Diseases*(Eastern Han4, Zhang1 Ji1 张机[Zhong4-Jing3 仲景]. He continues with his own way of translating, putting pinyin with tones first, followed by Chinese characters of 书名 meaning it is a book title, and finally the literal translation of the book title, together with the date when the book was written and its author's name both in pinyin and Chinese characters. PMPH's version is *Treatise on Cold Damage and Miscellaneous Diseases* (*Shāng Hán Zá Bìng Lùn*, 伤寒杂病论). As it usually does, this version begins with literal translation of the book title followed by pinyin with tones and Chinese characters. It is quite clear that this is the rule of translation for classics by PMPH. Simply put, the title of classics translated by PMPH contains three parts: meaning of the title in English (usually literally translated), pinyin with tones and Chinese characters. It is worth noting that *shanghan* is translated quite literally into cold damage.

• *Shennong Bencao Jing*

Shennong Bencao Jing is a Chinese book on agriculture and medicinal plants. Its origin has been attributed to the mythical Chinese sovereign Shennong, who was said to have lived around 2800 B.C. This book documents the comprehensive knowledge about 365 medicinal substances, including their taste, effects, and primary uses, as recorded by medical practitioners from the Warring States Period (476B.C.-221B.C.) to the Qin-Han Period (221B.C.-220A.D.). It represents the vast encyclopedic knowledge and intellectual contributions of ancient Chinese scholars in the field of pharmacology.

WFCMS does not include this classic in its catalogue. WHO's version is *Shen Nong's Classic of Materia Medica* (Shenongbencaojing). As can be seen, this English version includes transliteration of *Shen Nong*, and literal translation of *Classic and Materia Medica*. Once again, attached to the end is the pinyin. PMPH translates it as *Shen Nong's Classic of the Materia Medica* (*Shén Nóng Běn Cǎo Jīng*, 神农本草经). It is quite similar to that of WHO but with Chinese characters attached to the end as it usually does. In a word, for this classic, *bencao* is translated as materia medica. This is better than the word of "herbs", because materia medica refers to the branch of medical science concerned with the study of drugs used in the treatment of disease, including pharmacology, clinical pharmacology, and the history and physical and chemical properties of drugs. Herbs, however, are plants whose leaves are used in cooking to add flavor to food, or as a medicine. It turns out that Chinese materia medica uses not only plants, but also animals and minerals as its sources. Based on what is discussed here, materia medica stands out as a better version to translating *bencao*.

Apart from the above-mentioned exemplars, many other translations for TCM classics have emerged over the course of history. The ones discussed herein are prominent international standardized versions and those advocated by the esteemed TCM translator, Wiseman. Nevertheless, we enthusiastically urge you to delve deeper and unearth supplementary translations, while critically evaluating their individual merits and limitations.

Translating *Huangdi Neijing*

Huangdi Neijing is widely acknowledged as the most significant among the four classics of TCM. It also boasts the highest number of translation versions compared to the other three texts. As highlighted by Yang and Chen (2020), the first translation of *Huangdi Neijing* was recorded in 1925. Since then, a total of 24 versions have been produced up to the present time (Lan, 2004). Among them, fourteen are for academic research, nine for clinical application, and the remaining one for cultural promotion. The earliest translation of *Huangdi Neijing* was done by Percy M. Dawson and published in 1925 in *Annals of Medical History*. However, Dawson just translated excerpts of the book from the perspective of medical history. As for terminology translation, Dawson mainly adopted literal translation and free translation, except for the concepts of yin and yang. His negative sentiment towards this book and TCM is evident in the way he translated it.

Among the various versions, it is worth mentioning Paul Unschuld's translation. His version, entitled *Huang Di Nei Jing Su Wen: Nature, Knowledge, Imagery,* was published in 2003. Paul Unschuld is the Director of Institute of Medical History, University of Munich, Germany. His translation can be categorized as **compiled translation** (编译). Unschuld (2003) mentioned in the preface that "we aim to produce the first semantically correct complete SU WEN English version which can serve as a research tool for the original text". To accomplish this, he extensively referenced more than 3,000 papers and over 600 monographs as supplementary sources. Consequently, his translation project stands out as the most extensive endeavor of its kind in the Western world. Notably, it represents a unique integration of translation and research, with its content and style resembling that of textbooks published in China for TCM universities.

In 2005, Li Zhaoguo, a renowned Chinese scholar and translator devoted to the translation and dissemination of TCM across cultures, has published his version of *Huangdi Neijing*, entitled "*Yellow Emperor's Canon of Medicine: Plain Conversation*". Three years later, his version of "*Yellow Emperor's Canon of Medicine: Spiritual Pivot*" was published. Together, his version is considered as the first full English version of *Huangdi Neijing* done by scholars from China's mainland, a pioneering work, playing a pivotal role in TCM interculturalization. Professor Li Zhaoguo advocated the use of transliteration accompanied by annotations when there are no corresponding terms available. This approach is evident in his translation, for instance, where he rendered 神 as "Shen" with the annotation "Spirit", and 精 as "Jing" with the annotation "Essence".

The diverse English versions of *Huangdi Neijing* reflect a range of translation strategies, principles, and methods, each influenced by various factors such as sponsors, translators, target audience, academic and historical context, among others. While debates may arise concerning which version is superior, it is crucial to take into account all these factors. It is evident that there is still significant improvement to be made in accurately translating major medical works on TCM into foreign languages like English, Spanish, and others.

Activities

Comprehension Questions

1. Which classic is the most translated TCM book so far?

2. What is Dawson Percy's attitude towards TCM?

3. What are the features of Paul Unschuld's version of *Huangdi Neijing*? What are the underlying reasons?

4. Comment on Professor Li Zhaoguo's translation principle in dealing with terms without corresponding words of English.

5. Look for information of other TCM texts that are translated into English or other foreign languages, and report to the class.

Translation Analysis

Compare the following two translated versions. List their differences. After that, search for relevant information to analyze the possible factors causing these differences.

[Original Text]

今时之人不然也,以酒为浆,以妄为常,醉以入房,以欲竭其精,以耗散其真,不知持满,不时御神,务快其心,逆于生乐,起居无节,故半百而衰也。

——《素问·上古天真论》

[English Version A]

People nowadays, on the contrary, just behave oppositely. [They] drink wine as thin rice gruel, regard wrong as right, and seek sexual pleasure after drinking. [As a result] their Jingqi (Essence-Qi) is exhausted and Zhenqi (Genuine-Qi) is wasted. [They] seldom [take measures to] keep an exuberance [of Jingqi] and do not know how to regulate the Shen (mind or spirit), often giving themselves to sensual pleasure. Being irregular in daily life, [they begin to] become old even at the age of fifty. (Translated by Li Zhaoguo)

[English Version B]

The fact that people of today are different is because they take wine as an [ordinary] beverage, and they adopt absurd [behavior] as regular [behavior]. They are drunk when they enter the [women's] chambers. Through their lust they exhaust their essence, through their wastefulness they dissipate their true [qi]. They do not know how to maintain fullness and they engage their spirit when it is not the right time. They make every effort to please their hearts, [but] they oppose the [true] happiness of life. Rising and resting miss their terms. Hence, it is [only] one half of a hundred [years] and they weaken. (Translated by Paul Unschuld)

7.3   Cultural Default in TCM Translation

Culture is the total pattern of unique beliefs, customs, institutions, goals, and techniques that a society shares with its members. TCM has a long history and embodies rich traditional Chinese culture with distinct regional and national characteristics. In the context of TCM interculturalization, Chinese and English are two cultural systems that exhibit significant disparities in meaning. Consequently, when translating TCM classics into English, cultural default poses a huge challenge that needs to be addressed. If improperly handled, cultural default (文化缺省) can lead to misunderstandings that affect effective intercultural communication and hinder TCM interculturalization. Therefore, dealing with the challenge of cultural defaultduring the translation process from Chinese to English is of utmost importance for successful international promotion of TCM culture.

Definition and Function of Cultural Defaults

Cultural default often takes place due to the lack of shared cultural knowledge between the parties involved in intercultural communication (Shen Xiao, 2020). People who have the same cultural understanding have established specific cultural patterns influenced by historical background, traditions, and religious beliefs. Cultural default is the result of leaving blanks in these aspects by source language communicators or authors. When the target language communicators first encounter the language and culture of the other party, they may experience semantic gaps due to a lack of familiarity with the strangers' cultural traditions, thus encountering obstacles in visual reading or aural comprehension. The act of translation/interpretation is to fill in the missing elements between source language and target language by reducing the degree of deficiency as much as possible and achieving effective intercultural communication.

Cultural default plays an important role in TCM interculturalization. It functions in establishing coherence between the author and the reader by conveying cultural information that is presumed or omitted, thus ensuring continuity throughout the text. Readers are actively and constantly trying to figure out the hidden cultural implications by employing the cultural norms and frameworks of their own group, thus maintaining the cognitive comprehensibility of the text. When cultural norms and frameworks are misplaced, especially when incorrect cognitive information is used, it often results in misunderstandings, even if the conversation appears to be smooth on the surface. In other words, cultural default tends to create obstacles rather than dismantle the difficulties in intercultural transmission. Additionally, the aesthetic implication of cultural omissions out of cultural default should not be overlooked. Excluding cultural backgrounds usually contributes to concise writing and adheres to the principle of efficient communication. Cultural omissions also create "blanks" that encourage readers' imagination. When interpreting texts with cultural default, readers must rely on their own associations and imagination, draw upon their knowledge, engage in creative reading, actively participate in constructing meaning, and find delight in skillful interpretation. This may sound wonderful. However, these cultural omissions tend to discourage readers from other cultural groups to actively read and interpret the text.

Causes of Cultural Default

Cultural default in the translation of TCM classics is mainly caused by two factors: culture-loaded phrases and metaphors in TCM terminology (Li and Xie, 2021, p. 225).

Culture-loaded phrases are widely present in intercultural activities, which easily lead to misunderstandings when different ethnic groups and cultures interact with each other. They are manifested in the translation system as zero equivalent word, i.e., there is no counterpart corresponding to the cultural information carried by the source language vocabulary in the translated language (Bao and Bao, 2004, p. 10). To put it another way, **culture-loaded phrases** are words, phrases or idiomatic signs of things that are unique to the culture of a particular ethnic group and reflect the unique way of life that has gradually developed during its historical development and is not found in other ethnic groups (Li et al., 2023). Deeply influenced by ancient Chinese philosophy, history, and literature, TCM terminology and literature inherently comprise a significant number of culturally rich words. For example, the term "*shenming*" (神明) in the classic text *Suwen·Bazheng Shenming Lunpian* (《素问•八正神明论》) is a typical expression of culture-loaded phrases. In modern Chinese dictionaries, "*shenming*" means "the general term for gods". If it is translated directly into English as "deities" or "gods", it would result in misunderstanding. In TCM, the concept of "*shenming*" encompasses three distinct layers of meaning (Li *et al.*, 2021, p. 225): (1) spirit or consciousness; (2) natural phenomena such as sun, moon, stars, and their laws; (3) profound mysteries. The semantic correspondences of the term "*shenming*" in TCM, therefore, vary depending on different contexts. When used independently, "*shenming*" is commonly understood as referring to a "bright spirit". Nevertheless, given that the primary objective of the chapter "*Suwen · Bazheng Shenming Lun*" is to explain the impact of natural changes during the four seasons on the circulation of qi and blood, for better semantic accuracy, it should be translated as "Discussion on the Mysterious Influence of the Eight Directions on Acupuncture". Otherwise, cultural default takes place when English readers try to associate the influence of "*shenming*" with "supernatural being". This instance shows that the presence of culture-loaded phrases in TCM poses a challenge in translating TCM classics and many of them may contribute to cultural default.

Metaphor is not only a rhetorical tool, but also a cognitive pattern that is deeply rooted in culture and language. Metaphorical cognition forms the foundation of TCM reasoning, which emphasizes exploration rather than verification and recognizes analogy as a crucial characteristic of TCM terminology. By observing the inherent connections among universal phenomena, ancient Chinese people employed analogical methods to simplify complex problems into more general ones. The principles of yin-yang doctrine and five-phase theory exemplify this characteristic in various aspects. By observing the five primordial natural elements and their interconnected relationships, ancient Chinese people metaphorically described the interdependence among relationships between human organs by matching the five elements with the corresponding organs using concepts such as mutual generation, overcoming, restraining, multiplying, among others. This creative application of metaphor and analogy, collectively known as the image-thinking mode is another source of cultural misunderstanding out of cultural default in TCM inter culturalization.

In *Huangdi Neijing*, "*shanggong*" and "*xiagong*" use directional metaphors, referring to highly skilled and ordinary practitioners respectively. Similarly, the application of the terms "sovereign fire" and "ministerial fire" in TCM terminology demonstrates another clever use of metaphor. According to the *Dictionary of*

Traditional Chinese Medicine (Li *et al.*, 2009), sovereign fire and ministerial fire complement each other by nurturing the zang-organs and ensuring normal bodily functions. "Sovereign" represents a ruler and "minister" represents an assistant. "Fire" symbolizes the force behind growth and change. "Sovereign fire" directs growth and change, while "ministerial fire" follows its guidance, promoting transformations and development. These metaphors are vividly used to describe their relationship. A proper translation enables target readers to use a similar cultural framework for understanding, thus preventing potential misunderstandings caused by cultural differences.

Compensatory Strategies

The cultural gaps between the source language and target language create significant challenges for translation. Due to different cultural backgrounds, including values and thinking patterns, there is often a lack of shared cultural knowledge. Cultural information assumed or understood by the original author and readers may be unfamiliar or foreign to readers of the target language. If these shared pieces of information are not translated during the translation process, it becomes difficult for target language readers to form a coherent context, leading to misunderstandings or what is known as "semantic vacuum". In such a situation, it becomes necessary to bridge cultural gaps in translated texts in order to effectively convey the intended communication within the target culture. Translators often use two main strategies to address cultural gaps in translation: out-of-text annotation and in-text annotation. **"Out-of-text annotation"** refers to providing footnotes or endnotes alongside the main text, while **"in-text annotation"** involves indicating missing information directly within the main text itself through paraphrasing or combining literal translations with additional clarification.

Out-of-Text Annotation

Unschuld's annotated translation of "*Su Wen*" (2003) is a remarkable piece of work that extensively explores the sources and context of the text in its footnotes. By doing so, it successfully captures and reflects the original meaning and style of "*Huangdi Neijing·Su Wen*" to the maximum extent. To explore the original meaning of metaphorical expressions in ancient medicine, the translators refrained from using modern Western medical terminology to explain or rephrase a text written two thousand years ago. Instead, the translators carefully chose words based on a deep understanding of how ancient medical terms were originally formed. They also included annotations that help accurately portray the content of TCM. For example:

Original text:

食饮有节,起居有常,不妄作劳 (《素问·上古天真论》)

Translation:

[Their] eating and drinking were moderate.

[Their] rising and resting had regularity.

They did not tax [themselves] with meaningless work.

Footnotes:

Lin Yi et al., "Quan Yuanqi has 饮食有常节, 起居有常度, 不妄不作. The Tai Su (《黄帝内经太素》) has this wording, too. Yang Shangshan stated, 'They chose sound and form, as well as fragrant flavors, on the basis of li 礼, [that is,] they were not reckless(鲁莽的) in what they observed and heard. When they moved they did so in accordance with li; they never performed activities beyond their province.'" 2168/ 6 agrees with a lengthy discussion. Hu Shu, "The [wording in the] Quan Yuanqi edition and in the version of Yang Shangshan is correct. 作 is identical with 诈, 'to pretend,' 'to deceive.' 作 was read like 胙, zu, in antiquity (古代). The preceding three characters 者, 数, and 度 formed a rhyme [with 作] and they rhymed with 俱 and 去 below. When Mr. Wang changed 饮食有常节, 起居有常度 to 饮食有节, 起居有常, the sentence structure no longer juxtaposed(并列) true and false. When he changed 不妄不作 to 不妄作劳, he misread 作 as the 作 of 作为, 'to work.' Yang Shangshan in his comment on the Tai Su committed the same error. By linking 作 with 劳, Wang Bing completely distorted the meaning of the classic!" Following this argument, the passage should read, "In food and drinking they observed moderation. In rising and resting they observed regularity. Neither did they behave recklessly, nor did they commit any deceptive activities." (Unschuld and Tessenow, 2011, p. 31)

Apart from the addition of three words, namely "their", "their", and "themselves", the translation maintains consistency with the original text in both content and structure. However, in-depth explanations are provided in footnotes regarding different commentators on *Huangdi Neijing* including Lin Yi, Quan

Yuanqi, Yang Shangshan, Wang Bing etc., as well as their comments found in Tai Su edition. This footnote suggests that Wang Bing's alteration of "不妄不作" to "不妄不作" weakens certain semantic elements, thereby distorting the original meaning to some extent. Furthermore, this footnote offers a re-translation for the new interpretation, enabling readers to comprehend the multiple meanings or controversies that arise from this sentence. In doing so, it adds contextual depth to the understanding of the text.

In-Text Annotation

Maoshing Ni, a licensed acupuncturist and doctor of oriental medicine in California, US, approaches the translation of "Su Wen" from the standpoint of a clinical physician. Instead of relying on footnotes, Ni (2011) offered comprehensive explanations and translations within the text itself. The objective of this integration is to ensure that the translated version of "*Su Wen*" is clear, comprehensible, and readable. For example, in Chapter 3 titled "The Union of Heaven and Human Beings", there is a sentence that reads, "其生五,其气三." A literal translation of this sentence would be "It produces five, and its qi changes into three", which is almost incomprehensible for foreigners who are unfamiliar with TCM. Therefore, the author skillfully explains its meaning as follows, "These five elemental phases also correspond to the three yin and the three yang of the universe. These are the six atmospheric influences that govern the weather patterns that reflect in changes in our planetary ecology. If people violate or disrupt this natural order, then pathogenic forces will have an opportunity to cause damage to the body..." This interpretation helps readers understand the implied meaning and principles behind weather, which are derived from the concepts of the five phases and yin-yang theory. The translation becomes clear and straightforward.

Implications for TCM Interculturalization

Since the literature and classics of TCM hold a vast amount of traditional Chinese culture and its unique theories, translating TCM classics into English often involves cultural gaps, which poses challenges for intercultural understanding. Authors sometimes omit certain cultural information in their works, which encourages readers to actively interpret and engage with the text. However, these cultural omissions can lead to misunderstandings, especially when the cultural framework of the intended readers greatly differs from that of the authors. To address this, strategies such as out-of-text annotation and in-text annotation are utilized to compensate for the loss of cultural context, thereby facilitating TCM interculturalization.

Chapter Summary

- TCM language is characterized by two distinctive features: literariness and vagueness.
- The most prominent feature of TCM language lies in its being literary for TCM classics are full of various rhetorical devices such as simile, metaphor, metonymy, and parallelism.
- For TCM culture facilitators, it is advisable to use metonymy with care. Though some cognitive linguists argue that some metonymies are unlikely to cause difficulty in intercultural understanding, others do have greater potential to present compre hension difficulties between speakers of different cultures.
- Cultural default in the translation of TCM classics is mainly caused by two factors: culture-loaded phrases and metaphors in TCM terminology.
- Translators often use two main strategies to address cultural gaps in translation: out-of-text annotation and in-text annotation.

Checklist	Yes	No
Cognitive: I have mastered the core information		
Behavioral: I have the ability of putting what I've learned into practice		
Affective: I am willing to carry out what I've learned		
Moral: I will take the ethical consideration into account during practice		

Chapter 8

Nonverbal Communication: Action, Space and Time

Chapter Objectives

After reading this chapter, you should be able to:

◆ Define nonverbal communication and understand its function in human communication.

◆ Classify nonverbal communication and relate them to TCM interculturalization.

◆ Define the four diagnostic methods of TCM.

◆ Reproduce a scene of TCM diagnosis and treatment.

◆ Explore nonverbal communication strategies in TCM interculturalization.

─(Key Terms)─────────────────────────────

auscultation and olfaction

body language (kinesics)

contradiction

eye contact (oculesics)

facial expressions

gesture

inquiry

monochronic (M-time)

object language

observation

palpation or pulse-taking

paralanguage (vocalics)

polychronic (P-time)

repetition

spatial language (proxemics)

substitution

TCM diagnosis

time language (chronemics)

Quotes

"We should revitalize and further develop traditional Chinese medicine, giving it equal emphasis with Western medicine; promote complementary and coordinated development between Western medicine and TCM; and encourage the innovative transformation and development of TCM culture." (要着力推动中医药振兴发展,坚持中西医并重,推动中医药和西医药相互补充、协调发展,努力实现中医药健康养生文化的创造性转化、创新性发展。)

——2016 年 8 月 19 日习近平在全国卫生与健康大会上的讲话

"Inspection of the exterior manifestations will enable one to understand the interior conditions; diagnosis of the exterior manifestations will enable one to know the interior states. This is due to the fact that the functions of the internal organs often have their external manifestations." (欲知其内者,当以观乎外,诊于外者,斯以知其内,盖有诸内者形诸外。)

——《丹溪心法》(元·朱震亨)

"There is language in her eyes, her cheeks, her lips." (若人眼中、颊上、唇边莫不有话言。)

——William Shakespeare

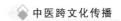
Before reading this section, please consider the following questions:

1. Have you ever heard of verbal and nonverbal communication? How do they differ from each other?

2. Do you agree that nonverbal communication is an inseparable part of TCM interculturalization? Why, or why not?

8.1 Essentials of Nonverbal Communication

Importance of Nonverbal Communication

Human communication is "a dynamic process in which people attempt to share their thoughts with other people through the use of symbols in particular settings" (Samovar *et al.*, 2017, p. 28). The two-way process as illustrated in previous chapters encompasses the source (encoder / sender), encoding, message (encoded thought), channel / medium, target audience (receiver / decoder), decoding, noise, context, etc. Traditionally, studies on the encoding process have mainly focused on verbal and written language, but over the last number of years the importance of nonverbal communication has gradually come into its own. That is to say, what is not said is sometimes as important as or even more important than what is said. On some occasions, people even express more nonverbally than verbally. For example, if you want to answer the teacher's questions during a lecture, you can let him or her know your intention with eye contact, facial expression, or just by putting up your hand.

Most people might not have realized the importance of those nonverbal means of communication and therefore ignored their full potential. Yet, communication theorists reveal that in daily face-to-face communication, less than 35% of the information is exchanged via speaking, and over 65% of the message is communicated by nonverbal means (Burgoon *et al.*,

2010). One study even goes further by claiming that 93% of the message is transmitted by voice tone and facial expression whereas only 7% is based on words (Mehrabian and Wiener, 1967). Though these research findings do not apply to most of our daily exchanges of information and even turn out to be "a faulty one" (Burgoon *et al.,* 2010, p. 4), we are at least reminded that we rely heavily on nonverbal cues to express ourselves and to understand others' communication. It follows that nonverbal communication also matters a lot to communicating traditional Chinese medicine (TCM) across cultures.

Defining and Classifying Nonverbal Communication

Nonverbal communication is present everywhere and runs through human communication. Like culture and communication, a single definition is never easy to compose. Jia *et al.* (2019) claimed that all intentional and unintentional, conscious and unconscious behaviors in interaction and communication, other than spoken or written words, are considered to be nonverbal. Likewise, Samovar and his colleagues deemed that nonverbal communication includes "all those nonverbal stimuli in a communication setting that are generated by both the source and his or her use of the environment, and that have potential message value for the source or receiver" (Samovar *et al.,* 2017, p. 297).

Let us pause for a while to decide if the following is considered a nonverbal stimulus.

- an upright posture
- coughing
- falling down in a hurry
- gazing with widely-opened eyes
- sitting in the first row because of a visual impairment
- wearing one black and one yellow training shoe

Some people may see these situations as communication,

while others may not. Burgoon *et el.* (2010) argued that in order to decide whether a certain instance of nonverbal stimuli can constitute communication, one has to make a distinction between information, behavior, and communication. Not every piece of information is accounted as behavior, let alone communication. To be communication, the behavior must be targeted to a receiver or receivers. Thus, we define nonverbal communication as a system of symbols, signs, and gestures other than language, which is developed and used by members of a culture to bring specific messages to expression.

Forms of Nonverbal Communication

In a broad sense, nonverbal communication covers the following areas: visual and auditory performance codes, body codes, contact codes, time and place codes (Burgoon, *et al.*, 2010). These are nonverbal codes based on the medium used to transmit signals.

Each of these areas include a couple of sub-areas. Below are some of the common topics most communication researchers are interested in:

- Body language (kinesics): postures, stance, gestures made by different parts of human body, facial expression, eye contact, physical appearance, adornment, and smell (olfactics).
- Paralanguage (vocalics): tempo, volume, silence, hesitation, pitch, etc.
- Time language (chronemics): time orientation, promptness, punctuality, etc.
- Spatial language (proxemics): distance kept between people, body touch (haptics).
- Object language: skin color, dress, cosmetics, etc.

In order to probe into the nature of nonverbal communication within the context of TCM interculturalization, and for the convenience of study, this chapter groups the above five areas into two broad categories: those that are primarily produced by human body and those that are mainly associated with environment and setting. The former category will be addressed in this section while the latter one will be discussed in section three of this chapter.

Cultural Differences in Nonverbal Communication

Edward Hall alerted us to the "silent" (Hall, 1959), "hidden" (Hall, 1966) and invisible aspects of culture and nonverbal communication (Hall, 1983); he warns us that much of our nonverbal communication is elusive (难懂的), spontaneous, and generally beyond our awareness and perception, unless they are unusual. Just like speech communication, nonverbal communication is full of cultural subtleties, and thus varies across cultures, with a small bunch of nonverbal signals being universal. Those strange gestures are harmless; they will catch your eyes for they are unusual, unknown, and therefore deserve exploring. What lies in the difficulty is that the same gesture is understood differently across cultures. It is easy for a mindless TCM culture facilitator to miss the point or misinterpret some nonverbal signals, thus unconsciously making social mistakes. The following part mainly compares and contrasts some of the most frequently used forms of nonverbal communication across the world, especially between China and English-speaking countries, against the backdrop of TCM interculturalization.

Kinesics

Kinesics, or the vernacular term body language, refers to any movement of any part of the body, excluding body contact. Being either voluntary or involuntary, it is perhaps the most commanding and influential of the nonverbal codes, because body movement is always visible, observable, and a lot of times meaningful. Research shows that an estimated "seven hundred thousand distinct elementary gestures can be produced by facial expressions, postures, movements of the arms, wrists, fingers, etc., and their combinations" (Pei, 1965, p. 19). Birdwhistell (1970), one of the pioneers of nonverbal communication research, even claimed that up to 250,000 hand gestures are possible. Krout (1954), much conservative, recorded 5,000 hand gestures in clinical situations.

These estimates demonstrate the wide range of nonverbal signals that can be used, especially considering that a person may display multiple behaviors on different occasions. For instance, there are many ways to show your approval to a friend. You can give a quick nod, nod vigorously, smile, combine a nod with a smile, give two thumbs up, or raise both arms with clenched fists. Each action conveys approval, but with slight variations, ranging from slim recognition to considerable enthusiasm. Cultural variability could complicate the issue still further. Trying to classify and list all nonverbal signals is a daunting task. The purpose of this part, therefore, is to call your attention to body language and master the basics of using and interpreting it while communicating TCM across cultures.

• Posture

David Brown is an American white working as a foreign teacher at a Chinese university. One day during the break between lectures, he rested his feet on the teacher's desk and closed his eyes to have a little nap. Several days later, rumor has it that he was rather vulgar. David was quite puzzled and asked one of his students what had happened. The class president told him some students thought he was showing his rudeness and arrogance by putting his feet on the desk. On hearing that, David realized he was absolutely wronged, and he told the whole class putting his feet on the desk in front of them meant he was comfortable with them.

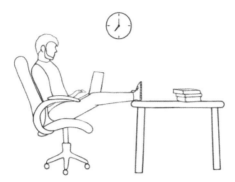

American's Putting his Feet on the Desk

In this case, both sides misunderstood each other by unconsciously adopting their own cultural standard: David Brown took it for granted that putting feet on the desk was practiced and understood across the globe, while Chinese students used Chinese norms to judge David's behavior, misinterpreting it as a highly improper and unfriendly behavior. If only one party had been more mindful. One should be attentive in Russia as well. For Russian people, behavior in public should be formal and respectful. Casual postures like standing with hands inserted into one's pockets, slouching postures, and putting feet up on the desk are not appreciated (Purnell, 2013).

Here is another story. Dr. Jiang, a TCM physician and lecturer, related his days working in South Africa. During a class demonstration on the role of interpreters in healthcare settings, Dr. Jiang set up himself and two other students in a triangle formation: He played the patient, one student was the physician, and the other student was the interpreter. Dr. Jiang asked the class what was wrong with the picture, intending to highlight the lack of eye contact between the healthcare provider and the patient. However, the first volunteer's comment surprised him. A student from Ghana pointed out that his folded arms indicated a challenge to the physician, explaining in Ghana, it is respectful to keep the hands behind the body. Another Vietnamese student joined the discussion and mentioned that keeping hands in the back is considered disrespectful in Vietnam. Similarly, students from the Republic of Korea and the Philippines agreed that folding hands in front shows respect, but with variations in the position: at waist level in Vietnam and down in the Philippines. Folding arms in front of one's body in public is quite common in China. It can mean a lot depending on the context. Overall, it is considered inappropriate to exhibit this posture in a formal situation. Hands clasped (without interlaced fingers) in front of the groin would be a better choice.

The above two stories inform us that in the process of cultural exchange, misunderstandings due to different interpretations of postures may occur at any time. Sometimes, unintentionally, we may offend someone with a gesture or other forms of body language. In such situations, the best approach is to apologize and ask them about the meaning in their culture. These moments can provide great opportunities to learn and share information about different cultural customs.

• Gesture

Before uncovering the colorful world of gestures, let us read a story that takes place in Los Angeles, US.

An Anglo patient named Jon Smith called out to Maria, a Filipina nurse, saying "Nurse, nurse." Maria approached him and asked politely, "How can I help you?" Mr. Smith motioned with his right index finger, gesturing for Maria to come closer. However, Maria became angry and asked, "What do you want?" Mr. Smith was confused by her sudden change in attitude. The problem is that the gesture he used, which means "come here", is considered offensive in the Philippines (and other parts of East and Southeast Asia, including China) when used towards people. It is typically meant to call animals. (In China, this gesture can be very provocative.) In the Philippines, the appropriate gesture to summon a person is to motion with the whole hand, palm facing inward and fingers pointing down.

Many US Americans are unsure about the meaning of the beckoning gesture in East Asian cultures, whether it means "come here" or "go away". Teresa, a Filipina nurse, experienced this confusion when she tried to call Nancy, an Anglo-American nurse, for help with a patient. Teresa motioned to Nancy with her hand, palm facing inward and fingers pointing down, signaling for her to come closer. However, Nancy simply smiled and waved back, thinking that Teresa was saying goodbye. This misunder standing left Teresa feeling confused and a little hurt.

Beckoning is among the most frequently used and the most important means in nonverbal communication, i.e., gesture. Many gestures are almost used, understood, and accepted universally across the world, for example, "handshaking" which is interpreted as friendliness, welcome, hospitality, etc. on diplomatic occasions. However, it is more likely that gestures are culture-specific, i.e., certain gestures belong to only some cultures. Even the frequency of using hand gestures differs across cultures. "Most US Americans gesture moderately when conversing and smile easily as a sign of pleasantness or happiness... A lack of gesturing can mean that the person is too stiff, too formal, or too polite" (Purnell, 2013, p. 22). However, from a Chinese perspective, US Americans may gesticulate too much. Very cautious approaches, therefore, must be taken in engaging in TCM interculturalization. The following table is a brief comparison of several gestures in China and English-speaking (or other) countries.

Table x A Brief Comparison of Some Gestures between China and English-Speaking Countries

Description	Gestures	In China	In English-speaking countries
Pointing Gestures		(Note: In Chinese culture, this sign is offensive)	Pointing to objects and even people with the index finger
		Pointing to objects or people with the entire hand, palm up	—

(To be Continued

中医跨文化传播

(Table x)

Description	Gestures	In China	In English-speaking countries
Beckoning Gestures		Hand extended toward others, palm down, with all fingers bent in a beckoning motion	—
		(Note: In Chinese culture, this sign is offensive)	Hand extended toward others, palm up, with fingers more or less together, and moving back and forth
A-OK gesture		Three; good; no problem	Good, no problem (Note: "money" or "coin" in Japan and the Repubic of Korea; "worthless" or "zero" in France; an obscene gesture in various places around the world)
Shaking head		Refusal; disapproval	In most English-speaking countries, it means disapproval, disagreement while in India, it may mean approval
The "Good-luck" Gesture		—	"Good luck to you" in the US; A religious symbol (because it resembles a partial cross) in some parts of the world; Representing being "close" or "best friends" in some cultures
Thumbs-up Gesture		Good; praise	Being good or for hitch-hiking in the US; "Speak up" or "turn up the volume" in parts of South America; An insult in many places (Iran, parts of South America and Europe), especially when the thumb is pumped up and down
Saluting with hands folded		Respect, good wishes, gratitude, congratulations, etc.	—

(To be Continued

Continued

Description	Gestures	In China	In English-speaking countries
The "V" Sign		Used when counting (meaning "two")	"Victory" or "peace" in many Western countries; If made with the open palm toward one's face, it is an insult in Australia, Great Britain, and South Africa
The "Hand Loose" Gesture		Used when counting (meaning "six") "Call me"	A common greeting in the Hawaiian culture and New Zealand

If all these terrify you in TCM interculturalization, and you think the safest way to avoid making mistakes is to simply tuck your hands into your pockets, then you may offend others too, because in countries like Belgium, keeping your hands in your pockets is considered rude.

• Eye Contact (Oculesics)

Many writers around the world romantically associate the eyes with the soul. Byron, for instance, extolled a soft and beautiful Italian lady in this way: "Heart on her lip and soul within her eyes." On the contrary, Shakespeare bestowed upon the eyes the ability to possess lethal power as Phoebe in *As You Like It* cried, "If mine eyes can wound, now let them kill thee." However, not many studies have explored cultural differences in eye contact. Hue, a Vietnamese nurse, had never realized that a basic gesture like eye contact could carry such different meanings in the US. She related a story during her stay in the US working as an intern.

Hue was one of the two new hires in Terry's unit. Both Terry, the mentor, and Sally, another nurse, came from the US. They had good communication with eye contact and trust. Sally felt comfortable asking for clarification when needed. However, the situation was different with Hue. Hue avoided eye contact, never asked questions. Whenever Terry asked if she understood something, Hue would nod in agreement, but later it would often become apparent that she did not understand. Terry felt frustrated and thought Hue did not like working with her. Terry considered stepping out of the mentoring role but decided to ask Hue's opinion first. Surprisingly, Hue wanted to continue with Terry as her mentor and even considered Terry the best nurse she had ever worked with. As they began to have a deeper discussion, both learned about each other's culture. Hue had intentionally avoided eye contact as a sign of respect. She refrained from asking Terry questions because she believed it would be impolite to question her mentor. Ironically, the behaviors that made Terry think she was failing with Hue were actually Hue's way of showing respect for Terry's higher position as a mentor.

Broadly speaking, people from individualistic cultures and collectivistic cultures differ in their perception of eye contact (Purnell, 2013). In individualistic cultures, regardless of social status, maintaining direct eye contact is expected without staring. Failing to keep eye contact can lead to perceptions of inattentiveness, untrustworthiness, lack of care, or dishonesty. Conversely, in certain collectivist cultures, prolonged eye contact can be considered offensive. Additionally, individuals of lower social or educational status are expected to avoid eye contact with superiors. Therefore, interpreting eye contact correctly within its cultural context is crucial for building relationships in TCM interculturalization and conducting accurate health assessments in healthcare settings.

In Chinese culture, people generally avoid long direct eye contact to show politeness, respect, and obedience. Similarly, in Guatemala, avoiding direct eye contact with others, including healthcare providers, is a sign of respect. It should not be misunderstood as avoidance, low self-esteem, or disinterest

(Purnell, 2013). Research also indicates that the Arabs tend to have more frequent and longer periods of eye contact compared to North Americans (Burgoon *et al.*, 2010; Samovar *et al.*, 2017). Of course, TCM physicians are an exception because observing the patient's eyes can help diagnose the disease; for example, if the whites of one's eyes turn yellow, it could mean inflammation, or something is wrong with his liver.

• Facial Expressions

While eye behavior has received less attention, facial expressions have been extensively studied for their cross-cultural similarities and differences. Darwin argued in his influential book that facial expressions of emotions are innate and universally understood (Burgoon *et al.*, 2010). Most researchers agree that expressions of happiness are universally recognized, with some lesser extent of agreement on sadness, anger, fear, surprise, and disgust. "Your face tells it all" is a daily verbal expression that can be verified in our interaction with other people. To Jun, it is not that simple, though.

Jun was a Chinese girl who was studying in the US. One day when she was having lunch in the school cafeteria, a young man asked if he could share the table with her. She agreed and they began to talk for a while. The young man told Jun his name was Fredriksen from Cyprus. He said he experienced a lot of difficulties along the way and finally arrived in the US. To Jun's surprise, Fredriksen started to sob during the narration of his sad story. Jun was quite puzzled and later she learned that in many Mediterranean cultures, people exaggerate signs of grief or sadness.

Jun's experience tells us that nonverbal signals like crying, smiling, and laughter appear to be universal, but also culturally tinted (轻微影响). Native Americans, for instance, while engaging with healthcare professionals who are outsiders, tend to communicate without displaying emotions, facial expressions, or gestures and avoid telling unpleasant news to prevent causing any emotional distress (Purnell, 2013). In cultures like Japan, China, and the Republic of Korea, it is common for people to remain calm even when they feel intense emotions such as anger, sadness, or happiness. On the other hand, Mediterranean cultures tend to express their feelings more openly, with animated facial expressions. It is not unusual to see men crying in public in those regions (Samovar *et al.*, 2017). No wonder Fredriksen burst into tears in front of his new friend.

When a TCM practitioner is working in the consulting room, he should observe the patient's face and try to assemble other evidence from the facial expression in addition to inquiry so as to figure out the true condition, because some people tend to conceal their sickness from doctors during verbal communication.

• Olfactics

Compared with animals, humans are far less competent in sense recognition, so you might be surprised that our olfactics, or the sense of smell, plays a role in social interaction. It is quite understandable because every person has odor preference, and people from different cultures may decipher smells differently.

Throughout history almost every culture has formed its own distinctive dietary habit. People in some parts of China like eating garlic; Japanese cuisine is noted for its freshness; Indians love curry, etc. Westerners, on the other hand, have a weakness for meat, especially beef and lamb; vegetables play only a minor role in their recipe. It is understandable, therefore, that body smell is also different: Arabs smell of onion and garlic, Europeans cheese and butter, Indians curry. As a result, each culture has developed a unique preference and dislike for certain smells. Some smells even have assumed very magic power. For instance, in Somalia, a country located on the east coast of Africa, "Incense is burned twice a day in order to protect the baby from the ordinary smells of the world, which are felt to have the potential to make him or her sick" (Purnell, 2013, p. 474).

Smell is important not just because it is related to our eating habits. "The air around us is filled with scents that express a variety of messages to us. Scents can communicate memories, fear, love, dominance, and excitement — and may even arouse powerful feelings about another person" (Richmond *et al.*, 2012, p. 11). This scent, to a great extent, can influence people's judgments they make about other people's attractiveness, thus influencing the willingness to communicate.

As one of the four basic diagnostic methods in TCM, olfactics has long been practiced by TCM physicians to gather patients' smell for accurate diagnosis. Diagnosis is determined by inspecting the patient's physical appearance, vitality, complexion, tongue, and senses, including scents. Excessive use of perfume by the patient can harm the accuracy of the diagnosis. TCM practitioners and TCM culture facilitators should take into consideration the language of scent in their intercultural activities.

Functions of Nonverbal Communication

It is evident that nonverbal communication plays an indispensable role in TCM interculturalization, with their various specific functions. In addition to expressing feelings and emotions, nonverbal signals also serve six major functions: **repetition**, **contradiction**, **substitution**, emphasis, complementation, and regulation (Chen, 2009a). To fully understand intercultural communication, it is essential to consider the role of nonverbal behavior and its functions.

A lot of times, we use nonverbal communication to reinforce what is said in verbal language. By repeating the message nonverbally, we give the audience another chance in another form to understand the message. For example, we nod as we say "yes". However, here is the rub. As nonverbal signals vary across cultures, confusion arises when the meaning deduced from the nonverbal signals are in conflict with the verbal messages. As people tend to trust more the nonverbal messages, the wrongly deciphered meaning from nonverbal communication has unintentionally contradicted the meaning. This leads to the second function, i.e., contradiction. In some situations, nonverbal behaviors can betray (无意中泄露) our real meaning. For instance, just before an important exam, when asked how well prepared you are, you reply with your voice quavering and hands trembling that you are relaxed and ready. Your gesture obviously betrays you. Or you may just look at your friends, saying nothing. However, your vacant eyes, weak breath, and sigh inform your friend that you are not ready. This is the third function of nonverbal communication, substituting for verbal messages. You are encouraged to explore the rest functions of emphasis, complementation, and regulation.

It should be noted that nonverbal communication seldom functions alone. It is usually studied and understood in relation to the verbal language that it accompanies. Therefore, in TCM interculturalization, we are supposed to employ either verbal communication or nonverbal communication or both flexibly and appropriately.

Activities

Comprehension Questions

1. In what way do postures and gestures help facilitate TCM interculturalization? Illustrate it with examples.

2. What is olfactics? How is it related to the diagnosis of TCM?

3. Explain the functions of nonverbal communication and support your answer with examples other than those mentioned in this section.

4. Smiling is well considered a universal language for indicating pleasure or friendliness. Yet, the use of a smile is also culture-dependent. Sometimes, Chinese people smile

or even laugh in an awkward situation, which could be misunderstood by people from another culture, say, the US Explore this theme in detail.

5.Haptics, or the study of touch, is also culturally conditioned. There is a strict rule for people of different sexes to touch in public in China, as Mencius once said, "Men and women should not touch hands when they give or receive things." A male TCM physician of the past usually placed a soft silk cloth on the patient's wrist before taking pulse to avoid directly touching the female's skin. First, do literature research to find out how male TCM physicians in ancient China diagnosed female patients, and then, collect information about the cultural variability in the preference of touch around the world.

Role Play

Directions: Non-native speakers seeking medical attention may find the experience particularly daunting. They may be limited to nonverbal communication to describe their symptoms, receive their diagnosis, and understand next care steps.

Role A: You are visiting Zambia and have begun to experience an illness. You go to the nearest medical facility and try to explain your symptoms to the doctor. Some of your symptoms are as follows.

Fever or chills	Headache
Cough	New loss of taste or smell
Shortness of breath or difficulty	Sore throat
Breathing	Runny nose
Fatigue	Diarrhea
Muscle or body aches	

You, as a patient, should explain your symptoms to your partner designated as a doctor without using English.

Role B: You are a local doctor who is trained in TCM as well as Western medicine. You are going to diagnose and present your patient with instructions for getting better without using English. After five minutes, have a conversation about the experience.

Guiding Questions

•Describe the experience.

•What frustrations did you encounter?

• What strategies did you use to try to communicate with each other?

• As the doctor in this scenario, what concerns did you have?

• As the patient in this scenario, how did you feel?

• How could this scenario change for the better?

Interview

Many people argue that theories about intercultural communication in books cannot catch up with the changes of cultures across the world; what is worse, the information taught in textbooks is sometimes wrong. First, collect nonverbal communication in various places (focusing on three or four countries or regions other than China) and then verify what you have collected by interviewing overseas students on your campus or in your city.

Case Study

Amir, a college student from Saudi Arabia was taking a Chinese Arts and Crafts class with other international students at a prestigious university in Scotland. During a group discussion, David, a native Scot, was sitting to the right of Amir. As David was talking to him, David placed his right ankle on his left knee. David noticed a definite change in Amir's conduct toward him. After class, David approached him and asked if he had done or said something that offended Amir. Amir told him that in the Arab culture, exposing the soles of one's shoes while directly speaking to someone is equal to giving them "one-finger salute". David apologized for his ignorance; Amir also apologized for his ignorance of David's ignorance. They ended up being friendly with each other for the remainder of the semester. They often had lunch together in the school cafeteria. They even hung out for the weekend several times. In the next semester, they did not have the same class. And Amir noticed that David was a little bit cold toward him. One day, they bumped into each other in the school corridor. When Amir was trying to have a quick chat with David, David obviously was not in the mood. Later that evening, Amir made a call to David, trying to invite him to a sports event, but David just declined. "David said we were friends. And I said friends are friends forever," Amir complained to Farid, another overseas student from Saudi Arabia.

Questions

1.In what way does a habitual conduct lead to intercultural misunderstanding? How is that misunderstanding solved? What lesson does this intercultural faux-pas offer us about communicating TCM across cultures?

2. What do David and Amir differ in terms of their attitude toward friendship? What do we learn from this case about how to make friends abroad?

Translation

Translate the following text into English.

文明的繁盛、人类的进步,离不开求同存异、开放包容,离不开文明交流、互学互鉴。历史呼唤着人类文明同放异彩,不同文明应该和谐共生、相得益彰,共同为人类发展提供精神力量。

——2017年12月1日习近平在"中国共产党与世界政党高层对话会"上的主旨讲话

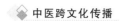

Before reading this section, please consider the following questions:

1. Have you ever heard of four TCM diagnostic methods? If yes, how much do you know about them? If no, try to get some information from the Internet.

2. How much do you know about channels and collaterals from TCM's perspective?

8.2 Four TCM Diagnostic Methods

Introducing TCM Diagnostics

TCM diagnostics is the study of theories, methods and diagnostic techniques used in the practice of TCM (Li and Wan, 2021). Throughout history, Chinese people have gradually developed medical practices in response to diseases and healthcare, contributing to the evolution of their healthcare system. As a bridge linking the basic theories of TCM and clinical practice, the rich content of TCM diagnostics constitutes the foundation of all branches of TCM.

A TCM physician makes diagnosis based on his sensory perceptions to gather clinical information and then analyzes and interprets this data without resorting to any modern instruments. It may sound unbelievable to an outsider. However, the underlying reason is quite simple (Zhang and Zhang, 2021): Within the framework of TCM, the human body is believed to be an organic whole, and all parts are interconnected by channels and collaterals. There is a connection between the internal and external aspects, as well as between the exterior and interior elements. Pathological changes inside the human body are reflected externally as abnormalities of the complexion, spirit, appearance of the tongue, and pulse. TCM physicians, therefore, can diagnose internal pathological changes by observing and analyzing external signs.

Fundamentals of TCM Diagnosis

The fundamentals of TCM diagnosis can be classified into three aspects (Li and Wan, 2021): (i) observing diseases by evaluating the human body holistically; (ii) analyzing comprehensively the data collected by diagnostic methods; and (iii) combining diagnosis of diseases with differentiation of patterns. Elaboration on these three aspects is as follows:

· Holistic Observation

When viewing the human body as an organic whole to diagnose illness or imbalances, a TCM physician keeps two points in mind. For one thing, attention is paid to the inter-relation and interaction between local pathological changes and maladjustments of the whole body. For another, the physician observes the patient in the context of his or her surroundings. When changes occur in the weather or environment, and the human body fails to adapt to these changes, pathological changes are likely to occur.

· Comprehensive Data Analysis

A TCM physician adopts a variety of methods to obtain clinical evidence such as questioning, inspection, auscultation (to discover the condition by listening), and olfaction (to check the condition by smelling), palpation or pulse-taking (to examine the human body by touching and taking the patient's pulse to arrive at a diagnosis). Because of the complexity of a disease and variety of manifestations, these methods can help a TCM physician avoid one-sided and false judgment and obtain the necessary and reliable clinical data.

· Differentiation of Syndromes

Pattern, or syndrome is a specific diagnostic concept in TCM. Roughly speaking, it is a pathological summary of the location, cause, nature, and condition of a disease at a certain stage and also a conclusion about the present pathological nature (Wang, 2007). Pattern Differentiation is a method of understanding and diagnosing disease by TCM practitioners. The diagnostic procedure involves an analysis of clinical data regarding symptoms, physical signs, and disease history, together with information obtained from the four diagnostic methods.

Four Diagnostic Methods of TCM

What are the four diagnostic methods of TCM? They are **inspection, auscultation and olfaction, inquiry** and **palpation** or **pulse-taking** (Shi, 2018). The four methods have their distinctive clinical functions and cannot be replaced by one another. Sometimes, false manifestations of a disease occur, which emphasizes the importance of integrating all diagnostic methods.

·Inspection

Inspection means that doctors directly observe the outward appearance to know a patient's condition. As the exterior and interior are closely linked to each other, any malfunction of the inner organs will be reflected through skin, tongue, face, nails, and even excrement.

·Auscultation and Olfaction

The method of auscultation and olfaction refers to the situation in which doctors listen to the patient while he is talking about his medical history, noticing any coughing, or checking the breathing. Meanwhile, TCM physicians sniff whether his mouth or body smells, including the sweat and phlegm. Information gleaned from these methods will be conducive to diagnosis and treatment.

·Inquiry

Inquiry means TCM physicians ask the patient various questions to know where and what the actual or potential problem is, to know the beginning and the development of the disease. Besides the general information about the patient's name, age, marital status, dietary habits, family history, etc., other commonly asked questions include: What symptoms do you have (The symptoms might be dizziness, pain, bowel movement, fever, sweat, indigestion and so on)? How long have you had these symptoms? What medicine did you take? Did you have any diseases before?

· Palpation or Pulse-Taking

To take the pulse and to use palpation, doctors note the pulse condition of patients by touching the wrist on both hands, and then to know the inner change of the human body. Altogether there are twenty-eight pulses (Li and Wan, 2021). When a person is in good health, the pulse is slow, steady, rhythmic, and strong. A rapid or a very slow pulse indicates presence of disease. The calm and strong pulse of a very sick person indicates a chance of recovery. However, if the pulse is fine and faint, almost imperceptible, it is a sign of grave consequences.

Differentiation of Disease and Pattern

The above four methods are essential to determine the cause of the disease from which an individual suffers. The external symptoms can often reflect a problem with the internal organs, which is mainly caused by yin-yang disharmony or qi stagnation. Since normality and abnormality are relative concepts, judgment is based on comparison. During diagnosis, it is important to make a comparison to find out the disorder.

TCM physicians believe that causes of symptoms are often attributed to exogenous evils (外邪) that invade the human body and disrupt its internal balance, thus leading to illness. Besides, illness can also arise inside the body and express itself through symptoms on the outside. A skilled TCM practitioner is able to distinguish where the origin of the problem comes from by using the four TCM diagnostic methods.

—[**Activities**]————————————————————————————————

Comprehension Questions

1.In what ways is TCM diagnostics important?

2.How much do you believe that the human body is an organic whole?

3.What are the four TCM diagnostic methods?

4.Which aspects are included in the inquiry process?

5.What are the differences between the syndrome and disease in TCM?

Role Play

Directions: According to your understanding of TCM, if a person has suffered from a common cold for two days, what clinical manifestations may be observed? What pulse condition and tongue coating may he or she have? Discuss these questions with your partners, and then role-play accordingly.

Role A: You are a patient from Italy who knows something about TCM, but has never visited a TCM physician before. Your limited information about TCM tells you that TCM is good for preventing diseases. You are not sure whether your cold can be cured by TCM. Moreover, you are worried about the herbs. Rumor has it that it contains some toxic substances. And it tastes bitter.

Role B: As an experienced TCM physician who once worked in England, you know how to dispel the illusion about TCM.

Translation

Translate the following text into Chinese.

Traditional Chinese medicine, abbreviated to TCM, is a scientific summary of the rich experience of the Chinese nation's struggle against disease for thousands of years. It is one of the oldest and strongest traditional medical systems in the history of the world. Deeply influenced by the thoughts of ancient Chinese philosophy and culture, TCM applies dialectical thinking to research on the law of a human being's life activities from a macroscopic and systematic point of view. Over the course of many centuries, TCM has gradually formed a unique theoretical system and diagnosing-treating techniques, which have made an indelible and substantial contribution to both the health and prosperity of the Chinese people.

Case Study

Case 1

The US writer Sanjay Surana tried TCM for the first time.

After playing soccer, I strained my right thigh. Back home I would have gone straight to a physical therapist, but I just recently moved to Singapore, and I had no idea where to go. I asked friends for recommendations, but the only one that I got was for a TCM center in the eastern part of the island. This friend had experienced a problem with his shoulder and was about to have surgery. He went to this particular TCM doctor for one visit, and the pain disappeared. "A miracle, I tell you, it was a miracle." With such strong praise, I had to give it a try.

"What is the problem?" he inquired. I explained. Perhaps I had gotten used to the soft approach administered by doctors in the US, but I wasn't prepared for what happened next. Rather than gently press my thigh to gauge where it was inflamed and where the muscles were out of whack, he pressed his thumb right into the core of the knotted area and started to dig and knead as though he were preparing dough to make pancakes. I yelped in pain, hoping he would stop and expecting his face to show some sympathy, but it was blank.

Then he asked me to rest the back of my hand on a little pillow that was on his desk. "Stick out your tongue." I stuck out the tip of it, not sure if that was enough. He pressed his two fingers on my wrist to feel my pulse.

"Hey, I'm still breathing. My heart is beating. I'm not dying," thought I with my tongue sticking out, not knowing what was going on.

"Small problem. Come." I hobbled behind him···

Questions

1. Why did Surana's friend praise TCM as a miracle?

2. How was Surana diagnosed by a TCM physician?

Case 2

Here is the story of TCM physician Wu, who has practiced TCM in New York City for 28 years. Before moving to the States, he had worked in China for 15 years. One of his patients, a man in his 50s, said that Wu is gifted and his talent unmatched.

The patient has visited Wu for the past 15 years whenever he needs routine help for wellness or to boost his immune system. He said Wu's ability to listen to his patients makes the doctor highly intuitive.

"I recently had severe back pain that came out of the blue. As soon as I walked into the doctor's office, he looked at me and said, 'How are you?' And before I could answer, he asked if I had back pain," the patient said. Wu, who plays down this ability, said, "I just use Chinese techniques, that's all. But I can watch your face, your walk, and your attitude to see who you are, your personality, and what is wrong."

His patients, who include a mix of Chinese and Americans, mostly arrive via word of mouth. Using acupuncture, the doctor inserts tiny, sterile, disposable needles in specific areas of a patient's body to target areas of pain or stress. He also uses small suction cups to draw blood to areas of the skin that have stagnation or blockages that need removing to improve qi, which in traditional Chinese culture is an active principle. For additional help, massage eases pain, and the effects and relief can be immediate.

The patient said, "Wu can 'scan' you in milliseconds and know exactly what's going on before you even communicate with him. I once experienced bloating, which I had never had before, but just one treatment from Dr. Wu resolved this issue."

Questions

1. How do you understand qi in TCM?

2. What TCM techniques do you think Dr. Wu would use when a patient limped into his clinic?

Group Work

TING ("聽") is the Chinese word meaning "To listen" — it describes a very complete way of listening so that your total focus is on the speaker. Often, when we are listening to another person, we are only partially listening while we are preparing our response. With TING, you are fully present to the speaker. The symbol on the left-hand side is ear ("耳"); the symbol on the lower half of the left-hand side is literally translated to "king" or "the dominant one" ("王"). The symbol on the right-hand side at the top is mind ("十"); below that is eye ("目"); the line below that is one, or "to become of one"; Heart ("心") is the bottom symbol on the right-hand side.

Work with your partners to discuss the meaning of each part that makes up the traditional Chinese character " 聽 ", and explain how this Chinese character helps one be an attentive or empathetic listener.

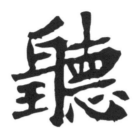

Debate

The following passage is on whether TCM is slow in efficacy when treating diseases.

TCM is believed to address the root causes of diseases, but it is often criticized for being time-consuming compared with Western medicine, which focuses on quick symptom relief. However, the effectiveness of TCM should be examined from two perspectives.

According to TCM theory, diseases occur due to imbalance between *yin* and *yang*. When the human body is invaded by pathogens, its healthy qi rises to resist them. This confrontation disrupts the balance of *yin* and *yang*, leading to various pathological changes. In some cases, with sufficient rest and nutrition, the body's strong healthy qi alone can overcome common ailments like wind-cold without the need for medication. However, if the body is fatigued or has some other diseases, the healthy qi weakens, allowing the disease to penetrate deeper into the organs. In such cases, treatment aims to replenish healthy qi and empower the body to fight the disease, which may require a longer course of treatment.

Do you think that TCM is slow in efficacy when treating diseases? Form teams with classmates who share the same side, with 2–4 members on each side. Give alternate speeches for and against the topic:

TCM is slow in efficacy when treating diseases.

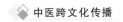

8.3 Time and Space Across Cultures

Beyond speech communication, there are messages that our body sends out constantly. Sometimes the body message reinforces the verbal message, sometimes the body message is sent to challenge the verbal message, and sometimes the body message is perceived to augment, or even to regulate the conversation. In addition to these means of nonverbal communication, environmental language also speaks and affects communication to a great extent. By environmental language, we mean both the physical and psychological environments, including time, space, interior decoration, play a role in communication.

Time Orientation (Chronemics)

We often hear that people in those industrialized countries have a very strong sense of punctuality, while people in some Asian and African countries are said to be less time conscious. Indeed, different cultures have different perceptions of time. The study of time — how people perceive it, use it, and understand its passage — is called chronemics. A very well-known time framework is put forward by Hall (1983) who argued that cultures organize time in one of two ways — either monochronic (M-time) or polychronic (P-time), which represent two approaches to perceiving and utilizing time.

M-Time stresses schedules and promptness; it features one event at one time. In M-Time culture, time is perceived as a linear structure, which goes from the past and will keep going to the future without stop. People who observe M-Time consider time as a commodity, so it can be measured, saved, lent, lost, and sold. Since "Time is money", it should be used wisely. The primary emphasis is usually on completing the task or achieving a goal within a certain period of time. Northern American and Western European cultures are typical of M-Time cultures. They expect meetings and classes to start on time (within a minute, or so). Patients are expected to arrive at the clinic at the appointed time within one or two minutes.

P-Time culture, on the other hand, is less strict about the use of time. People from such a culture are more flexible and schedule several events at the same time.

In other words, they seem to have the ability to "multitask". Most Asian and Latin American cultures are P-Time cultures. They think of time as "more holistic, more fluid, and less structured" (Burgoon *et al.*, 2010, p. 195). For instance, "Some Mexicans and Mexican Americans perceive time as relative rather than categorically imperative. Deadlines and commitments are flexible, not firm. Punctuality is generally relaxed, especially in social situations" (Purnell, 2013, p. 377). Healthcare facilities that utilize an appointment system for patients may need to make accommodations to see patients who arrive without a scheduled appointment.

Time language can shed light on TCM interculturalization. TCM practitioners and TCM culture facilitators should know how to accommodate participants from both T-time and P-time cultures. When treating foreign patients, TCM physicians should be tolerant of the patients' being late, for they may come from a P-Time culture. Also, TCM physicians are supposed to give the consulting room exclusively for patients from an M-Time culture, for they tend to do one thing at a time, and nine out of ten, privacy is their top concern.

A word of warning: Do not think of P-time culture and M-time culture as two battalions of time orientations, but rather two ends of a time orientation continuum. Like the cultural framework of high-context and low-context orientation (Hall, 1976), they can exit within one culture. For example, in an educational setting, some students prefer to do many homework assignments at the same time while others choose to finish one by one.

Spatial Language (Proxemics)

Humans are social animals. We like to spend time together with our family members, friends, and workmates. As little kids, we prefer to huddle together with our parents, later with our playmates. At the same time, humans are also territorial animals. We tend to set aside a place of our own even in our house. The use of space functions as a very important system in every culture. However, each culture differs in terms of need for personal space and the messages used to indicate territoriality. There is an invisible bubble surrounding us when we are communicating with other people. It helps define who we are and how we feel comfortable without being threatened or warmly received without being kept aside. While some scholars make a distinction between territory and personal space, defining territory as "a fixed geographic area that is occupied, controlled, and defended by a person or group as their exclusive domain" (Burgoon *et al.*, 2010, p. 159) but personal space as "an invisible, adjustable bubble of space that people carry around with them" (Burgoon *et al.*, 2010, p. 159), it is the invisible personal space that is elusive and therefore deserves further attention.

Edward Hall, who coined the term proxemics "for the interrelated observations and theories of man's use of space as a specialized elaboration of culture" (Hall, 1966, p. 1), has suggested that people in the US interact within four spatial zones or distance ranges: intimate, personal, social, and public. The following data is based on Hall's (1959) research of US Americans.

Table x North American Zones of Space

Spatial Distance Zone	Spatial Distance	Usage	Other Characteristics
Intimate distance	0–45 centimeters	for lovers, family members, etc.	Reserved for private, informal interaction with people we like and trust; smell and feel of others; eye contact unlikely exception: in a dentist's or barber's
Personal distance	45–80 centimeters	most common when friends and relative converse	Eye-contact is preferable in individualist cultures; Touch is possible
Social distance	1.3 meters 3.0 meters	for people who work together, or people doing business	More formal tone; Eye contact likely
Public distance	farther than 2 or 3 meters	generally for speakers in public or teachers in classroom	Subtle details lost; Only obvious attributes noticed

When interacting with multicultural patients and staff, it is necessary to respect personal space. In individualistic cultures, the typical conversation distance is at least half a meter. Though most European countries belong to individualistic cultures, the personal bubbles become smaller and smaller from north Europe to south Europe (Lustig and Koester, 2010). Therefore, when a Spaniard and a Finn engage in an informal conversation, their different cultural norms regarding personal space become apparent. The former prefers to be closer, while the latter tries to maintain a comfortable distance by moving backward. This mismatch can lead to negative perceptions: The Finn may think that the Spaniard is invading their space, while the Spaniard may see the Finn as distant and unfriendly.

The short personal distance preferred by the Spaniard, in the eyes of a Chinese, is still considered too long because collectivistic cultures require less personal space during conversations, as they perceive physical closeness as a positive reflection of emotional intimacy (Hall, 1959). Therefore, it is important for healthcare practitioners to be aware of these differences, as some patients may feel offended if a healthcare provider stands / sits too far away or too close.

Decorations of TCM Clinics

Culture can be reflected in seating arrangements too — another part of spatial language. Americans tend to talk with those opposite them rather than those seated or standing beside them. In China, meetings often involve individuals sitting beside each other. Seating arrangements can also be applied to TCM clinics. The desks or chairs in the consulting room can be arranged and displayed according to the local cultural norms. "Sitting behind a desk to interview or assess a client is often unacceptable for many non-Western immigrants, minorities, and strangers" (Leininger and McFarland, 2002, p. 127). Surely, we can adhere to Chinese culture while practicing TCM overseas: maintaining the traditional Chinese way of arranging furniture in TCM clinics in foreign countries. If necessary, Corporate Identity System can be employed to standardize the furniture arrangement of TCM clinics across the globe. This is an interdisciplinary area that requires knowledge from arts, TCM, local culture, and personal preference. Balance should be stricken so that the essence of TCM can be retained, personal preference is considered, and cultural diversity is respected.

Chapter Summary

- Communication theorists reveal that in daily face-to-face communication, less than 35% of the information is exchanged via speaking, and over 65% of the message is communicated by nonverbal means.
- Nonverbal communication is conceptualized as a system of symbols, signs and

gestures other than language, which is developed and used by members of a culture to bring specific messages to expression.

- In a broad sense, nonverbal communication covers the following areas: visual and auditory performance codes, body codes, contact codes, time and place codes.
- Kinesics, or the vernacular term "body language", refers to any movement of any part of the body, excluding body contact.
- In addition to expressing feelings and emotions, nonverbal signals also serve six major functions in the communication process: repetition, contradiction, substitution, emphasis, complementation, and regulation.
- The fundamentals of TCM diagnosis can be classified into three aspects: (i) observing diseases by taking the human body holistically, (ii) analyzing comprehensively the data collected by diagnostic methods, and (iii) combining diagnosis of diseases with differentiation of patterns.
- Four diagnostic methods of TCM are inspection, auscultation and olfaction, inquiry, and palpation or pulse-taking.
- Environmental language such as time, space, and interior decoration also speaks and affects communication.
- Edward Hall proposed that cultures organize time in one of two ways — either monochronic or polychronic, which represents two approaches to perceiving and utilizing time.
- Edward Hall, who coined the term proxemics "for the interrelated observations and theories of man's use of space as a specialized elaboration of culture", has suggested people in the US interact within four spatial zones or distance ranges: intimate, personal, social, and public.

Checklist	Yes	No
Cognitive: I have mastered the core information		
Behavioral: I have the ability of putting what I've learned into practice		
Affective: I am willing to carry out what I've learned		
Moral: I will take the ethical consideration into account during practice		

Part Four

Health

Chapter 9

Perceptions of Health and Illness Across Cultures

Chapter Objectives
After reading this text, you should be able to:

◆ Define different paradigms of worldview and healthcare belief systems.

◆ Describe and evaluate the effect of cultural diversity in the causes and prevention of illness.

◆ Summarize TCM's perspective on illness prevention.

◆ Isolate some commonly found communication barriers in health communication.

◆ Learn how to overcome cultural barriers in health communication.

Key Terms

biomedical

body constitution

causes of illness

family role

health communication

health literacy

holistic

humoral theory

linguistic and non-linguistic barriers

magico-religious

medical culture

prevention of illness

self-disclosure

uncertainty

Quotes

"We need to uphold the beauty of each civilization and the diversity of civilizations in the world. Each civilization is the crystallization of human creation, and each is beautiful in its own way." (坚持美人之美、美美与共。每一种文明都是美的结晶,都彰显着创造之美。)

——2019年5月15日习近平在亚洲文明对话大会开幕式上的演讲

"All things are nourished together without their injuring one another. The courses of the seasons, and of the sun and moon, are pursued without any collision among them. The smaller energies are like river currents; the greater energies are seen in mighty transformations. It is this which makes heaven and earth so great." (万物并育而不相害,道并行而不相悖。小德川流,大德敦化,此天地之所以为大也。)

——《礼记·中庸》

"To effectively communicate, we must realize that we are all different in the way we perceive the world and use this understanding as a guide to our communication with others." (人们认识世界的方式各异。对此,我们必须知晓,并应用于实践,才能达到有效沟通。)

—— Anthony Robbins

Before reading this section, please consider the following questions:

1. How much do you know about the causes and prevention of illness from the perspective of Western medicine?

2. Have you ever heard of nine body constitutions?

9.1   Worldview and the Healthcare Belief System

This is a true story that happened in a traditional Chinese medicine (TCM) clinic. A young man came in and sat in front of the doctor. When asked about his issues, he quietly replied, "Kidney deficiency". The experienced doctor understood him easily and, after checking his tongue and pulse, prescribed a formula to tonify (滋补) his kidney yang, with the diagnosis of "kidney yang deficiency" (肾阳虚).

To someone unfamiliar with TCM or Chinese culture, this diagnosis might seem strange. In China, it is widely believed that poor sexual function is connected with kidney deficiency. This belief stems from the idea that kidneys play a role in sexual health and reproduction. However, for Westerners who associate kidneys solely with urinary (泌尿的) functions in biomedicine, the connection between kidneys and sex can be difficult to understand without a detailed explanation. So, if a TCM physician links sexual problems to kidney issues, communication may become ineffective. As a result, there could be difficulties in healthcare delivery.

People from different cultures have varied perspectives on illness, healthcare, and death. This can be challenging for both patients and healthcare providers. To address these challenges, healthcare professionals need to develop good intercultural communication skills, with a fundamental understanding of how culture, healthcare, and communication are connected. We begin with the discussion of the influence of worldview on healthcare system in this section, followed by perceptions of health and illness in Section Two, and concluded by topics on health communication across cultures.

Introducing Worldview

In everyday conversations in China, people often discuss "three views", i.e., philosophy of life, worldview, and values. These three concepts are closely interconnected. Philosophy of life influences an individual's actions on a personal level, and values reflect collective beliefs about what is important or unimportant, good or bad, normal or abnormal, and so on (For more information, please consult Chapter 5). The English term "worldview", directly translated from the German word "Weltanschauung", was coined by Immanuel Kant in 1790, who defined it as the perception of the world (Naugle, 2002). Although Kant only used the term once and considered it of minor significance, it quickly evolved to represent an intellectual understanding of the universe from a human perspective. Nowadays, it is widely considered as "the way a people interpret reality and events, including their self-image and their relationship with the world around them" (Bailey and People, 2014, p. 34). Worldview encompasses a comprehensive philosophy of how the world functions and how individuals fit into it. Questions about truth and its discovery are integral to one's worldview.

Every individual possesses their own worldview, but within each culture, a dominant and influential worldview emerges that shapes the collective understanding of reality. Similar to culture, worldviews operate automatically and unconsciously. Since culture plays a significant role in shaping diverse perspectives on the world, our perceptions of health are also influenced by culture through the representation of worldview. Therefore, we will focus on how worldview influences the healthcare belief system in the rest part of this section.

Varieties of Worldview

Many factors contribute to the formation of a person's worldview, including their religions, national history, personal experiences, and thinking patterns. Religious beliefs are often an important factor in how people see the world, since every culture begins with an attempt to understand the world around them, and this eventually leads to the development of religion. However, religion is not the only contributor that shapes our worldview when it comes to health and disease. Different ways of thinking, such as whether someone sees the world in a holistic or dualistic way, can greatly affect how they view illness and how they believe it should be treated. By exploring these different worldview patterns, we can better understand how worldview plays a role in shaping communication and behavior in healthcare settings.

·Dualistic vs. Holistic Worldview

The common notion of environment being separate from humans comes from the nature vs. culture dualism (二元论), where humanity is set in opposition to everything else. This conception of environment as something that is relevant to human existence stems from anthropocentrism (人本中心论), "which places humanity at the center stage of everything" (Thin, 2010, p. 233). Dualism, which is mostly seen in the Western world, is an oversimplified way of thinking, and it creates a division between humans and nature. Dualistic worldview enforces the idea that humans are distinct from the natural world. People with this worldview are taught that they should dominate and shape nature to meet their individual needs and desires.

While dualism provides a clear and logical way of thinking, it is important to recognize that the world is complex and not everything can be seen in black and white. Many situations are interconnected and have mutual influences on each other. This is why different cultures adopt different ways of thinking. For instance, Eastern cultures often embrace a holistic worldview, which is influenced by their historical background as agrarian civilizations.

· Mechanistic vs. Non-mechanistic Worldview

The second division arises between mechanistic and non-mechanistic perspectives of the world. Western cultures commonly adopt a mechanistic worldview known as mechanism (机械论). This ideology is rooted in atomism, which asserts that atoms serve as the fundamental building blocks of the universe and that properties of matter stem from properties of atoms. It seeks to comprehend or reduce all motion within the world to mechanical motion, such as atoms shifting from one position to another.

"American thought patterns prioritize rationality over mysticism, and they predominantly embrace a mechanistic conception of the universe. The foundational premise (前提) upon which this entire worldview is constructed is the belief that the universe operates as a physical system functioning in a definitive manner according to scientific laws... Due to their perception of the universe as a mechanism, Americans inherently hold the belief that individuals possess the capability to manipulate it" (Hoebel and Frost, 1976, pp. 147-148).

However, the Eastern perspective on reality and truth differs greatly from that of the Western viewpoint. The non-mechanistic worldview has historically emerged in countries like India, Japan, and China. For instance, ancient Chinese culture regards qi as the fundamental essence of the world, considering everything to be composed of qi. This belief system suggests that all elements in the world share a common composition, allowing for interaction through the medium of qi. This approach can be described as dialectical materialism or, in other words, non-mechanism. This dialectical viewpoint embodies a holistic, interconnected, and dynamic understanding of problems.

Cultural Diversity in the Causes of Illness

After a brief introduction to the worldview, we will explore the impact of diverse healthcare belief systems on the understanding of the causes, treatment, and prevention of illnesses. According to Eipperle and Andrews (2020), healthcare belief systems can be classified into three main categories: biomedical, magico-religious, and holistic. As you encounter these varied beliefs, we encourage you to think of how the dimensions of dualistic vs. holistic and mechanistic vs. non-mechanistic worldviews greatly contribute to the diverging perspectives individuals from different cultures hold regarding healthcare. By doing so, you will gain an insight into the challenges that TCM culture facilitators encounter when communicating TCM principles across different cultural contexts.

Most healthcare practitioners in Western cultures are trained under the **biomedical** model of health and illness. This approach emphasizes biological concerns and is primarily interested in abnormalities in the structure and function of body systems as well as in the treatment of disease. Followers of this approach believe that the biomedical model, which diagnoses diseases based on a person's deviation from established norms in biomedical science, is more genuine and important than psychological and sociological explanations of illness. The purpose of treatment, whether it involves surgery, medication, or therapy, is to bring the person back to the accepted standard determined by scientific norms (Magner and Kim, 2018). "Patients are expected to use information seeking and problem solving in preference to faith in God, patience, and acceptance of one's fate as primary coping mechanisms" (Purnell, 2013, p. 172).

The **holistic** healthcare perspective is based on the belief that humanity is an integral part of the universe. Everything, including humans, animals, plants, or even the stars is interconnected and interdependent. Many people of Asian descent (for example, Chinese, Filipinos, Koreans) do not believe they have control over nature. They have a perspective that focuses on people adjusting to the physical world instead of trying to control or overpower the environment. Traditional Asian teaching stresses a harmonious relationship with nature in which the forces of yin and yang are kept in balance. Yin represents a negative, inactive, feminine principle, while yang represents a positive, active, masculine force. Yin and yang combine to produce every occurrence in life. Consequently, many Asians believe that an imbalance in this combination causes illness. They need to stay in balance with their environment and maintain harmony with the world around them.

Traditional Egyptian and Iranian medical beliefs are based on the Hippocratic **humoral theory** that specifies four humors of the body, which are blood-hot and wet, yellow bile-hot and dry, phlegm-cold and wet, and black bile-cold and dry. "The key to humoral theory is balance and moderation. The belief is that too much of any one category can cause symptoms of being overheated or chilled" (Purnell, 2013, p. 467). An imbalance of one of the four body humors is seen as the cause of illness.

The **magico-religious** healthcare tradition is centered on the idea that a supernatural force exists out there that dominates the world, including human beings. One of the oldest and most prevalent beliefs regarding the origin of illness is the concept of the "evil eye" (Purnell, 2013). This belief suggests that someone can cause harm or bring about misfortune to another person simply by looking at them intently or staring at them. "Cuban families may use an azabache, or other types of amulets (护身符) for various protective purposes. The azabache is a black stone placed on infants and children as a bracelet or pin to protect them from the evil eye" (Purnell, 2013, p. 210). In Native

American cultures, people have strong beliefs in fate and do not question the reasons for getting sick. They accept illness and even death as part of the cycle of birth and rebirth (Danielson *et al.*, 1998).

Cultural Diversity in the Prevention of Illness

There is no doubt that no one wants to get ill. However, what can we do for our body and health? What does it mean to stay healthy? Cultures reflect various degrees of diversity in their beliefs and practices about what can be done to prevent illness. Unlike the causes and treatment of illness, where the approaches are rather systematic, in the prevention of illness, people from many cultures employ a combination of biomedical, holistic, and magic approaches.

In the US and other highly technological cultures, for instance, good health is based on annual physical examinations, immunizations at a specified time, exercise, and good nutrition (Samovar *et al.*, 2017). Yet, many people also follow health practices that may include stress-reducing massage and the use of a variety of natural supplements to keep fit. In addition, they may seek treatments from TCM as preventive measures.

In Mexican and Puerto Rican (波多黎各的) cultures, it is widely believed that good health can be attributed to luck or as a reward from God for virtuous behavior. As a result, many individuals rely on various objects for protection. Amulets or charms, often engraved with magical symbols or phrases, are commonly used to safeguard against illnesses (Leininger and McFarland, 2002).

Although many cultures practice preventive measures, prevention is a totally new concept for others. "Some Guatemalans relate their illness to punishment or impending death to God's will and refuse intervention or heroic measures to reverse the outcome" (Purnell, 2013, p. 465).

TCM's Perspective on Illness Prevention

It is well-known that TCM aims to prevent rather than to treat illness. Some 2,000 years ago, the idea that "prevention is better than cure" was recorded in *Huangdi Neijing,* one of the four TCM classics. The end of the second chapter of this canon says "the sages did not treat those already ill, but treated those not yet ill; they did not put in order what was already in disorder, but put in order what was not yet in disorder" (是故圣人不治已病治未病，不治已乱治未乱). When the sages treat, they do it before the symptoms are completely reflected on a person, which emphasizes the idea of prevention rather than treatment. If we do not actively seek treatment until the disease is fully developed, it is equivalent to digging a well when we are thirsty. Isn't that a little too late?

Professor Wang Qi (2021) from Beijing University of Chinese Medicine, master of Chinese Medicine (国医大师), academician, introduces the concept of **body constitutions** (体质), the prevention and treatment of related illnesses according to the different types of body constitutions as well as their respective health management.

According to Professor Wang Qi, there are nine body constitutions: yin-deficient, yang-deficient, blood stasis, phlegm-dampness, dampness-heat, qi-deficient, balanced, inherited special, and qi-stagnation constitution. Different body constitutions have their own unique body physique (体格), physiological, and psychological characteristics, pathological reactions, and predisposition (倾向). Therefore, understanding body constitution helps TCM physicians find the most suitable and appropriate treatment and health management methods to achieve a most favorable curative effect and maintain good health.

The immense work stress and fast-paced life in modern life are the main culprits that cause people to overlook their mental and physical health, resulting in subhealth (亚健康), which may continue to develop into illnesses, if left uncared for. Hence, early prevention and treatment are the key to optimal health. As an increasing number of diseases and illnesses, say, heart attack or high-blood pressure, are starting to attack even the younger population, it is important that we make use of TCM to maintain our health. It is also meaningful to let people in other parts of the world know the feasibility of applying TCM in their health management. However, before we move on to the cultural influence on health communication, it is important to note that some beliefs and practices may seem unusual. To make TCM interculturalization effectively, one has to respect and keep a mindful attitude toward the "unusual" healthcare system which in fact has been practiced for a long time.

Activities

Comprehension Questions

1. How do Western cultures view the causes of illness?

2. How do Asians understand the causes of illness?

3. What are different ways of preventing illness in different cultures?

4. Can you offer an example of how people around you prevent illness?

5. What are the nine body constitutions in Chinese? Try to explain with specific examples how to prevent illness by applying Professor Wang Qi's theory of body constitution.

Translation

Translate the following text into English.

上古之人,其知道者,法于阴阳,和于术数,食饮有节,起居有常,不妄作劳,故能形与神俱,而尽终其天年,度百岁乃去。今时之人不然也,以酒为浆,以妄为常,醉以入房,以欲竭其精,以耗散其真,不知持满,不时御神,务快其心,逆于生乐,起居无节,故半百而衰也。

——《素问·上古天真论》

Case Study

Case 1

This is a story about an American lady named Linda.

"My cousin Lily is an American lady who moved to China a few years ago. When she got pregnant, she decided to go back to America to deliver her baby after realizing all the differences in healthcare. In China, doctors refuse to tell you the gender of your baby, and they make you deliver your baby in the same room where other women are in labor, which are practices that are not very common in the US. What's more unbelievable is that in China, most women follow the Chinese tradition that they should be confined to their homes for one month. And during that one month, they should not take a bath, no air conditioning, or no tooth brushing. It is terrible."

Questions

1.What seems to be bothering Lily?

2.What advice would you give to Lily if she wanted to stay in China to give birth?

Case 2

The following is the story of Mingming, a Chinese immigrant to the US.

The longer I stay in the US, the more differences I find between American and Chinese healthcare practices. For instance, some elderly people spend the rest of their lives in nursing homes even if they have children. However, in China, children have the responsibility to take care of their elder parents. Sending one's parents to nursing homes, although not illegal, is considered by the general public as a very bad practice. Another difference I found is that, in the US, abortion is a very controversial topic; however, in China, it is commonly considered just as a medical practice and is not associated with moral judgments in general.

Questions

1.What seems to bother Mingming?

2.What do you think can explain Mingming's trouble?

Before reading this section, please consider the following questions:

1. Have you ever heard of someone who was once received by doctors whose culture is different from yours? Share the story with your partners.

2. What factors would influence the accuracy of medical history during history-taking?

9.2   Intercultural Barriers to Effective Health Communication

Defining Health Communication

Topics of communication vary, one of which is health-related issues. Examples of health communication abound: calling your mom on the phone for advice about your headache, noticing signs on the food package in the supermarket that show the number of calories in each service, hearing emergency TV or radio broadcasts from a local public health official about what to do during a typhoon, flood, or snowstorm. Simply put, **health communication** "is the study of messages that create meaning in relation to physical, mental, and social well-being" (Harrington, 2015, p. 9). If we narrow down the health message to TCM related information and broaden the context where health communication takes place to incorporate cultural variability, then, a new angle of understanding TCM interculturalization is to be found. Instead of perceiving it from the perspective of intercultural communication, one can approach the essence of TCM interculturalization from the framework of health communication across cultures.

The diversity of the population and culture in a healthcare context makes it necessary for healthcare workers to deal with patients from different cultural backgrounds. The delivery of healthcare around the world presents a unique challenge. Part of this challenge is, of course, cultural. In order to cope with this diversity, satisfactory ways of caring for all members of society must be discovered and practiced during the promotion of TCM interculturally.

Barriers in Health Communication

Health issues are never just about illnesses and diseases. There is a long way to go from birth to death, and many complex health-related problems occur in between. In this modern era of globalization, the interaction in the healthcare context on the choice of healthcare system is by no means personal, but a lot of times, social. Fostering strong intercultural sensitivity helps TCM practitioners and TCM culture facilitators better get connected with the audience. Family roles, self-disclosure (自我表达), linguistic and non-linguistic messages are three prominent cultural barriers in a healthcare setting, which, if poorly handled, could severely hinder effective communication.

Firstly, the issue of **family roles** in health communication is relevant because cultures assign specific roles to various family members. These roles provide guidelines for family members on how to perceive and communicate about healthcare matters. Many cultures have clear distinctions between what is considered appropriate behavior for men and women. Therefore, as medical workers, understanding patterns of family dominance is crucial in order to make informed decisions to whom they are addressing. Sometimes, patients themselves may be accustomed to being accompanied by a relative who speaks on behalf of him or her. For example, among many Mexican Americans, the elderly are valued for their folk care knowledge and experience. "When there is an illness, members of the family will usually go to the elder mother first" (Leininger and McFarland, 2002, p. 366). Interestingly enough, Mexican American community is also viewed as a male-dominated society; the male may consider it to be rude if a medical worker turns to the mother and asks questions about a child's illness.

Saudi culture is heavily male dominant as well. In Saudi Arabian culture, men take on the responsibility of serving as an intermediary between the outside world and their wives (Galanti, 2015). At the doctor's, it is common for men to answer all the questions on behalf of their wives. When dealing with patients from these and similar cultures, TCM practitioners should expect the wife to transfer all questions to her husband, who may consult with his wife about her health status before answering the question. The practitioner who ignores the husband and seeks information directly from the wife runs the risk of raising feelings of personal humiliation and disrespect for the husband. In some cases, routine procedures can be delayed, while in other cases, the patient's life may be in danger. Judging whether this indirect information eliciting (引出信息) procedure is moral or not might end up being ethnocentric, i.e., evaluating the feasibility from the standpoint of one's own cultural framework (For more information, please consult Chapter 12).

Secondly, cultural norms may also influence **self-disclosure**, or how much patients are willing to tell during history-taking. Proper healthcare demands that patients trust the healthcare professionals so that both parties can exchange essential medical information. Yet, cultural rules can have a strong influence on patients' self-disclosure and communication. It makes a big difference if the patient is willing to share. Women from Middle Eastern and Latin American cultures, for instance, may be reluctant to discuss domestic violence with strangers (Galanti, 2015). Additionally, culture often determines who can discuss what with whom. Some women from Mexico and Latin America, for example, may feel embarrassed or shy when talking about female problems (Purnell, 2013). Frequently, they will refrain from discussing birth control or childbirth with doctors. In that case, it is important not to push too much. Otherwise, health communication will not be successful. Among the Chinese, too much talk about personal matters is often considered in poor taste. Chinese women, therefore, tend not to talk about or discuss female problems. The above examples demonstrate that not all patients are willing to talk to healthcare providers with the same degree of openness. Understanding these cultural variations in communication and self-disclosure can help professionals gather important information about patients' health. Though inquiry is a very important diagnostic technique for TCM physicians to collect information about patients' medical history, it should be used wisely and gradually in cultures where it takes time to establish mutual trust between doctors and patients.

Lastly, **linguistic and non-linguistic barriers** apply to the healthcare context as well. Language barriers and the need for interpreters complicate medical interactions. Literal translation often does not convey the true meaning of a communicated message. Think for a moment about the potential confusion if a TCM physician speaks of a woman's "*yinqu*", a TCM term that often refers to privacy, such as the genitals and sexual activity, to someone whose culture does not use this euphemism. A literal translation of the phrase "hidden twist" may render nothing at all.

Besides language issue, nonverbal messages can also be troublesome. Cultural diversity in nonverbal behavior can affect health communication, and often does. Nonverbal behavior sometimes has clear meaning, but it is frequently ambiguous. People in one culture often use nonverbal behaviors — distance, eye contact, gestures, and so on — that are misunderstood by people in other cultures. Healthcare practitioners and patients often communicate their beliefs, feelings, and attitudes about illness and treatment nonverbally. While it would be ideal if TCM healthcare providers were knowledgeable about the nonverbal behavior of all cultures, it is at least reasonable to ask that you learn more about the meaning and use of nonverbal behavior across cultures!

Implications for TCM Interculturalization

In health communication, culture intervenes at every step of the way. As should be evident by now, cultural miscommunication has become a major problem in a healthcare setting. On many occasions, ignorance of culture can lead to a false diagnosis (Qureshi, 1994). Only by taking a full history and being sensitive to a patient's culture can a doctor make an accurate diagnosis, understand patterns of illness in various cultural groups, and isolate diseases which may or may not be specific to a particular cultural group.

The globalization of TCM culture has a long history. Its medical theories and skills have been widely spread to Central Asia, West Asia, and other regions. Nowadays, many people are willing to accept cupping, acupuncture, and other related treatments. Yet, it is still a challenge for TCM to be fully endorsed by people of diverse cultural backgrounds. One thing is for sure: Respect for cultural diversity in the healthcare system is a must. Mainstream healthcare providers in Western countries have been trained under, are familiar with, and most of the time believe in biomedical healthcare system. It is difficult for them to adapt to non-mainstream healthcare systems. For TCM to become part of the mainstream medical culture, a critical issue to address is to identify the enculturation (文化适应) of health belief in the world, in other words, how to coexist with local healthcare systems without losing the essence of TCM. If the global acceptance of TCM is a goal in the 21st century, then TCM physicians and TCM culture facilitators must be aware of potential problems related to cultural differences in health communication.

Activities

Comprehension Questions

1.What is necessary for healthcare workers to deal with patients from different cultures?

2.Besides illnesses and diseases, what other issues is health concerned with?

3.What are three cultural barriers in a healthcare setting? Do you know other factors?

4.What should a TCM physician do if he wants to talk to an African American family about treatment options?

5.Medical jargon is notorious for being incomprehensible, even to native speakers, let alone foreigners. Think of some medical terms that are confusing to nonprofessionals. Use both Western medicine and TCM as examples.

Survey

Almost everyone has to visit a doctor at least once in their lifetime. In each hospital, there are some rules about how to receive a patient, collect fees, or admit a patient. Foreigners in a host country can encounter a lot of difficulties in these procedures. Sometimes, they are even frustrated with the formalities of buying flu medications. Conduct a survey among foreigners in your city to find out their difficulties in a healthcare setting and provide some useful suggestions accordingly.

Case Study

The following is a story shared by a couple: The husband is Korean, and his wife is Chinese.

Not long after they got married, the wife became pregnant. One day, the wife asked her husband for a glass of water. The husband hurriedly took out the bottled water from the refrigerator and gave it to his wife. The wife looked very unhappily and barked at him, "Why did you give me ice water?" The husband couldn't understand why his wife was reacting so strongly. Many people in the Republic of Korea like to drink cold water and feel that hot water does not quench their thirst. Chinese people value TCM culture and believe that drinking cold water does harm to their health.

Questions

1.What should the Korean husband and Chinese wife do in their future life?

2.What do you think is important for this interracial marriage?

9.3   Improving Multicultural Health Communication

Challenges in Multicultural Health Communication

When considering multicultural issues, what often comes to mind are racial and ethnic distinctions among individuals. Yet, as Gillmor (2001) aptly indicates, "there is a distinct **medical culture** that can be extremely confusing and frightening to those on the outside. After all, humans are naturally inclined to fear illness because it is a situation when humans don't function normally" (p. 19). The specialized language used by TCM staff often makes their communication difficult to understand for many people. Besides, before the wide application of electronic medical history, patients barely understood their medical records simply because doctors' handwriting was beyond recognition. That could hamper effective information exchange.

Personal considerations like uncertainty in illness and health literacy influence health communication as well. People face **uncertainty** in different aspects of life, such as illness. They will try to manage and deal with this uncertainty, which can have both positive and negative effects. In addition to this psychological skill, another skill is also important for making informed decisions and achieving positive health outcomes. This skill, called **health literacy** (健康素养), refers to "the capacity to obtain, process, and understand basic health information and services needed to make appropriate health decisions" (Head and Cohen, 2015, p. 187). People who have low health literacy may not understand the information about their health, including a diagnosis, given by healthcare providers.

Failure to consider cultural diversity would pose even greater challenges for the promotion of TCM interculturally. Some of these challenges and measures to overcome difficulties are covered in other chapters of this book. We present two of them here in a way that highlights how they can be of great help for effective TCM interculturalization in a healthcare context.

Recognizing Diverse Medical Systems

The first step in overcoming cultural barriers is to recognize that many cultures may have several medical systems running together. In China, for instance, both traditional medicine and Western medicine are practiced. In other words, the combination of TCM and Western biomedicine has been very successful. It is effective and feasible to utilize the same approach to medical treatment in other parts of the world. This is the hard data that can be used as evidence to promote TCM across cultures. TCM culture facilitators can design basic courses or workshops on the history and successful cases of TCM to foster a shift in the participants' mindset, boosting their health literacy.

For TCM practitioners, successful treatment of patients requires that TCM practitioners acknowledge patients' beliefs concerning the causes, treatment, and prevention of illness. Otherwise, it may be very difficult to persuade an outsider to take TCM as a medical option. No single healthcare system in the world is powerful enough to deal with every kind of illness successfully or equally effectively. Each one has its strengths and weaknesses. If the patient believes in certain kind of healing system that is not TCM, it is advisable for healthcare providers to listen and offer advice on the integrative method.

Admittedly, being sensitive to patients' beliefs requires a great deal of information. Besides cultural understanding and awareness of communication patterns, it is also essential to have specific knowledge about the individual. When you begin to engage a new patient, it can be helpful if you determine how much "TCMized" the patient might be, i.e., how much your new patient welcomes TCM. Some of the following questions will help this process:

- What language(s) is/are spoken by the patient?
- What cultural traits does the patient possess?
- Is the patient representative of the culture where she or he comes?
- What are the traditional concepts of disease and health held by the patient?
- What types of medicine is practiced by the patient's culture?
- What is the patient's attitude toward healthcare?

Avoiding Ethnocentrism

Besides, another key move for you to do is to recognize ethnocentrism. Ethnocentrism — the universal tendency of human beings to think that their ways of thinking, acting, and believing are the only right, proper, and natural ways (For more information, please consult Chapter 12) — can "be a major barrier to providing culturally competent care" (Purnell, 2013, p. 7). Up till now, we have explicitly and implicitly emphasized one important fact: You must recognize that there is no one single answer to all health problems. When you behave as if you believe that your culture possesses that single answer, your ethnocentric logic comes into play. Avoiding ethnocentrism demands that you consider the cultural backgrounds of both patients and practitioners. In so doing you become culturally sensitive to the healthcare expectations held by people whose cultural background is different from your own.

Unconscious ethnocentrism in a healthcare setting sometimes takes place out of good intention, which usually leads to unexpected negative consequences. Galanti (2015) recorded an incident between a group of US American doctors and Magdi Bal, a 27-year-old woman from Saudi Arabia, and her father's controlling role in her medical decisions. Magdi needed surgery that could make her unable to have children, but her father refused to let her sign the consent form. The doctors were upset because they believed the surgery might save Magdi's life if she had uterine cancer.

Magdi let her father make decisions for her because in Saudi culture, fathers are in charge of their daughters until they get married. If Magdi could not have children, her father believed that she would not get married. In that case, she would become a burden to the family. The doctors went ahead with the surgery without compromising (破坏) Magdi's ability to have children, as her father desired. Afterward, the doctors and nurses discussed the case and were angry with Magdi's father for not caring about his daughter's health. Some were also upset with Magdi for not standing up for herself. One staff member, Danielle, said that women should not be seen only as baby-makers and that their worth should not depend on having children. This is a typical example of being ethnocentric. After letting out their frustration, these medical workers realized that it was not their role to criticize. The patient had the right to choose someone else to make decisions for her, and they recognized that their own values differed from hers. "In other words, they achieved a measure of cultural relativism" (Galanti, 2015, p. 134).

Cultures differ in the way they explain, treat, and prevent illness. Healthcare practices must accommodate a culturally diverse group of patients. Issues related to family roles, self-disclosure, language, and nonverbal communication can influence effective communication in a healthcare setting. If TCM is to be successfully recognized across cultures, TCM practitioners and TCM culture facilitators must acknowledge diverse medical systems, different approaches to treatment, and be aware of ethnocentrism. Apart from these two suggestions, it is not wise if you assume that the information discussed in this section applies to all people associated with a particular culture. Otherwise, you fail to acknowledge individual and contextual differences. It is a long journey to develop proficiency in intercultural competence. By implementing the above suggestions, you will overcome cultural barriers and improve health communication.

Chapter Summary

- Different cultures have different ideas about the causes and prevention of illness.
- People from many cultures employ a combination of biomedical, holistic, and magico-religious approaches to prevent illness.
- The purpose of treatment within the framework of biomedical healthcare system is to bring the patient back to the accepted standard determined by scientific norms.
- From the perspective holistic model, an imbalance in the combination of yin and yang, or four humors, causes illness.
- A supernatural force dominates the world and causes illness to human beings from the angle of magic model.
- Family roles, self-disclosure, and linguistic and non-linguistic messages are three prominent cultural barriers to effective communication in a healthcare setting.
- For TCM to become part of the mainstream medical culture, a critical issue to be addressed is to identify the enculturation of health belief in the world.
- Besides cultural factors, other challenges in multicultural health communication include difficult medical culture and personal considerations like uncertainty and level of health literacy.
- It is important to recognize that many cultures may have several medical systems running together.
- Avoiding ethnocentrism demands that you must consider the cultural background of both patients and practitioners.

Checklist	Yes	No
Cognitive: I have mastered the core information		
Behavioral: I have the ability of putting what I've learned into practice		
Affective: I am willing to carry out what I've learned		
Moral: I will take the ethical consideration into account during practice		

Chapter 10

TCM Around the World: Past and Present

Chapter Objectives

After reading this chapter, you should be able to:

◆ Describe the history and status quo of TCM across five continents,

◆ Outline TCM education in Japan, the Republic of Korea, US, UK, Brazil, Russia, India, and South Africa,

◆ Understand the challenges and prospects of TCM in the above countries,

◆ Develop a sense of patriotism for the glorious contribution of TCM to global health.

┌─────────────┐
│ **Key Terms** │
└─────────────┘

acupuncture diplomacy

acupuncture fever

BRICS

Confucius Institute for Chinese
   Medicine (South Africa)

Dongui Bogam

Dr. B. K. Basu

Eclectic School

Goseiha School

James Reston

Jianzhen

kampo

Ke Dihua

Kohoha School

Legislations on TCM

Lu Yigong

Luo Dinghui

Mei Wanfang

Sasang Medicine

St. Petersburg's TCM hospital

The Confucius Institute for TCM (UK)

UFG Confucius Institute

─┤Quotes├──

"The combination of teaching Chinese language, traditional Chinese culture and modern Chinese medicine helps open a new channel for Australian people to become acquainted with Chinese culture, serving as a bridge to connect hearts and foster friendships between two nations." (中医孔子学院把传统和现代中医药科学同汉语教学相融合,必将为澳大利亚民众开启一扇了解中国文化新的窗口,为加强两国人民心灵沟通、增进传统友好搭起一座新的桥梁。)

——2010 年 6 月 20 日习近平出席(澳大利亚墨尔本)中医孔子学院授牌仪式时的讲话

"China acknowledges the important role of the World Health Organization and is ready to continue to strengthen cooperation between the two sides, to promote the development of integrated Chinese and Western medicine and TCM overseas, to facilitate the entry into the international market of more Chinese-produced medicinal products, and to jointly assist African countries in the prevention and treatment of diseases and in their health systems development, with a view to making a greater contribution to the promotion of global health and the attainment of the United Nations Millennium Development Goals." (中方重視世界衛生組織的重要作用,願繼續加强雙方合作,促進中西醫結合及中醫藥在海外發展,推動更多中國生產的醫藥產品進入國際市場,共同幫助非洲國家開展疾病防治和衛生體系建設,爲促進全球衛生事業、實現聯合國千年發展目標作出更大貢獻。)

——2013 年 8 月 20 日習近平在人民大會堂會見原世界衛生組織總幹事陳馮富珍時的談話

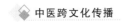
Before reading this section, please consider the following questions:

1.How much do you know about traditional Korean medicine?

2.What is your opinion on the prospects of TCM in Asia?

10.1　TCM in Japan and the Republic of Korea

Traditional Chinese medicine (TCM), as an eminent (突出的) representative of Chinese culture, has been practiced for thousands of years and has saved millions of lives in China and across the globe. It has not only made remarkable contributions to the prosperity of the Chinese nation, but also exerted a positive impact on the advancement of world civilization. The enduring vitality of TCM culture lies in its openness and inclusiveness, which inject a sense of vigor and vitality into the development of global medicine, particularly within the realm of Asian medicine.

With a cultural bond spanning over 2,000 years, Japan and the Republic of Korea, as neighboring countries to China, have fostered extensive cultural exchanges with China, especially in the field of traditional medicine. This fruitful integration has built trust in TCM among the Japanese and the Republic of Korean peoples, leading to a growing number of students traveling to China to study this ancient practice. Simultaneously, the export of Chinese medicine to these nations has experienced a steady annual increase. This section aims to provide a concise overview of the historical background and current state of TCM in these neighboring nations, in the hope of offering valuable insights into the development of traditional medicine within the modern context, serving as a source of guidance and knowledge for practitioners and policymakers alike.

TCM in Japan

In Japan, traditional medicine is known as **kampo**, which owes its origins to the theories and classics of TCM. Its primary treatment methods encompass herbal medicine, acupuncture, and massage derived from TCM techniques. These practices hold immense importance in the field of medical treatment in Japan.

• Beginning of Kampo

The exact date of the introduction of TCM to Japan is unclear, but it is generally accepted that it was introduced from the Korean Peninsula in the early 5th century (Zhang Y J, 2021). In 562 A.D., Zhicong (知聪) of ancient Wu kingdom, transported TCM classics such as *Huangdi Neijing, Shennong Bencao Jing*, along with many TCM medical tools, to Japan, and began to teach the art of Chinese herbs processing. During the Asuka Period in 600 A.D., Prince Shotoku (圣德太子) dispatched envoys (特使) to the Sui Dynasty for the purpose of studying Buddhist scriptures and cultural practices. They also acquired knowledge of TCM, which they brought back to Japan. In 754 A.D., Jianzhen (鉴真), a prominent monk of the Tang Dynasty, took a great many TCM books and medicines to Japan. This event greatly advanced the development of Japanese medicine, and Jianzhen continues to be respected as the ancestor of kampo in Japan. Subsequently, during the Song, Yuan and Ming Dynasties, as Chinese and Japanese monks engaged in more frequent cultural exchanges, alongside other forms of communication, additional knowledge about TCM found its way into Japan (Zhu *et al.*, 2019).

• Goseiha School and Kohona School

The story of the birth of kampo medicine can be traced back to one influential figure named Tashiro Sanki (田代三喜) who had a strong connection with China. Reportedly, he traveled to China in the year 1487 to study TCM (Zhu *et al.*, 2019). Following 11 years of extensive research and learning, he returned to Japan and established the Goseiha School of kampo, which was based on the medical doctrines of Li Dongyuan (李东垣) and Zhu Danxi (朱丹溪), the leading TCM physicians of the Jin and Yuan Dynasties (1115-1368). The school paid special attention to the Yin-yang, five-phases, and meridian theories.

In Mid-Edo Period, a new medical school of kampo known as the Kohoha School came into existence. Prominent figures associated with this school were Gotō Gonzan (后藤良山) and Yoshimasu Tōdō (吉益东洞). They held contrasting views to the Jin-yuan medical theory, emphasizing instead the guidance of Zhang Zhongjing's principles. Their approach involved supporting yang, subduing yin, and reviving ancient classic formulas.

• Eclectic School and Western Medicine

During the later years of the Edo Period, a significant development took place in the field of kampo medicine. Many practitioners began to merge the perceived strengths of the Goseiha and Kohoha schools, giving rise to the Eclectic School, which successfully integrated the perceived advantages of the Goseiha and Kohoha schools, emphasizing *Shanghan Zabing Lun* as the core theory and supplementing it with *Huangdi Neijing*. This integration of theories eventually paved the way for the fusion of kampo and Western medicine during the later period.

After 1868, the new government actively promoted Western medicine and placed great emphasis on its advantages. As a result, kampo hospitals were closed down, greatly impeding the development of Japanese kampo medicine during this period.

After Second World War, kampo medicine experienced a revival in Japan, marking the beginning of a new era. In 1967, the health insurance authorities introduced a reimbursement system for kampo drugs. Initially, reimbursement was available for 147 drugs, and by 1987, this number had increased to about 200.

• Revival of Kampo and its Collaboration with China

For over 100 years, starting from 1883, the Japanese

government had excluded kampo education from the public education system. However, in 2001, there was a gradual reintroduction of kampo education into formal medical teaching (Fan and Zhang, 2020). By 2022, approximately 80 medical colleges and universities in Japan were offering courses on various aspects of kampo, covering fundamentals, prescription, and medicinal materials. Despite this progress, there is still no inclusion of kampo medicine in the national medical qualification examination, and there are no dedicated (专门) kampo doctors. Instead, kampo courses serve as an auxiliary (辅助) component within Western medicine education, with limited coverage of basic knowledge and clinical practice. To practice kampo medicine, doctors must obtain bachelor's degrees in Western medicine and be qualified to practice Western medicine. Consequently, kampo remains a complementary part of Japanese medical education.

Currently, a limited number of kampo clinics have been established within hospitals, while private clinics or hospitals offering acupuncture and physiotherapy treatments can be found in various locations. The availability of kampo services is expanding, leading to an increasing number of Japanese people utilizing kampo prescriptions. Another clear indication of kampo's thriving growth is the production and sales of kampo medicine, which receives significant support from the Japanese government and is regulated by laws. With the integration of modern science, technology, and advanced sales methods, kampo has not only gained widespread popularity within Japan but also across the globe.

TCM in the Republic of Korea

In the Republic of Korea, the preferred English term for what is commonly known as Chinese medicine in most parts of the world is Oriental medicine (Baker, 2003). Traditional Korean medicine (TKM), which originated from TCM, has developed some of its own features in diagnosis and treatment. Since the late 6th century A.D., the classic works of TCM such as *Huangdi Neijing* and *Shanghan Zabing Lun*, were gradually introduced to the Korean Peninsula (Li, 2015). Subsequently, they were integrated with local traditional medicine, leading to the development of a distinctive TKM.

Over the years, Koreans enhanced the medical theory and clinical guidance from those classical works by incorporating more recent Chinese publications, as well as Korean texts that offered local alternatives to the Chinese ingredients in TCM prescriptions. Most of these books were used in court, and therefore were too bulky for easy use. However, in 1613, a compact guide to medical theory and practice was made, i.e., **Dongui Bogam** (*Principles and Practice of Oriental Medicine*《东医宝鉴》), which is considered as the greatest original contribution to the development of oriental medicine. Having been read by both Confucian scholars and physicians, *Dongui Bogam* played a pivotal role in shaping medical thought and practice throughout the entire Joseon Dynasty (1392-1910) and continues to exert its influence to this day. The global significance of this work in medical history was duly acknowledged in 2009, when UNESCO included *Dongui Bogam* in the Memory of the World Register.

During the late 19th century, Western medicine made its way to the Republic of Korea, which prompted the Korean government to adopt a policy of coexistence between oriental medicine and Western medicine. Consequently, these two medical systems began to develop independently. Despite facing suppression in 1910 due to national policies, oriental medicine experienced a revival in 1951 when the Republic of Korean government issued a decree that granted equal status to oriental medicine and Western medicine within its borders. In 1964, a six-year oriental medicine education program was established. To better represent its cultural identity, oriental medicine was officially renamed TKM in 1986 (iFeng, 2006), and since 1987, TKM has been covered by the National Health Insurance in the Republic of Korea.

• Sasang Medicine

After years of adjustment and development, the theory of TKM, which is rooted in TCM, has gradually evolved into a medical system with distinct Korean characteristics. Among these developments, the most renowned is Sasang Medicine (四象医学), a theory proposed by the 19th century philosopher and medical scientist Lee Je-Ma (李济马). Sasang Medicine divides human beings into four Sasang constitutional types, recommending utilizing type-specific medical herbs and acupuncture to achieve safer and more effective treatments.

The concise and practical nature of Sasang Medicine is considered its most significant advantage (Choi *et al.*, 2012). Doctors can select appropriate drug prescriptions based on an individual's Sasang constitutional type determined by their physique. As a result, it has been widely explored and clinically applied in hospitals and medical fields, gradually becoming the essence of modern TKM.

• TKM Education

Over the past few years, the Korean government has been actively promoting TKM and integrating it into formal university education (Han *et al.*, 2016). There are now more than ten full-time TKM universities that offer bachelor's, master's, and doctoral degrees. These universities follow a standardized six-year curriculum. Although these universities place a strong emphasis on providing students with a solid foundation in medical theory, the duration allocated to clinical practice is relatively limited. As a result, it is often essential for students to gain practical experience through off-campus training or by attending seminars related to their field before they can start practicing medicine.

In the Republic of Korea, there are more than 20 hospitals dedicated to TKM, along with 3,000 clinics and numerous scientific research institutions where extensive research has been conducted on the pharmacology of drugs. The WHO has established 27 collaborating centers worldwide for traditional medicine, two of which are located in the Republic of Korea (Yu et al., 2017). Additionally, several Korean academic organizations and industry associations focused on Korean medicine have been established, which play a crucial role in supporting government management, facilitate academic exchanges, and promote widespread awareness and understanding of TKM.

China, the Republic of Korea, and Japan are three neighboring countries that are separated only by a narrow strip of water. Historically, Japan and the Republic of Korea had a close vassal (附庸国) relationship with China, which explains the strong ties between the three nations. Cultural exchange, including the exchange of medical and health management practices, must have been quite frequent. The theories and practices of TCM that were transmitted to these two countries are part of a larger traditional Chinese culture, encompassing Chinese philosophy, particularly Confucian ideals, festivals, religion, and the rest. Kampo in Japan and TKM in the Republic of Korea share a common feature—they derived medical theories and practices from China while also adapting to local needs.

Activities

Comprehension Questions

1. Please select one of the three schools of kampo in Japan to describe its history of development, and if applicable, explore any connections it may have with TCM.
2. Who is recognized as the originator of Sasang medicine in the Republic of Korea?
3. Jianzhen is more renowned for his contribution to the Buddhist culture in Japan than

for his introduction of TCM to Japan. Find more information about how Jianzhen helped spread TCM in Japan.

4.What is your opinion on the localization of TCM in the Republic of Korea?

5. Find more information about the current status of kampo medicine on the international market.

Translation

Translate the following text into English.

亚洲先人们早就开始了文明交流互鉴。现在,"一带一路""两廊一圈""欧亚经济联盟"等拓展了文明交流互鉴的途径,各国在科技、教育、文化、卫生、民间交往等领域的合作蓬勃开展,亚洲文明也在自身内部及同世界文明的交流互鉴中发展壮大。

——2019年5月15日习近平在亚洲文明对话大会开幕式上的主旨演讲

Debate

Read the following statements.

UNESCO included *Dongui Bogam* in the Memory of the World Register in 2009. Some scholars argue that this book is a compilation of medical theories and practices taken from various TCM classics, therefore lacking specificity to the Republic of Korea. However, Korean scholars assert that *Dongui Bogam* is a result of local adaptations and interpretations of TCM.

What do you think of it? Do you consider *Dongui Bogam* primarily as a Korean translation of TCM, or do you believe it to be a distinct and unique medical document representing TKM?

Form teams with classmates who share the same position, with 2-4 members on each side. Give alternate speeches for and against the topic.

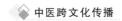

Before reading this section, please consider the following questions:

1. Which report from *The New York Times* in 1971 sparked significant interest in acupuncture among the American people?

2. What is your opinion on the fact that acupuncture enjoys greater acceptance in Western countries compared to herbal medicine?

10.2 TCM in the US and the UK

The United States and the United Kingdom are considered the birthplaces of Western medicine. Continental European countries also contributed to the development of biomedicine. However, it was the scientific revolution, notably the biomedical breakthroughs in the US, that played a crucial role in propelling modern Western medicine forward. This revolution led to the replacement of ancient Greek health management and the spread of Western medicine worldwide. It is hard to imagine the challenges faced by TCM practitioners in the US and European countries. Still, TCM gradually finds its way into the UK. and the US. The introduction of TCM to these two countries, particularly acupuncture, is truly remarkable. This section provides a preliminary overview of TCM development in two major English-speaking countries: the US and the UK, with a primary focus on the period following the founding of the People's Republic of China.

TCM in the US

•Early Contact

The introduction of TCM to the US can be traced back to the mid-18th century (Zhang D Q, 2021). In 1784, some Chinese medicinal materials began to be shipped directly to the US. During the early 19th century, some TCM books written by European medical scientists were published and subsequently brought to the US. Notably, in 1822, an editorial on acupuncture was published in an American medical journal, emphasizing the need to recognize and value its astonishing power. In 1825, Benjamin Franklin Bache, a renowned chemist and physician in the US, translated Morand's *Memoir on Acupuncture* from French into English and published it for clinical use, thus becoming the first person to release an English version of acupuncture monographs in the US (Zhang D Q, 2021). As the gold rush era unfolded in the 1850s, a significant number of Chinese immigrants arrived in the US, bringing acupuncture and Chinese herbs with them. However, these practices remained confined to the Chinese community and were not widely known among other American people. Some first-generation Chinese immigrants established TCM pharmaceutical shops, where they not only provided Chinese Americans with TCM services but also offered Chinese herbs for sale.

Prior to the biomedical breakthrough that revolutionized Western medicine, there were hardly any therapeutic differences between TCM and Western medicine. However, TCM did not receive widespread recognition not only due to cultural diversity in healthcare management but also possibly because of political disputes between the two countries. In 1971, just one year before President Richard Nixon's visit to China, James Reston, a senior reporter from *The New York Times*, experienced acute appendicitis (阑尾炎) in China and had to have his appendix removed at Peking Union Medical College Hospital. After the surgery, he received acupuncture for pain relief and thus had the opportunity to witness acupuncture anesthesia (麻醉), which left a lasting impression on him. Immediately after returning to the States, James Reston published an article titled "Now about my Operation in Peking", creating a sensation and greatly contributing to the popularization of acupuncture among the American people. The publication of this article has since become a historic symbol of **"acupuncture fever"**, sparking widespread interest in acupuncture, cupping, and other TCM techniques in the US (Shi and Zhang, 2022).

• Legislation on TCM

Legislating acupuncture in the US is a challenging process (Lin, 2001). In January 1973, Mr. Lu Yigong (陆易公), a renowned acupuncturist from Hong Kong, was invited to deliver a series of acupuncture lectures in New York City. However, he was arrested by the NYPD for engaging in illegal activities. Mr. Lu Yigong, taken aback by this turn of events, decided to actively contribute to the promotion of acupuncture legislation. After learning that legislators in Nevada were preparing to enact new laws, Mr. Lu Yigong, with the assistance of Arthur Steinberg, a retired lawyer, provided on-site acupuncture treatments to 60 state lawmakers in a convention hall in Nevada. These treatments yielded highly positive results. Eventually, these efforts contributed to the formal legislation of acupuncture in Nevada. This significant milestone played a crucial role in the development of TCM in the States, serving as a foundation for subsequent actions such as including acupuncture in the medical insurance system and recognizing acupuncturists as physicians.

The year of 1973 also witnessed the establishment of the first Chinese medicine association in the US, namely, the California Institute of Traditional Chinese Medicine and Acupuncture. Its primary mission is to promote understanding of acupuncture within American society and advocate for acupuncture legislation at the state government level (Liu and Zhou, 2023). In April 1996, the Food and Drug Administration (FDA), a governmental organization in the US, officially approved acupuncture needles as medical devices (Wang, 2016). In October 2018, former U.S. President Donald Trump signed H.R.6 into law, granting approval to acupuncture as an evidence-based and effective therapy for opioid (阿片类药物) replacement. This historic event marked the first-ever recognition of acupuncture in federal law (Liu Yingying and Zhou, 2023). As of 2020, 48 states and Washington DC have passed acupuncture laws, ensuring the legal use of acupuncture in these places (Cui *et al.*, 2020). However, the legislation regarding acupuncture is not uniform across all states, and currently, there is no federal law that specifically addresses the legality of practicing acupuncture. Additionally, moxibustion, which is often used in conjunction with acupuncture, still lacks legal recognition. The journey towards complete legalization of acupuncture as a legitimate treatment remains a considerable challenge.

The legislative journey of herbal medicine in the US has also faced challenges. In recent decades, as Chinese medicines gained recognition in the US medical market, the federal government has established a series of laws and regulations regarding Chinese herbal medicines. In 1994, the US enacted the *Dietary Supplement Health and Education Act* (FDA, 2023), which allowed Chinese herbal products to legally enter the U.S. market as dietary supplements, while drugs derived from animals were prohibited for internal and external use. In 2004, the FDA released the updated *Guidance for Industry Botanical Drug Products*, which provides specific guidelines for herbal drugs applying for clinical trials (FDA, 2020). According to the FDA's *Guidance of Industry on Complementary and Alternative Medicine Products and Their Regulation* (2006), Chinese herbal products are classified as dietary supplements and thus cannot be labeled as "treating diseases". Although some TCM treatments have progressed to phase II/III clinical trials, only *Danshen Drops* (复方丹参滴丸) has completed phase III trials. Other treatments, such as *Guizhi Fuling Capsules* (桂枝茯苓胶囊) and *Lianhua Qingwen Capsules*, are still undergoing phase II trials with very few promising results for further development. Despite the various real-world clinical benefits of TCM, it remains extremely challenging to demonstrate their compelling safety and effectiveness within the current clinical evaluation system. So far, only a few Chinese compound medicines have obtained clinical trial approval from the FDA (You *et al.*, 2022).

• Education of TCM

Compared with other Western countries, the US has a relatively systematic and comprehensive education system for TCM. Since the establishment of the New England School of Acupuncture in 1975, 56 Chinese medicine colleges or schools in the US have obtained national certification from the Accreditation Commission for Acupuncture and Oriental Medicine (Wei *et al.*, 2017). This specialized accreditation (认证) agency, recognized by the US Department of Education, is aimed to ensure the quality of teaching and research in the field of TCM. Each year, more than 2000 students pursue their bachelor's, master's, and doctorate degrees in TCM or acupuncture, which are offered by specialized schools and colleges such as the New England School of Acupuncture, the New York College of Traditional Chinese Medicine, and the American College of Traditional Chinese Medicine. Additionally, some comprehensive universities, including Harvard University and Yale University, offer TCM courses within their medical colleges. Upon graduation, most students from these institutions are eligible to take the certification examination conducted by the National Certification Commission for Acupuncture and Oriental Medicine or their state's acupuncturist certification examination, enabling them to become certified acupuncturists.

TCM in the UK

• Overview of TCM History in the UK

Since it was first introduced to the UK in the late 17th century, TCM has a history of over three hundred years in the UK. The British have a long-standing tradition of using herbs, making it relatively easy for them to accept Chinese herbal medicine. In

1821, British surgeon John Churchill published a paper on the use of acupuncture for treating diseases, marking the earliest documentation of acupuncture therapy in Britain (Chen Y *et al.*, 2019). In the 1960s and 1970s, some British individuals traveled to China for short-term studies and learned basic acupuncture techniques. Upon returning to the UK, they established acupuncture clinics in London and other cities.

In the 1970s, several Chinese doctors who had received formal education in TCM arrived in Britain and established TCM clinics in the Chinatowns of London and Manchester. One notable doctor was **Luo Dinghui** (罗鼎辉). After graduating from Guangzhou University of Chinese Medicine, Luo Dinghui gained experience working in a TCM hospital for several years. Upon arriving in England in 1983, she rented a storefront in Chinatown and opened her clinic called "Hong-Ning Herbal Medicine" (康宁堂), where she provided treatment to patients using Chinese medicine prescriptions. During that time, Luo Dinghui successfully treated numerous British children suffering from eczema (湿疹), an ailment considered challenging to address using Western medicine. Her success even prompted renowned David Atherton , a British dermatologist (皮肤科医生) to refer his patients to her clinic (Sheehan and Atherton, 1992).

News media and academic reports have helped promote TCM in the UK. British mainstream media, such as *The Guardian*, *The Observer*, or BBC, all competed to report on Luo Dinghui's TCM clinic. Even prestigious journals like *The British Journal of Dermatology* and *The Lancet* reported her TCM treatment of skin diseases, causing a huge sensation in the UK (Xia, 2017). In 1982, Mei Wanfang (梅万方), a Chinese British based in London, established an acupuncture clinic named AcuMedic that quickly gained widespread recognition in the UK. By the 1990s, many famous people had visited his clinic for medical treatments, with Princess Diana (1961-1997) being the most notable (Wu *et al.*,

2013).

During the late 1980s and early 1990s, as China's reform and opening up deepened, an increasing number of Chinese people, including TCM physicians, went to the UK (Chen Y *et al.*, 2019). TCM played a crucial role in cultural exchange by gradually altering the perception of Chinese people held by the British. It showcased that Chinese people could excel not only as chefs but also as exceptional doctors. While many European countries at the time prohibited the import of Chinese patented medicine, the UK government displayed tolerance and allowed the sale of Chinese herbal medicine products. Recognizing the opportunities, some businessmen embarked on opening Chinese medicine shops one after another. These shops generated substantial profits by selling Chinese patented medicine and offering services like acupuncture, cupping, massage, and moxibustion. From 1995 to 2005, several chain companies emerged. TCM shops have become prevalent in large supermarkets and shopping malls.

The British government's tolerance has facilitated the robust growth of TCM. However, due to the lack of supervision, the development of TCM has become somewhat uncontrollable. In response to the disorderly expansion of TCM clinics, the British government decided in 2004 to implement the EU Traditional Herbal Medicinal Products Directive, which was later modified in 2020 (MHRA, 2020). This directive (命令) mandates (规定) that herbal products be registered with authorization from the European Union member states. Only after obtaining approval can these products be sold and used as medicines in the EU market. The UK government permitted a 10-year transition period from 2004 to 2014. According to this directive, all imports of Chinese patented medicines have to obtain a license, with the prerequisite being a comprehensive ingredient test for the drug. The cost of this test is prohibitively high, deterring (使却步) both TCM manufacturers who are not very interested in exploring the

British market, and owners of TCM clinics in the U.K. who cannot afford the expense (Ye, 2016). Consequently, by the end of the transition period, only one Chinese medicine, namely Phynova Joint and Muscle Relief Tablet (凡诺华缓解关节肌肉疼痛片), had been registered in the UK. However, there is always a silver lining. "It is possible to demonstrate that almost any traditional Chinese medicine can successfully pass scientific tests conducted by Western science. That is the only way TCM will ever achieve full acceptance in Western markets," stated Robert Miller, the chief executive officer of Phynova (Liu, 2015).

The unforeseen financial crisis in 2008 dealt a devastating blow to the TCM industry in the UK. The exclusion of Chinese medicines and acupuncture from the coverage provided by the National Health Service in the UK, coupled with the worsening unemployment rate, forced many British individuals to remove TCM services from their family budgets. Another setback for the TCM business was the British government's restrictions on the import of Chinese patented medicine, which constitutes a significant portion of revenue for TCM shops. As a result, many TCM clinics were unable to sustain their operations, while a few managed to endure the challenges and survive.

•TCM Education

Since the introduction of TCM to the UK, TCM clinics initially had no worry about the adequacy of TCM physicians. This was because there were not many patients, and typically the clinic owners themselves were qualified TCM physicians who could train their children to follow in their footsteps. However, as the demand for TCM services increased, TCM clinics started to become concerned about how to recruit TCM physicians. "Prior to the 1990s, TCM education in the UK primarily relied on private Chinese medicine schools, most of which focused solely on teaching acupuncture and did not cover other TCM treatment methods" (Chen Y *et al.*, 2019, p. 690). Several medical associations are established by TCM practitioners in the UK in order to provide a platform for academic exchange. In 1980, the British Medical Acupuncture Society (BMAS) was formed in London with the purpose of establishing a nationally recognized and authoritative academic association for acupuncture. During the next two years, BMAS actively participated in the WHO's research on acupuncture standardization and made significant contributions to the standardization of meridian abbreviations. The Council for Complementary and Alternative Medicine, another association established in 1986, has played a crucial role in the development of TCM in the UK by providing a platform for communication and collaboration between different traditional medicine and modern medicine practices (Ye, 2016).

Currently, there are four universities in the UK that offer education in acupuncture and Chinese medicine, including the Chinese Medical Institute and Register, the University of Westminster, Middlesex University, and London South Bank University (Liu and Denge, 2014). Two events in particular should be highlighted. First, Beijing University of Chinese Medicine and Middlesex University co-organized a TCM program in 1997, which was the first five-year program of its kind in Europe. Second, the Confucius Institute for Traditional Chinese Medicine was established at London South Bank University, the first official institute of its kind in the world. This institute offers full-time undergraduate and postgraduate degree programs in TCM (with an emphasis on acupuncture and moxibustion). Graduates receive degree certificates recognized by the U.K. education system, and they can establish their own private clinics or practice locally after graduation.

Activities

Comprehension Questions

1.What is the legislative process for acupuncture in the US?

2.How do celebrities like US swimmer Michael Phelps help publicize TCM?

3.Why is the UK regarded as a paradise for the promotion of TCM?

4.Why is it difficult for three TCM drugs and three herbal formulas (三药三方) to pass clinical trials in the US?

5.What are the similarities and differences between the UK and the US in terms of TCM localization?

Case Study

Case 1

Doctor Xu Chaoji's excellence in TCM saved patients in Australia.

Xu Chaoji, who had worked as a doctor in Shanghai for 15 years, relocated to Australia. In 1989, he established a TCM clinic in Australia. Over the past 30 years, Doctor Xu has treated a multitude of patients, including both Chinese and notable local figures such as politicians, celebrities, and businessmen. Among these cases, he takes particular pride in successfully treating several patients with severe brain injuries.

In 2019, there was a remarkable case involving Zhang Jingting, a Chinese student studying in Australia. Zhang had suffered a significant brain injury in a car accident and was admitted to the best hospital in western Australia. Despite receiving a week of treatment, Zhang remained unconscious, with ongoing bleeding in her brain and multiple organs. Seeking additional help, Zhang's family turned to Xu Chaoji for assistance. Xu's initial treatment focused on reducing the pressure in Zhang's brain. During the second treatment session, Dr. Xu was delighted to observe signs of spontaneous breathing in the patient. However, the attending doctor suggested that Zhang was likely to enter a vegetative state. Undeterred, Dr. Xu persisted with his treatments, working tirelessly during the day, and meticulously planning the treatment strategy at night. He faced immense pressure throughout the four-month treatment period. Gradually, the patient's condition stabilized, and Zhang Jingting became well enough to return to Beijing for rehabilitation. Zhang's family later informed Dr. Xu that she was able to get out of bed and walk around. Both Zhang and her parents were hopeful for further recovery (Wang Chuanjun, 2019).

Questions

1. How would you evaluate the benefits and drawbacks of acupuncture treatment based on this specific case?

2. If one of your closest friends were to suffer from a condition similar to the case mentioned above, would you consider recommending acupuncture treatment? Why or why not?

Case 2

Mr. George Green is a Caucasian math teacher who has no idea about what coin cupping is. The following is what happened to his sick pupil and him.

A Vietnamese girl named Kathy Dinh was in her first year at an American elementary school. She was not feeling very well one morning, so her mother rubbed the back of her neck with a coin. She then felt well enough to attend school. Later in the day, however, she began to feel worse and told Mr. Green. They rushed to the school infirmary. When the nurse discovered the welts on Kathy's neck, she immediately assumed she was seeing a case of child abuse. Mr. Green was confused. He personally knew Kathy's parents and did not expect such a terrible thing could happen to Kathy. Yet, the evidence was strong enough to prove that the Dinhs were abusing their daughter. Mr. Green conscientiously reported the Dinhs to the authorities.

Questions

1. Why did Mr. Green inform against the Dinhs?

2. What suggestions do you give to Mr. Green if he notices anything unusual about his health in the future?

Group Work

1. Imagine yourself as a reporter from a local TV station with the objective of promoting TCM overseas through short videos. Your assignment is to create a 10-min video showcasing the story of Luo Dinghui, a TCM physician practicing in the UK.

2. Please collaborate in groups to research information about Dr. Lin Ziqiang (林子强) and his contributions to the legislation of TCM in Australia. Present your findings to the class.

Action Points

1. With the guidance of your instructor, work in groups or pairs to conduct a small research project on TCM in a specific country or region that is not covered in this chapter. Present your findings to the class.

2. Work in groups or pairs and imagine that you are planning to start a TCM-related business in a foreign country. Choose a country and research the local business customs and professional etiquette, evaluating how they may differ from your own culture. If possible, look into the TCM legislation in that country. Brainstorm ideas on how to approach business interactions in this new cultural setting. Present your business plans to the class.

10.3 TCM in Brazil, Russia, India, and South Africa

BRICS in Brief

The term **BRICS** stands for Brazil, Russia, India, China, and South Africa. Originally, it was referred to as BRIC, which was coined by Jim O'Neill, an economist at Goldman Sachs, an American multinational investment banking firm, in 2001(Chen, 2023). South Africa joined the group in 2010, resulting in the term being revised to BRICS. The BRICS functions as a loosely organized alliance, aiming to enhance economic cooperation among member nations and elevate their economic and political influence on a global scale.

During the special press conference of the 15th BRICS Leaders' Meeting, which took place in Johannesburg, South Africa, in August 2023, the BRICS extended a warm welcome to its new member countries. This marks the second and largest expansion of cooperation within the BRICS framework. The prospects for further active cooperation among the BRICS member countries appear promising. Given the close ties between other member states of BRICS and China, it is valuable to allocate time and resources to discuss TCM in the original four member states, apart from China itself.

TCM in Brazil

Brazil, the fifth largest country in the world, is characterized by its vast territory and comparatively low population density. In Brazil, basic health services are made accessible to every citizen through the Unified Health System (SUS), which provides medical insurance.

The introduction of TCM to Brazil can be traced back to the early 19ᵗʰ century when over 2,000 Chinese immigrants arrived in the country. However, at that time, the dissemination of TCM was constrained due to challenges such as language barriers and limited channels for communication.

It was not until in the 1960s that the growth of TCM in Brazil truly began, driven by Asian immigrants, including those from Japan. This marked a significant milestone for TCM in Brazil. In 1961, the first acupuncture clinic was established, followed by the formation of the Brazilian Acupuncture Association in 1972 (Wang R T, 2021). Notably, Brazil officially recognized the legal status of acupuncturists in 1977, further enhancing the promotion and acceptance of TCM.

During the 1980s, China's reform and opening up policy had a positive impact on the foreign relations between China and Brazil. This development served as a catalyst (促进因素) for the remarkable progress of TCM in Brazil. In response to this growing interest in TCM, the Brazilian Federation of Physicians took an active step to establish the Brazilian Association of Acupuncturists in 1984. The primary purpose of this association is to provide training, facilitate academic exchange, offer consultation services to patients, and offer guidance to acupuncturists. This establishment played a crucial role in fostering collaboration and knowledge sharing between practitioners from both countries, further contributing to the advancement and acceptance of TCM in Brazil.

In 2006, natural therapies such as acupuncture and herbal medicine were officially adopted by the SUS. The number of acupuncture sessions provided through the SUS increased by almost seven times within a span of five years. By 2011, approximately 270, 000 acupuncture sessions were conducted in Brazil, compared to just about 40, 000 in 2007 (Wang R T, 2021). The growing popularity of acupuncture in Brazil earned praise even from Brazilian politicians. Former President Luiz Inácio reportedly expressed his confidence in the efficacy of TCM after being successfully treated for arthritis in his shoulder joint by a TCM physician. Following this experience, he is said to have taken his TCM physician along during his overseas visits (He and Liang, 2016). This anecdote highlights the increasing acceptance and recognition of TCM practices in Brazil.

Overall, Brazil's vast territory, combined with the provision of basic health services through the SUS, creates favorable conditions for the development and implementation of TCM practices since the legislation on acupuncture in 2006 (He and Liang, 2016). So far, 29 TCM diagnostic methods are covered by the SUS (Wang R T, 2021). There are currently ten Confucius Institutes in Brazil, one of which is established within Federal University of Goiás (巴西联邦戈亚大学) (UFG) in cooperation with two universities in China. **UFG Confucius Institute** is unique because it is the only university in Latin America to offer not only language and culture courses but also classes in TCM, which helps facilitate TCM interculturalization.

TCM in Russia

Russia holds significant importance as a country in the Belt and Road Initiative, and its understanding of TCM is earlier than that of many other European countries. The introduction of TCM, including acupuncture, to Russia can be traced back to around 1000 years ago during the Northern Song Dynasty (960-1127), through folk exchanges and international trade. Throughout the Ming Dynasty (1368-1644), such cultural exchanges and communications experienced a consistent and steady growth (Yang *et al.*, 2012).

With the establishment of diplomatic relations between China and the Soviet Union in the 1950s, acupuncture experienced rapid progress. Numerous training courses for acupuncturists became available in various cities such as Moscow and St. Petersburg during the 1960s. In 1976, acupuncture, moxibustion, and other natural therapies were categorized collectively as reflex therapy (反射疗法). Notably, since 1997, doctors specializing in reflex therapy have been officially enlisted onto the professional board of doctors and pharmacists (Zhang J B, 2021).

St. Petersburg's TCM hospital, established in 2016 by BUCM in cooperation with Russian (medical) universities, marks itself as the first general hospital of TCM in Russia (Lan *et al.*, 2023). This hospital holds significant importance as a cultural exchange platform for both countries, featuring a medical team comprising distinguished experts from China and Russia. Especially during the COVID-19 pandemic in Russia, BUCM took active measures by organizing online lectures on pandemic prevention specifically designed for the hospital. Furthermore, BUCM developed comprehensive guidelines on TCM health management during the pandemic, available in both Chinese and Russian languages, which offer professional TCM strategies to combat the pandemic, benefiting both the Russian population and the local Chinese community.

Chinese herbal medicine has gained significant recognition and development in Russia as well. In 1773, Russian doctors conducted a study and reported on the collection and application of herbal medicine, many of which originated from TCM (Yang, 2018). In the 1880s, Russian adventurers began cultivating Chinese herbs in St. Petersburg. The cultivation of Chinese herbs gained momentum after China and Russia engaged in international cooperation in TCM, with Russia allowing Chinese farmers to plant Chinese herbs within its borders in 2015. It is predicted that by 2035, Russia's annual export of raw herbal materials to China will reach $100 billion, accounting for 25% of the raw medicinal market in China (Hu, 2017). The collaboration in Chinese herb cultivation between China and Russia not only promotes bilateral trade but also facilitates the promotion and dissemination of TCM in Russia. This, in turn, further supports the legislation of TCM in Russia.

TCM in India

India, located in South Asia, is a federal parliamentary republic and has the second largest population on earth. Traditional medicine is deeply embedded in India's history, with Ayurveda (阿育吠陀医学), naturopathy (自然疗法), yoga, and other practices occupying a prominent place. In TCM, the concept of "unity of heaven and man" embodies the ancient idea of naive materialism (朴素唯物主义), aiming to reconcile the relationship between humans and nature and seeking ways to prevent and cure diseases. In contrast, Indian Ayurvedic medicine is based on the philosophical foundation of "Brahman and I are the same" (梵我一如), representing objective idealism (客观唯心主义). It focuses on maintaining human health, easing patients' suffering, and ultimately achieving enlightenment through understanding and connection with God. Given this sharp contrast, it is not difficult to envisage the challenges that lie ahead when one tries to introduce the theories and techniques of TCM into India (Teng and Zhang, 2021).

TCM found its way to India as early as the 2nd century B.C. through religious exchanges and trade activities. However, it was not until in the mid-20th century that TCM experienced a resurgence in India. The revival of TCM in modern times, especially acupuncture, is closely tied to the Indian medical mission dispatched to China during the China's War of Resistance against Japanese Aggression.

Overall, significant achievements have been made in terms of medical exchanges between China and India, especially in the field of acupuncture. The practice of acupuncture has contributed to fostering a sense of friendship between India and China. According to Dr. Mrigendranath Gantait (Xinhua, 2022), the president of Acupuncture Association of India, acupuncture was first introduced to India in 1959 by **Dr. B. K. Basu** (巴苏华) in Kolkata, the capital city of West Bengal state. Dr. Basu accompanied Dwarkanath Kotnis, widely known as **Ke Dihua** (柯棣华) in China, during his time in China from 1938 to 1943 to provide aid to wounded soldiers as part of the Indian medical mission (Shao *et al.*, 2009). In 1959, he was offered an acupuncture training course by the Chinese government. During his stay in China, Dr. Basu not only focused on learning Chinese but also underwent comprehensive training in acupuncture and moxibustion. After returning to India, he established an acupuncture clinic in his hometown and designed training programs for medical students, practitioners, and health workers in the field of acupuncture. In 1973, Dr. Basu was once again invited to China to learn innovative techniques in acupuncture anesthesia. Upon his return to India, his trip was hailed as **acupuncture diplomacy** by the Indian media, receiving widespread praise across the country. Dr. Basu also played a crucial role in establishing the Acupuncture Association of India, generously donating his house and savings to support the development of acupuncture (Bakshi *et al.*, 1995).

Acupuncture is currently undergoing rapid development in India, with certain state governments officially recognizing its practice. Recently, the central government of India also granted official recognition to acupuncture as an independent therapeutic system within the country's healthcare system (Elahee *et al.*, 2019). During his attendance at the G20 Hangzhou Summit in China in 2016, Mr. Narendra Modi, Indian Prime Minister, expressed a strong desire to integrate acupuncture into India's healthcare system. He questioned why TCM could not be utilized by Indian citizens when yoga was popular in China (Elahee *et el.*, 2019). Thanks to his enthusiasm and the increasing popularity of acupuncture among Indians, the Indian government officially declared acupuncture as a healthcare therapeutic system in 2019, marking a significant milestone in its development in India.

It is worth mentioning that the official recognition of TCM in India has an impact on its status in neighboring countries such as Bangladesh and Nepal. It is reasonable to expect that the popularity and recognition of TCM will also gain momentum in these countries.

TCM in South Africa

South Africa is a country situated at the southern tip of the African continent. It is characterized by a relatively small population and its linguistic diversity, with eleven official languages recognized within its borders. It holds the distinction of being one of the earliest countries to officially recognize TCM. Throughout the years, TCM practitioners in Africa have gained a strong reputation for their effective TCM therapies, often successfully treating challenging diseases such as malaria.

Almost 300 years ago, during the Qing Dynasty (1644-1911), 21 craftsmen were sent to South Africa, some of whom were TCM practitioners. Towards the end of the 18th century, TCM began to establish itself in South Africa when more than 2, 000 Chinese workers, employed by Britain, eventually settled as immigrants (Guo, 2002). However, TCM then went through a period of slow development, during which there were only around 40 small-scale TCM clinics in South Africa, primarily located in large cities. Since establishing diplomatic relations with China in 1998, South Africa has witnessed significant improvements in the development of TCM. In 2000, the South African government underwent the legislative process to recognize the legality of TCM. As a result, TCM physicians have been regulated by the Allied Health Practitioners Council, which reports to the Department of Health in South Africa. Meanwhile, TCM medicines are regulated under the Complementary Medicines Regulations of the South African Health Products Regulatory Authority Act (Hou and Bao, 2012).

In addition to medical legislation, the development of local medical education is vital. Otherwise, relying solely on employing TCM practitioners from China would be unlikely to meet the growing demand for TCM services among the local population. In 2005, a TCM acupuncture program was developed in South Africa, signifying the integration of TCM into the country's higher education system. Ten years later, in 2015, with the global popularity of learning Chinese, South Africa began incorporating Chinese language education into its national education system. In 2019, **the Confucius Institute for Chinese Medicine** was launched at the University of Western Cape in Cape Town, which is the fruit of the collaboration among the University of Western Cape, Zhejiang Normal University, and Zhejiang Chinese Medical University, the first of its kind in Africa. It plays a significant role in promoting educational and cultural exchanges between China and Africa, particularly in the field of TCM in South Africa. In 2021, the University of Johannesburg (UJ) established the Acupuncture Center and Museum in partnership with Fujian University of Traditional Chinese Medicine. The center aims to provide access to TCM, offering educational resources to students and the general public.

This initiative made UJ the only university in South Africa to offer bachelor's, master's, and doctoral programs in acupuncture (Xinhua, 2021). Over 1,000 students expressed interest; unfortunately, only 45 students were accepted in the first batch of acupuncture students. To accommodate more students, more similar exchange programs have been established between UJ and Fujian University of Traditional Chinese Medicine, as well as UJ and Zhejiang Chinese Medical University (Jia, 2022).

Being the most prosperous and advanced economy in Africa, South Africa assumes a prominent position in foreign affairs on the continent. The successful collaboration between South Africa and China in TCM has established a noteworthy precedent for future partnerships for China with other African nations. This collaboration serves as a means to promote the spread of TCM throughout Africa. However, fully integrating TCM into the mainstream healthcare, incorporating its knowledge into modern practices, and ensuring its adherence to contemporary safety and efficacy standards are challenging tasks that are still far from being accomplished (Gasiorowski-Denis, 2016).

Challenges and Prospects of TCM in BRICS

TCM has made significant progress within the BRICS member countries. However, there are still challenges and issues to overcome. For instance, though it is encouraging to know that except for Russia, acupuncture is legalized in Brazil, India, and South Africa, it is only in Brazil that Chinese herbal medicine is incorporated into its national health insurance system. Furthermore, although Brazil and South Africa have relatively stable local educational programs for nurturing TCM practitioners, most training programs in Russia and India are established primarily by Confucius Institutes which offer only basic courses on TCM.

In order to tackle these challenges, it is crucial to actively pursue comprehensive legislation for TCM within the BRICS member countries. We firmly believe that with the unwavering (坚定不移的) efforts of the Chinese government and the strong support from TCM enterprises, the future of TCM within the BRICS nations holds considerable promise. Interestingly, the acronym "BRICS" sounds like "brick", which is a fundamental building material, symbolizing the vital and essential roles these emerging countries play in the world economy. Therefore, the acceptance of TCM in these emerging markets holds significant importance for TCM Interculturalization. Although there is still a long road ahead before TCM becomes fully integrated into the national healthcare systems of these countries, progress is being made day by day.

Chapter Summary

- In Japan, traditional medicine is known as kampo, which finds its origins in the theories and classics of TCM.
- During the history of kampo, three noticeable schools have evolved, namely, Goseiha School, Kohona School, and Eclectic school.
- Formerly known as oriental medicine, traditional Korean medicine, which originated from TCM, has developed some of its own features in diagnosis and treatment.
- James Reston's report on the miraculous acupuncture aroused "acupuncture fever", sparking widespread interest in acupuncture, cupping, and other TCM techniques in the US.
- Mr. Lu Yigong, a renowned acupuncturist from Hong Kong, with the assistance of Arthur Steinberg contributed to the formal legislation of acupuncture in the state of Nevada.
- As of 2020, 48 states and Washington DC in the US have passed acupuncture laws, ensuring the legal use of acupuncture in these places.
- Luo Dinghui, a Chinese born TCM physician, rented a storefront in Chinatown and opened a clinic called Hong-Ning Herbal Medicine, which is the first TCM clinic in the UK.
- The Confucius Institute of TCM was established at London South Bank University, the first official institute of its kind in the world.
- In 2006, natural therapies such as acupuncture and herbal medicine were officially adopted by the SUS in Brazil.
- St. Petersburg's TCM hospital, established in 2016 by Beijing University of Chinese Medicine in cooperation with Russian (medical) universities, marks itself as the first general hospital of TCM in Russia.
- The practice of acupuncture has contributed to fostering a sense of friendship between India and China. Dr. B. K. Basu and his colleague Dwarkanath Kotnis are among those ardent proponents of acupuncture in India.

- In 2000, the South African government underwent the legislative process to recognize the legality of TCM.
- In 2019, the Confucius Institute for Chinese Medicine was launched at the University of Western Cape in Cape Town, which is the fruit of the collaboration among the University of Western Cape, Zhejiang Normal University, and Zhejiang Chinese Medical University, the first of its kind in Africa.

Checklist	Yes	No
Cognitive: I have mastered the core information		
Behavioral: I have the ability of putting what I've learned into practice		
Affective: I am willing to carry out what I've learned		
Moral: I will take the ethical consideration into account during practice		

Chapter 11

National Policies and TCM Education

Chapter Objectives

After reading this chapter, you should be able to:

◆ Understand the elements and principles of the Belt and Road Initiative.

◆ Be aware of the importance of national policies to TCM interculturalization.

◆ Outline the status quo of international students pursuing TCM in China.

◆ Understand basic structure of undergraduate TCM programs for international students.

◆ Develop a strong sense of patriotism and pride in being Chinese.

Key Terms

---

closer people-to-people ties

financial integration

infrastructure connectivity

China's Law on TCM

motivations for studying TCM

policy coordination

principles of BRI

the Belt and Road Initiative (BRI)

Outline of the Strategic Plan on the Development of TCM

TCM program length and curriculum

unimpeded trade

Quotes

"We should promote the high-quality development of traditional Chinese medicine and its industry, and make full use of its unique advantages and role in preventing and treating diseases. To contribute to building a healthy China and realizing the Chinese dream of great national renewal." (推动中医药事业和产业高质量发展,推动中医药走向世界,充分发挥中医药防病治病的独特优势和作用,为建设健康中国、实现中华民族伟大复兴的中国梦贡献力量。)

——习近平对中医药工作作出的重要指示(据新华社北京 2019 年 10 月 25 日电)

"China will continue to expand its high-level opening up to the outside world, steadily expand the institutional opening up of rules, management and standards, implement the national treatment of foreign-funded enterprises, and promote the high-quality development of the Belt and Road Initiative." (中国将继续扩大高水平对外开放、稳步拓展规则、管理、标准等制度开放,落实外资企业国民待遇,推动共建"一带一路"高质量发展。)

——2022 年 1 月 17 日习近平在 2022 年世界经济论坛视频会议的演讲

"The statement 'I am a foreigner, but not an outsider' by Ma Wenxuan, a young man from Kazakhstan who actively supported the fight against the epidemic in Shaanxi, has deeply resonated with numerous Chinese individuals. These heartwarming anecdotes have evolved into a touching harmony, symbolizing the shared experiences and close connections between China and the people of Central Asian nations." (在陕西支援抗击疫情的哈萨克斯坦小伙马文轩的一句"我是外国人,但不是外人",感动了无数中国人。这样的暖心故事汇成了中国同中亚国家人民同甘共苦、心心相印的动人交响曲。)

——2022 年 1 月 25 日习近平在中国同中亚五国建交 30 周年视频峰会上的讲话

Before reading this section, please consider the following questions:

1.How much do you know about the Belt and Road Initiative?

2.How do government policies either support or hinder TCM interculturalization?

11.1   National Policies and TCM Interculturalization

As traditional Chinese medicine (TCM) continues to advance within the framework of the Belt and Road Initiative (BRI), people worldwide have benefited from it. By September 2022, TCM had spread to 196 countries and regions, establishing itself as a vital area of cooperation between China, ASEAN, the European Union, the African Union, the Shanghai Cooperation Organization, BRICS and other regional or international organizations. TCM now increasingly serves the populations living along the Belt and Road. These countries and regions hold excellent prospects for TCM development. TCM is a valuable asset not only for the Chinese nation but also an essential force in maintaining global public health. Since TCM interculturalization is a national effort as well as an individual one, it is reasonable to understand some of the key policies and agendas established at the national level. This section, therefore, is designed to provide a glimpse of how national policies such as BRI are helpful in promoting TCM across cultures.

BRI at a Glance

In September and October 2013, during his visits to Kazakhstan and Indonesia, Chinese President Xi Jinping proposed the initiative of collaboratively establishing the Silk Road Economic Belt and the 21st Century Maritime Silk Road (Xi, 2018). This initiative, known as **the Belt and Road**, consists of two main components: the land-based Silk Road Economic Belt, which encompasses six development corridors, and the 21st Century

Maritime Silk Road.

The Chinese government released the "Vision and Actions on Jointly Building Silk Road Economic Belt and 21st Century Maritime Silk Road" in March 2015, officially kicking off BRI. Two years later in 2017, the first Belt and Road Forum for International Cooperation ("一带一路"国际合作高峰论坛) was organized. Additionally, China has hosted various notable events such as Boao Forum for Asia (博鳌亚洲论坛) Annual Conference, Qingdao Summit of the Shanghai Cooperation Organization(上海合作组织青岛峰会), the 2018 Beijing Summit of the Forum on China-Africa Cooperation (2018年中非合作论坛北京峰会), China International Import Expo (中国国际进口博览会), and the third Belt and Road Forum for International Cooperation. During the past ten years, BRI has won positive responses from numerous countries and international organizations, drawing global attention.

BRI has its origin in China; however, it is a global endeavor. It draws upon historical foundations while having a forward-looking orientation. While its primary focus is on Asia, Europe, and Africa, it remains open to partnerships with all nations. This initiative encompasses diverse countries and regions, varying stages of development, distinct historical traditions, different cultures, religions, customs, and lifestyles. It stands as a peaceful development initiative, fostering economic cooperation rather than being driven by geopolitical (地缘政治) or military alliance. All countries are welcome to participate in this initiative based on their own will.

BRI adheres to the spirit of broad consultation, joint contribution, and shared benefits. It embodies the essence of the Silk Road, characterized by peace, cooperation, openness, inclusiveness, mutual learning, and mutual benefit. This initiative places emphasis on policy coordination, infrastructure connectivity, unimpeded trade, financial integration, and people-to-people connections. It has successfully transformed ideas into tangible actions, turning vision into reality. As a result, the initiative has become a widely embraced public endeavor welcomed by the international community.

Elements of BRI

Since its inception in 2013, BRI has made solid progress. Remarkable advancements have been achieved, including several notable early outcomes. Participating nations have gained tangible advantages, leading to a growing appreciation for and engagement with the initiative.

• Policy Coordination

Policy coordination stands as a vital assurance for this initiative, acting as an essential prerequisite to joint actions. During the past ten years, China has carried out thorough coordination with participating nations and international organizations, leading to a wide consensus on global cooperation toward building BRI. Within BRI framework, all participating nations and international organizations have exchanged views on economic development plans and policies, abiding by the principle of seeking common ground while reserving differences. They have discussed and agreed upon economic cooperation plans and measures.

The Chinese government has signed cooperation agreements with 152 countries and 32 international organizations. BRI has broadened its scope from Asia and Europe to Africa, Latin America, and the South Pacific.

• Infrastructure Connectivity

Infrastructure connectivity holds a prominent position on the agenda of BRI. Member countries have made joint endeavors to construct a comprehensive and multi-tiered infrastructure framework, with railways, roads, shipping, aviation, pipelines, and integrated space information networks as its focal points. This framework is rapidly taking form and has significantly lowered the costs associated with the transportation of goods, capital, information, and technologies across regions. It has effectively facilitated the smooth movement and efficient allocation of resources among various areas. Consequently, it will contribute to achieving mutually beneficial cooperation and fostering common development.

Over the past decade, infrastructure connectivity has witnessed remarkable improvements, resulting in enhanced accessibility and smoother transportation. Several significant projects have been successfully completed, including the China-Europe liner and the China-Laos railway. Specifically, the China-Europe liner has established 84 operational routes, connecting 211 cities across 25 European countries (Cai, 2018).

• Unimpeded Trade

One of the significant objectives of BRI is to promote unobstructed trade. The dedicated efforts made towards this initiative have resulted in the liberalization and facilitation of trade and investment within the participating countries and regions. This approach has effectively reduced the costs associated with trade and business while unleashing growth potential, thus enabling participants to engage more broadly and deeply in economic globalization.

Between 2013 and 2022, China's trade in goods and non-financial direct investment with participatory countries has experienced an average annual growth rate of 8.6 percent and 5.8 percent, respectively. Additionally, the total two-way investment between China and these countries has surpassed US$270 billion.

• Financial Integration

Financial integration stands as a crucial foundation of BRI. In order to expand the avenues of diverse financing and offer stable, transparent, and high-quality financial support, international multilateral financial institutions and commercial banks have played an innovative role. Their contributions include exploring investment and financing models, thereby providing valuable assistance to BRI.

China, as the initiator and a significant participant in BRI, has been actively establishing and expanding numerous financing platforms to support the high-quality development of this initiative. Both China Development Bank (CDB) and Export-Import Bank of China have been improving their awareness and capabilities to effectively serve the BRI projects.

During the first five years, CDB provided financing exceeding US$190 billion for over 600 BRI projects. As of the end of 2020, eleven Chinese-funded banks had successfully established 80 first-tier branches in 29 countries along the BRI, while three Chinese-funded insurance companies had established seven business organizations in Singapore, Malaysia, and Indonesia. Moreover, a total of 48 banks from 23 countries and regions along the route have established branches and representative offices in China.

In November 2014, China established the Silk Road Fund with a capital of US$40 billion. Then, in December 2015, the Asian Infrastructure Investment Bank, the world's first multilateral financial institution primarily focused on infrastructure investment, was formally established. It gained recognition with 104 member countries officially joining in December 2015 (Wang W, 2023).

• Closer People-to-People Ties

People-to-people connections play a vital role in the high-quality advancement of BRI, serving as a central role for achieving the other four links, i.e., policy coordination, facility connectivity, unimpeded trade, and financial integration (Wang, 2022). Prioritizing people's livelihoods, people-to-people communication upholds the core concept throughout the process of building BRI. It focuses on people's interests, well-being, and aspirations, with the primary objective of promoting the welfare of individuals.

The aspiration for a peaceful and prosperous life is a shared dream among all nations. In the past ten years, countries involved in BRI have actively engaged in diverse forms of diplomatic activities and cultural exchanges across various domains. These efforts have fostered mutual understanding, recognition, and established a robust cultural groundwork for the future development of the initiative.

The ultimate goal is to foster better socio-economic development in the countries and regions, strengthen scientific and cultural cooperation, safeguard peace and security in those areas, and enhance the living and working conditions of their residents. To fulfill this objective, we must promote joint construction efforts, create job opportunities, eradicate poverty continually, enhance the overall quality of life, and uplift people's well-being and property.

Principles of BRI

The current global landscape is marked by significant developments, transformations, and adjustments. Amidst these changes, peace, development, and cooperation remain the most crucial themes of our time. As China continues to pursue BRI, it will inevitably face challenges and obstacles, alongside unprecedented opportunities and prospects for development.

As China is committed to nurturing BRI, it is believed that with time and the dedicated efforts of all participating stakeholders, this cooperation will become more profound, concrete, stable, and expansive. BRI will pave a path of peace, prosperity, openness, sustainable development, innovation, cultural connectivity, and good governance (Chen, 2018). It will also promote more inclusivity, balance, and universal benefits within economic globalization. Five principles have been strictly abided by in the construction of BRI, which are as follows.

• Road of Inclusiveness and Openness

BRI is not an exclusive and closed small "Chinese circle", but an open and inclusive regional cooperation initiative. Today's world thrives on openness, which fosters progress, while closure leads to backwardness. We firmly believe that openness helps to identify and seize opportunities which can be utilized and transformed into new ones.

The primary objective of BRI is to transform global opportunities into opportunities for the participants, and vice versa. This understanding and vision shape the initiative's orientation towards openness, aiming to construct an open, inclusive, balanced, and diverse region. This objective is pursued by strengthening the development of transportation, energy, and network infrastructure, facilitating the orderly and unrestricted flow of economic factors, efficient resource allocation, and deep market integration. Additionally, BRI aims to expand regional cooperation on a wider, higher, and deeper scale, establishing an open, inclusive, balanced, and comprehensive framework for regional economic cooperation, which helps address the challenges of economic growth and balance.

Consequently, BRI represents a diversified, open, and inclusive cooperative endeavor. Its remarkable characteristic lies in its commitment to openness and inclusiveness, setting it apart from other regional economic initiatives.

• Road of Practical and Equal Cooperation

BRI serves as a platform for practical cooperation, rather than a geopolitical tool exclusively for China. The Silk Road spirit, characterized by peace and cooperation, openness and inclusiveness, mutual learning and mutual benefit, has become a shared historical treasure of humanity. BRI upholds this spirit and principle, representing a significant endeavor of our time. Through comprehensive and multidimensional exchanges and cooperation among participating countries, and by fully tapping into their respective development potential and comparative advantages, BRI has fostered a mutually beneficial and win-win regional community encompassing shared interests, destiny, and responsibilities. In this framework, countries are equal participants, contributors, and beneficiaries. Therefore, equality has been deeply embedded in BRI from its inception.

Equality, an important international norm adhered to by China, serves as the fundamental basis for the construction of BRI. Lasting and mutually beneficial cooperation can only be achieved through an approach based on equality. The emphasis on equality and inclusiveness within BRI has reduced resistance to its promotion, enhanced the efficiency of its collaborative development, and facilitated practical implementation of international cooperation initiatives.

At the same time, the construction of BRI is inseparable from a peaceful international and regional environment. Peace represents an essential attribute of the Belt and Road Initiative and serves as an indispensable factor for its smooth progress. These considerations dictate that BRI should not and cannot be reduced to a tool for political rivalry among major powers, nor should it replicate (复制) outdated geopolitical games.

• Road of Open and Fair Discussion

BRI is a collaborative development endeavor focused on open discussions and resource sharing, rather than being solely a foreign aid program led by China. The construction of BRI is advanced through specific projects based on bilateral or multilateral connections, and it is a development plan formulated after thorough policy communication, strategic alignment (战略对齐), and market operations.

"The Joint Communiqué (联合公报) of the Roundtable Summit of the Belt and Road Forum" in May 2017 highlighted that BRI is a collective development initiative (Xinhua, 2017). The

Joint Communiqué also emphasized the fundamental principles for constructing BRI, including adherence to market principles. This entails recognizing the market's role and the importance of enterprises as primary actors, ensuring that the government plays an appropriate role, and BRI aims to promote open, transparent, and non-discriminatory government procurement processes.

These principles demonstrate that the driving force behind the construction of BRI is not just limited to the government, but also involves enterprises. The fundamental approach relies on following market rules and realizing the interests of participating parties through market-oriented operations. The government's role is to establish platforms, create mechanisms, guide policies, and fulfill other directional and service-oriented functions.

• Road of Complement to Existing Mechanisms

BRI serves as a complement to existing mechanisms rather than a substitute. The countries participating in the BRI possess evident differences in comparative advantages and strong potential for complementarity. Some countries are rich in energy resources but lack development efforts, while others have abundant labor but insufficient job opportunities. There are countries with big market but a weak industrial base, and countries with a strong demand for infrastructure construction but limited funds.

China, as the world's second-largest economy with the highest foreign exchange reserves, boasts increasingly advantageous industries, extensive experience in infrastructure construction, robust equipment manufacturing capacity, high quality products, cost-effectiveness, and comprehensive advantages in terms of capital, technology, human resources, and management. This presents practical needs and great opportunities for China and other participants in BRI to achieve industrial alignment and complementary advantages.

Therefore, the central focus of BRI is to promote

infrastructure construction and connectivity while aligning with the policies and development strategies of the member countries. It is evident that BRI seeks to complement existing regional cooperation mechanisms rather than replace them, emphasizing mutual assistance and cooperation.

• Road of Bridge to Promote Humanistic Exchanges

BRI serves as a bridge to promote humanistic exchanges, not as a trigger for a clash of civilizations. Although BRI spans different regions, cultures, and religious beliefs, it does not provoke a clash among civilizations. Rather, it fosters exchanges and mutual understanding.

While BRI promotes infrastructure development, strengthens cooperation in production capacity, and aligns development strategies, it also prioritizes people-to-people exchanges. BRI upholds the spirit of the Silk Road and engages in extensive cooperation in fields such as science, education, culture, health, and people-to-people exchanges. This has made BRI more deeply rooted in public opinion and firmly grounded in society.

BRI aims to transcend cultural barriers through cultural exchanges, overcome the clash of civilizations through mutual understanding, and transcend the superiority of civilizations through coexistence among them. By doing so, it builds new bridges for people in the countries involved to strengthen their exchanges and enhance their understanding. BRI also weaves new bonds to facilitate dialogue, exchanges, and interaction among different cultures and civilizations, while promoting mutual understanding, respect, and trust among all nations.

BRI and TCM

Over the past few years, General Secretary Xi Jinping has consistently stressed the importance of enhancing collaboration in TCM. This message has been conveyed at more than 30 international events. Additionally, he has observed the signing ceremonies of several bilateral cooperation agreements focused on TCM. Examples of such agreements include those between China and Kyrgyzstan, China and Ukraine, China and Australia, China and Nepal, as well as China and Brazil. These efforts have elevated TCM's significance as a vital contributor to diplomatic endeavors and its role in fostering a global sense of shared destiny among all humanity.

Furthermore, the release of *Development Plan for TCM within the Framework of BRI* (2016-2020) (NATCM, 2016), and the subsequent development plan of *Promoting the High-quality Integration of TCM into the Framework of BRI* (2021-2025) (NATCM, 2021), have made significant improvements to the overall strategy for incorporating TCM into the project. These plans have not only enhanced the top-level design of integrating TCM with BRI but have also provided blueprints for its future development.

The top-level design of BRI has effectively improved the integration of TCM within the project and has laid out a comprehensive plan for its expansion in the context of BRI. To facilitate the growth of trade in TCM services, various measures have been taken. For instance, TCM has been successfully included in 16 free trade agreements, and the establishment of 31 national export bases for TCM services has been undertaken. Moreover, active participation has been demonstrated in the establishment of domestic pilot (试点的) free trade zones. Finally, efforts have been made to promote the integration and development of TCM in conjunction with health tourism and forest recreation.

TCM Interculturalization as a National Policy

In order to overcome obstacles that hinder the development of TCM, specific national policies and measures have been formulated to achieve a breakthrough. Thirteen policies and measures are designed to promote the inheritance and advancement of TCM. State Council of People's Republic of China or the President has issued five policies from a national guidance perspective.

The development of TCM has been addressed through various major plans, with the ultimate goal of establishing a TCM healthcare system that incorporates technology and innovation. *Law of the People's Republic of China on TCM* (中华人民共和国中医药法), the first specialized law in this field, has been instrumental in offering robust legal protection for the healthy growth of TCM since its implementation in July 2017, which presents an opportunity to enhance and improve TCM. Efforts are being made to elevate the quality of TCM healthcare services to meet the medical needs of people throughout China. Collaboration across all aspects will continue to support the innovation and preservation of TCM, as specified in the policies and measures.

The Outline of the Strategic Plan on the Development of Traditional Chinese Medicine (中医药发展战略规划纲要) (2016-2030) (State Council, 2016a) encompasses a majority of the crucial aspects related to TCM, such as medical services, scientific innovation, and industry transformation. More detailed management policies are under way for the development of each specific area. Additionally, overseas development and collaboration with foreign nations would expand the scope and scale of TCM services. Guided by the principle of creative transformation and innovative development, there should be extensive promotion of TCM culture. Above all, the training of a skilled team of TCM professionals will serve as the cornerstone for the revitalization of TCM.

By 2030, the TCM medical and healthcare service system is hoped to cover every community in China with modernized medical equipment, high-level professionals and safe, efficient

TCM drugs (State Council, 2016b). Consequently, with the boost of Chinese national power, TCM would be accepted all over the world, not only as a carrier of Chinese culture but also as a medical science to prevent and cure diseases.

Implications for TCM Interculturalization

The tide of world development continues to flow. BRI reflects the prevailing trend of human history, for the Initiative embodies values and development concepts that meet the demands of human society, with the aim of creating a global community with a shared future. It fulfills the aspirations of people in participating countries to share development opportunities and improve their quality of life. Undoubtedly, as time progresses, BRI will demonstrate even greater vitality and creativity. With comprehensive plans and concrete measures in place, it will yield long-term benefits as we persist in pursuing higher-quality and advanced development.

BRI will contribute significantly to the establishment of a world characterized by lasting peace, common security and prosperity, openness and inclusiveness, as well as a clean and beautiful environment. It will make a substantial contribution to the construction of a global community with a shared future. Together with BRI and other policies at the provincial and national levels, TCM interculturalization has won the national endorsement, which is greatly helpful in communicating TCM across cultures.

---| **Activities** |--

Comprehension Questions

1.Please introduce the origin of BRI in your own words.

2.2023 marks the 10th anniversary of the proposal of BRI. What positive changes has the BRI brought to world development? Choose one area and report to the class.

3.Among the five features of BRI, which one impresses you the most? And why?

4.In what way(s) does *China's Law on TCM* contribute to the development of TCM around the world?

5.Can you offer some statistics to show the achievements of TCM interculturalization because of BRI?

Role Play

Suppose you were a TCM culture facilitator with a six-month long-term visiting program in a certain country or region along the BRI route. Select a country or a region, design your own visiting plans and schedules, and do the role-play with your classmates in 15 minutes.

Before reading this section, please consider the following questions:

1.Why do people choose to study abroad? What challenges do international students face when studying abroad?

2.What are the most popular majors for international students in China and in the US respectively? And why?

11.2   International Students of TCM in China

Surge in the Pursuit of Higher Education in China

When considering overseas education, the majority of individuals typically think of selecting prestigious universities, many of which are located in the US and Europe. While this idea held true in the past decades, there has been a noticeable shift in recent years. With the rapid advancement of higher education in China, people from around the world have started to be drawn to China. Statistics in 2018 (MOE, 2019) shows that nearly half a million international students from 196 countries and regions enrolled in 1004 higher education institutions across China. It is important to note that the COVID-19 pandemic significantly impacted global mobility, leading to a reduction in the number of overseas students in China. However, as border controls gradually eased, the trend has started to rebound (回 升). International students opt for a diverse range of academic programs, with the top three being Clinical Medicine, International Economics and Trade, and Chinese Language.

In recent years, World Education Services, a non-profit organization that provides educational services, has observed an almost 100 percent surge in applications from students seeking credential evaluations for TCM qualifications obtained in China (Zheng and Lee, 2016). It appears that an increasing number of international students is turning to China as their preferred destination for studying TCM, rather than enrolling in TCM programs offered in other countries. Our goal in this section, therefore, is to delve into this phenomenon and explore the underlying reasons behind this surge, while also providing a concise overview of the TCM education in China.

Motivations for Studying TCM in China

In 2022, approximately 8, 000 international students enrolled in TCM programs in China (Zhang *et al.*, 2023). The majority of these students came from other Asian nations. Notably, most international students enrolled at the bachelor's level. The following table displays the number of international students who are studying at four TCM universities in China.

Number of International Students of TCM in China in 2018 (MOE, 2019)

	Total	Bachelor's	Master's	Doctoral	Others
University A	3022	1207	165	45	1605
University B	1638	458	191	51	938
University C	1523	527	158	216	622
University D	1005	506	123	164	212

•Influence of TCM on the World Medical Community

The reasons behind the growing interest of international students in pursuing TCM education in China are difficult to pinpoint (明确指出) precisely. However, it is likely that several factors, both within and outside China, contribute to this phenomenon. One possible factor is the surge in public awareness of TCM following the receipt of the 2015 Nobel Prize in Medicine by Chinese scientist Tu Youyou. Professor Tu's research into Chinese herbal medicine led to the discovery of artemisinin, a potent anti-malarial compound. The Nobel committee's recognition of Tu's work marked a significant milestone for the development of TCM. Marta Hanson, professor of history of medicine at Johns Hopkins University, noted that the Nobel Prize had not previously considered traditional medical knowledge as a potential recipient (Gibbons, 2016). Tu's award represents a shift in this perspective since this recognition is part of a broader trend of seeking scientific explanations for ancient remedies, particularly as the effectiveness of antibiotics diminishes.

• Governmental and Institutional Efforts

The attraction towards China, in comparison to other countries offering TCM training, also stems from various other factors. One significant factor is China's active endeavor, through its "Study in China" initiative and others, to establish itself as a prominent destination for international students. Additionally, the Chinese government recognizes TCM as a substantial economic driver. To further stimulate growth, the government has implemented several crucial policies and plans for the advancement of TCM (NATCM, 2016 and 2021; State Council, 2016a and 2016b). These policies and plans both at the national and provincial levels set ambitious goals for the industry, aiming to make it one of the key pillars of Chinese economy while promoting excellent TCM education and practices across the globe. As reported by the director of the National Administration of TCM, the total estimated value of TCM in 2022 was approximately RMB 400 billion (Editors, 2023). As part of TCM endeavor, TCM universities are pushing forward with establishing TCM overseas centers where research and education related to TCM is encouraged.

Lastly, China's status as a better place for learning TCM has its real attraction. Researchers (Jiao *et al.*, 2011) evaluating TCM in a local and international context deemed TCM education in China more authentic. They also noted that TCM education in other countries often places a predominant emphasis on acupuncture while overlooking other vital practices like materia medica. As TCM universities in China firmly uphold the excellence of tradition in nurturing qualified TCM physicians, even people from Japan and the Republic of Korea, where TCM is well-preserved and deeply ingrained in people's minds, are eager to learn TCM in China. This phenomenon is not limited to these regions alone, as people worldwide show a keen interest in gaining TCM education from China.

• International Demand for TCM Practitioners

The demand for proficient TCM practitioners is steadily increasing in the US, which can be attributed to the growing acceptance of complementary and integrative health interventions by mainstream societies. Many highly reputable institutions, including the MD Anderson Cancer Center, the Memorial Sloan Kettering Cancer Center, and the Cleveland Clinic, have established integrative medicine centers featuring herbal clinics, massage therapy, acupuncture, and other such therapies (Zheng and Lee, 2016). The National Center for Complementary and Integrative Health (NCCIH) has been working towards promoting the integration of complementary therapies alongside Western medicine instead of replacing the former by the latter. The center's latest strategic plan for 2021-2025 (NCCIH, 2020) has expanded the definition of integrative health to include Whole Person Health (全人健康), empowering individuals, families, communities, and populations to improve their health by taking into account various interconnected factors such as biological, behavioral, social, and environmental aspects. This new concept of health is in line with TCM philosophy, which also considers the interconnectedness of many factors, just like biochemical indicators.

Another significant factor contributing to the increasing demand for qualified TCM practitioners in the US may stem from a nationwide opioid epidemic, leading to a surge in emergency room visits, overdose (过量用药) deaths, and associated costs. In recent years, the US government has been actively seeking solutions for managing chronic pain without relying on opioids. In March 2016, the Interagency Pain Research Coordinating

Committee, comprising representatives from various US agencies such as the Department of Defense, Centers for Disease Control and Prevention, FDA, scientists, patient proponents and members of the public, released a National Pain Strategy, which recommends the development of a patient-centered system for managing chronic pain, incorporating TCM techniques, notably acupuncture, among other solutions (Zheng and Lee, *et al.*, 2016). Two years later in 2018, the *Support for Patients and Communities Act* was enacted, granting approval to acupuncture as an evidence-based and effective therapy for opioid replacement (Liu and Zhou, 2023).

On a global scale, the demand for TCM practitioners, specifically acupuncturists, is also climbing steadily thanks to TCM legislation. Since 1985, Australia has witnessed a growing demand for TCM. The first TCM law in the world was established in Australia in May 2000. The road to national legislation on TCM became smoother, culminating(达到高潮) in TCM's incorporation into the *Health Practitioner Regulation National Law Act* in 2012 (Lin, 2016). Many people in South Africa have long utilized herbal medicines and natural remedies, which makes it easier for South African people to embrace TCM. The legal recognition of TCM in 2001 in South Africa has created favorable conditions and opportunities for the promotion of TCM practice and culture. In Brazil, acupuncture has been practiced by physicians in public hospitals since 2006, after it was added to the national medical insurance policy. As a result, TCM therapies have become an increasingly popular choice for individuals seeking medical treatment (CNS, 2021). These three countries located in three different continents have paved the way for wider recognition of TCM by other nations, leading to the boost of medical needs from the local people, thus creating a shortage of qualified TCM practitioners.

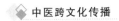
TCM Education in China

In 1956, the Ministry of Education in China established four colleges specializing in TCM in four cities: Beijing, Shanghai, Guangzhou, and Chengdu. That year is viewed as a watershed (转折点) in the formalization of TCM education in China. Sixty years later, China has 44 TCM colleges/universities and 409 universities that offer TCM programs. Among the 44 TCM higher education institutions, 25 universities offer master's programs and 22 offer PhD programs (NATCM, 2022).

• Admissions Requirements for International Students

Bilingual curricula in English and Chinese or Chinese alone are offered by most bachelor's level TCM programs for international students. Some schools also provide a portion of the curriculum in Japanese. Admission to these programs is based on high school GPAs and, depending on the language of instruction, performance on standardized language exams. For programs taught in Chinese, admission criteria include performance on the Chinese Proficiency Test (HSK), an international standardized test that assesses Chinese language proficiency in an academic setting. Non-native English speakers seeking admission to English language programs are evaluated based on their performance on either TOEFL or IELTS, both of which gauge (判定) English language proficiency in an academic context (MOE, 2020).

A few universities that accommodate international students have supplementary admission criteria. Take Shandong University of TCM for example, where applicants are required to submit a brief self-introduction video in addition to their academic transcripts and HSK results (SDUTCM, 2023).

• Program Length and Curriculum

The majority of accredited (官方认可的) bachelor programs in TCM typically span five years of study (as most medical programs do in China), although students have the flexibility to complete their studies over a period of seven or even eight years if they choose. In general, undergraduate students need to fulfill a credit requirement ranging from 220 to 280 credits. This includes a clinical internship (实习) of one year or 800 hours of practical experience. International students pursuing a bachelor's degree are typically taught separately from their Chinese counterparts. In some universities, they are also incorporated into standard cohorts (一群人) of Chinese students.

The program, which is governed by a panel of experts at the provincial and national levels, follows a rigorous structure, where students are required to take specific courses during designated semesters. Approximately 30 percent of the curriculum focuses on foundational courses in basic science and medical education. TCM theory courses, which include TCM classics, constitute 20 percent. Clinical practice courses, including TCM diagnosis, patient communication, and internships, form another 20 percent of the program's requirements. The remaining 30 percent of courses are elective, enabling students to expand their understanding of medical foundations, TCM practical skills, or even enhance their Chinese language proficiency. All of the theoretical courses are designed to be finished during the first four years. The final year is dedicated to completing an internship and undertaking graduation exams. After successfully completing their studies, students are awarded a Bachelor of Medicine in TCM. In China, this degree is acknowledged as the first professional qualification, granting individuals the right to practice TCM within the Chinese Mainland upon completion of clinical residency training (住院医师规范培训).

At the postgraduate level, Master of Medicine and Doctor of Medicine in TCM are widely acknowledged as the most common TCM degrees. Typically spanning three years respectively, these advanced degree programs are primarily designed for students inclined towards research or aspiring for faculty positions as well as for clinical practice. Students who pursue these higher-level

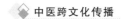
programs have already obtained bachelor's degrees in TCM.

Owing to favorable policies such as BRI, TCM has experienced significant growth both in China and overseas. As a result, the number of international students enrolled in TCM programs in China is expected to rise. These graduates have an important role to play as TCM cultural ambassadors, sharing their knowledge about the effective use of TCM in treating illnesses and promoting Chinese culture after they return to their homelands.

Activities

Comprehension Questions

1. What are some of the factors that contribute to the growing number of international students pursuing TCM studies in China?

2. Some argue that the current undergraduate TCM programs, which typically last around five years, may not provide enough time for students to fully master the necessary skills. They point out that in ancient China, TCM disciples were required to learn under their masters' guidance for extended periods of time before becoming independent TCM physicians. What is your perspective on this issue?

3. Can you provide concrete instances to demonstrate how national and provincial policies are instrumental in attracting international students to pursue TCM education in China?

4. What are some potential challenges that international students may face when studying TCM in China? Please provide specific examples if possible.

5. As is discussed in the passage, international students either study alone or mix with Chinese students in their study. Which one do you think is better? And why?

Action Points

1. Create a survey targeting international students of TCM in your local city, with a particular focus on their experiences and challenges encountered in this field. Prepare a poster presentation based on the instructions provided by your teacher.

2. Conduct research to investigate the recruitment methods employed by TCM

universities for international students. Analyze and compare the enrollment advertisements of each university, offer some suggestions if necessary, and deliver an oral presentation of your findings to the class.

Case Study

Miss Wang, a Chinese teacher of acupuncture and moxibustion, reflects on her teaching experience at Confucius Institute for Chinese Medicine in the UK.

I have noticed some cultural differences between Chinese and British classrooms. When it comes to my teaching style, I've realized that I tend to teach in a more straightforward and fast-paced way in the UK compared to what I did in China. There is a certain expectation in the UK for this style of teaching. However, I also understand that British students have their own unique ways of learning. For example, some students are comfortable speaking up right away, while others take more time to think before participating. So, I always need to consider this balance between culture and individuality in my teaching experience in the UK.

Questions

1.How does Miss Wang adapt to the local culture in her teaching methods?

2.What can be learnt from Miss Wang's flexibility in her teaching?

Chapter Summary

- In September and October 2013, during his visits to Kazakhstan and Indonesia, Chinese President Xi Jinping proposed the initiative of collaboratively establishing the Silk Road Economic Belt and the 21st Century Maritime Silk Road.

- The Belt and Road Initiative had its origins in China; however, it is a global endeavor. It draws upon historical foundations while having a forward-looking orientation. While its primary focus is on Asia, Europe, and Africa, it remains open to partnerships with all nations.

- The BRI places emphasis on policy coordination, infrastructure connectivity, unimpeded trade, financial integration, and people-to-people ties.

- The BRI will pave a path of peace, prosperity, openness, sustainable development, innovation, cultural connectivity, and good governance. It will also promote more inclusivity, balance, and universal benefits within global economic globalization.

- International students opt for a diverse range of academic programs in China, with the top three being Clinical Medicine, International Economics and Trade, and Chinese Language.

- In recent years, World Education Services has observed an almost 100 percent surge in applications from students seeking credential evaluations for TCM qualifications obtained in China.
- In 2022, approximately 8,000 international students were enrolled in TCM programs in China. The majority of these students came from other Asian nations. Notably, most international students enrolled at the bachelor's level.
- The reasons behind the growing interest of international students in pursuing TCM education in China are threefold: (i) the increased influence of TCM on world medicine; (ii) governmental and institutional efforts; (iii) international demand for TCM practitioners.
- Currently, China has 44 TCM colleges/universities and 409 universities that offer TCM programs. Among the 44 TCM higher education institutions, 25 universities offer master's programs and 22 offer PhD programs.
- Bilingual curricula in English and Chinese or Chinese alone are offered by most bachelor's level TCM programs for international students. Some schools also provide a portion of the curriculum in Japanese. Admission to these programs is based on high school GPAs and performance on standardized language exams.
- The majority of accredited bachelor programs in TCM typically span five years of study (as most medical programs do in China).

Checklist	Yes	No
Cognitive: I have mastered the core information		
Behavioral: I have the ability of putting what I've learned into practice		
Affective: I am willing to carry out what I've learned		
Moral: I will take the ethical consideration into account during practice		

Part Five

Action

Chapter 12

CIntercultural Challenges: Recognizing and Dealing with Differences

Chapter Objectives

After reading this chapter, you should be able to:

- ◆ Define and discuss the nature of ethnocentrism.
- ◆ Describe the dimensions of stereotyping and provide examples of stereotypes (e.g., racial and ethnic, language, gender, religious).
- ◆ Identify ways to combat ethnocentric tendencies and stereotypes.
- ◆ Explain the notion of culture shock, its symptoms, and some basic causes.
- ◆ Compare the U-curve model of adaptation with the W-curve model.

── **Key Terms** ──────────────────────────────

ambivalence stage

cultural relativism

culture shock

ethnocentrism

frustration/hostility stage

honeymoon stage

in-sync adjustment stage

rebound/humorous stage

reentry culture shock stage

resocialization stage

stereotype

U-curve and W-curve

Quotes

"To uphold and develop Marxism, we must integrate it with China's fine traditional culture. Only by taking root in the rich historical and cultural soil of the country and the nation can the truth of Marxism flourish here."（坚持和发展马克思主义,必须同中华优秀传统文化相结合。只有植根本国、本民族历史文化沃土,马克思主义真理之树才能根深叶茂。）

——习近平总书记在中国共产党第二十次全国代表大会上的报告

"Yellow Emperor asked: 'When the same kind of diseases are treated by different physicians with different ways, the diseases can all be cured, and what is the reason?' Qibo answered: 'It is due to the different conditions of the localities...'"（黄帝问曰:医之治病也,一病而治各不同,皆愈何也? 岐伯对曰:地势使然也。）

——《素问·异法方宜论》

"Stereotypes are perpetuated by those who believe in them and those who place their faith in them."（坚信者持守之,依赖者推崇之,刻板效应才得以延续）

——Chinua Achebe, modern African writer

Before reading this section, please consider the following questions:

1.What does "stereotype" mean to you?

2.Have you ever been stereotyped by or stereotyping others?

12.1   Stereotype and TCM Interculturalization

Misunderstanding Guasha

Nicola Dall'Asen, the news editor at Allure.com, is talking about her experience with guasha.

"Since the first time my fingertips felt the cold, smooth surface of a guasha tool, one belief about it has been pounded into my head more than any other: It can make a double chin disappear like a magician. Though I've never been actively looking for it, I can't stop the flood of guasha and other types of facial massage content that has snaked its way onto my For You page multiple times a day for the past couple of years. An overwhelming amount of that content focuses on reducing the appearance of or trying to eliminate a double chin."(https://www. allure.com/story/gua-sha-for-double-chin)

It is well-known in the community of traditional Chinese medicine (TCM) or among most Chinese people that guasha is first and foremost a healing technique that is meant to restore the imbalance between yin and yang in one's body. Loosely translates as "to scrape (刮)" in English, guasha is the practice of using a flat tool against the skin to target stagnation and help restore the flow of qi, which is vitality energy in the body and has a close relationship with blood flow. Western culture has largely disregarded that concept and opted for techniques that prioritize striking visual outcomes, even if it means compromising the true intentions and effectiveness of traditional guasha. Typing guasha on TikTok, the app's suggested search terms encompassed common phrases like "guasha routine" and "guasha tutorial", but it also provided additional phrases like "guasha for double chin" and "guasha for slim face". Maybe, guasha accidentally helps to make your chin thinner and prettier. However, when this by-product or unexpected result becomes increasingly popular, it will stay firm among the public, replacing its real function. Then, things could become nasty. People no longer think of guasha as a therapeutic method, but only associate it with aesthetic power. That is a huge stumbling block to TCM interculturalization. In the next two sections of this chapter, we focus on two barriers to intercultural activities: stereotype and ethnocentrism that people have during intercultural interactions.

Defining Stereotype

Simply put, stereotype refers to the fixed impression of a certain group of people formed by social classification according to gender, race, age, or occupation. In intercultural communication, it can relate to some inflexible statements about a category of people, which are then applied to all group members without regard for individual differences (Allport, 1954). It is a normal cognitive process when meeting strangers. After all, we are living in such a big world, which is too complex and too dynamic for us to comprehend everything in detail. For instance, we often say that Chinese people have a rich cultural heritage and value family; Japanese people are known for their strong work ethics and attention to detail; the French are often associated with their appreciation of art, cuisine, and romance, and the English are recognized for their politeness and love for tea. These positive generalizations may become the basis for further communication. However, this characterization refers to a very small number of people who are represented in a specialized context. Because stereotyping narrows our perceptions and often tends to be negative, it sounds like a kind of gossip about the world, a gossip that makes us prejudge something or someone before we ever lay eyes on them.

Jackson (2014) summarized how stereotyping leads to intercultural barriers as follows:

- Stereotypes can deceive us into accepting a widely held belief as true, even though it may not reflect reality.
- Stereotypes can make us stubbornly stick to our initial judgments about a certain group, ignoring any evidence that goes against our preconceived notions, even if we happen to come across someone who is different.
- Stereotypes are hard to change because we learn them from important people and the media when we were young, so even if they do not match what we see and experience later, it is difficult to let go of them.
- When we stereotype, we mistakenly assume that everyone in a group is the same and we ignore the fact that individuals within that group can be different from one another.
- Stereotyping can lead to using disrespectful language, making broad assumptions, and causing inequality. Examples include sexist language, racism, and age-based discrimination.

Dimensions of Stereotype

Stereotypes may vary in four dimensions: direction, intensity, accuracy, and content (Chen, 2009a).

The direction of stereotypes refers to the positive and negative aspects of statements. People may say that TCM is effective, safe, and inexpensive. People may also say that TCM is unscientific, unproven, and dangerous.

The intensity of stereotypes shows how strongly someone believes in something. "Acupuncture is very useful in reducing pains" is an example of an intense stereotype. "Chinese herbal medicine is quite popular in the West. You can buy all sorts of herbs online and sellers have sprung up in malls around the world" is another example of an intense stereotype.

Stereotypes also differ in accuracy. Stereotypes, while often exaggerated and oversimplified beliefs, are not always false. Some of them may contain partial truths, while others might be partially inaccurate.

Finally, stereotypes may vary in their specific content. Not everyone from the same cultural group shares the same stereotypes about the same people. Initially, some British people may be frightened away from acupuncture, thus forming some negative impressions of it. Gradually, further contact with acupuncture may ease some unfavorable opinions. Both favorable and unfavorable tags can be attributed to acupuncture by people from the same culture.

Commonly-held Stereotypes of TCM

Currently in the US and some other countries in the world, there are four main common misconceptions or stereotypes about TCM because of ignorance or unconscious prejudice. Let us discuss them one by one.

Common stereotype number one: It is either TCM or Western biomedicine when someone is sick. Many people who do not fully understand TCM have this false idea that TCM and Western biomedicine are natural enemies. They believe one has to rely completely on either way of treating illness, and there is no middle ground in between. Actually, TCM and Western biomedicine are not enemies but allies. Both have their strengths and weaknesses. Biomedicine is more suitable for serious illnesses like cancer, acute diseases, and surgical procedures, whereas TCM is more applicable to disease prevention and chronic illnesses, say, headache and natural pain management. Hence, it is great to integrate both medical systems into one, drawing on the strengths of each medical system to restore your health. In China, as well as in many other countries around the world, it is quite popular to visit doctors who are both knowledgeable about Chinese and Western medicines.

Common stereotype number two: Acupuncture is painful. Acupuncture involves needles, leading people to believe that it will be painful. The truth is that the needles are about as thin as human hair and while you may feel them entering, they do not hurt. Some patients barely feel anything when the needles are entering. Additionally, studies show that acupuncture can help ease common symptoms such as chronic pain, depression, and anxiety, without the risk of side effects.

Common stereotype number three: TCM is exotic (异类). Sometimes when people hear the term traditional Chinese medicine, they think of foreign ingredients that are unapproachable. This is simply not the case. TCM focuses on the body and energy as a whole system, which includes acupuncture, herbal medicines, tuina, lifestyle changes, exercise, and diet. Many of the herbal remedies are commonly found in your own kitchen, for instance, ginger, ginseng, or mushrooms.

Common stereotype number four: TCM is baseless and unproven. People in the West tend to believe that biomedicine and science are always best friends and TCM are always left out. Some patients would be frightened off by TCM physicians who are trying to tell them that the imbalance of yin and yang within their body is the cause of a certain kind of disease, or that it is the disruption of qi that leads to illness. It sounds rather superstitious for those people who are only familiar with evidence-based medicine. It is quite understandable. After all, biomedicine and science were developed in conjunction with each other. The evidence-based Western medicine is made popular and accepted by people in the US and some other countries because it is in line with their local culture. People with little knowledge of traditional Chinese culture may well be confused and frustrated, and sometimes even shocked by TCM. Nowadays, there are numerous studies and random clinical trials that prove the efficacy of TCM therapies.

The misunderstandings and criticisms are related to the difficulty of testing the efficacy of TCM. TCM is personalized to each individual and its treatment is therefore seldom the same between any two patients, whereas doctors and scientists trained in Western medicine tend to prefer evidence gained from randomized clinical trials. In addition, TCM terms are not easy to understand. Many TCM terminologies are obscure, lacking clear and accurate explanation, which will inevitably affect the spread and development of TCM culture on a world scale. Lastly, it takes a while for TCM as a medical system to be scientifically proven because the underlying cultural assumptions such as the perception of the world, of body, and the relations between nature and humans, which help develop and nurture TCM are completely different from Western cultural values.

Overcoming Stereotyping

It is normal for us to make generalizations to navigate our complex world. However, if we are not careful, this habit can turn into stereotyping. What stereotypes have you met in your life? What beliefs did you encounter about people from different languages and cultures that you now realize were stereotypes? Additionally, think about how you use language. Do you or your friends use terms or tell jokes that could be offensive to people from other cultures? In what situations have you used the norms of your own culture to judge and understand the actions of individuals who come from different cultures (including language)?

To help overcome stereotyping, Ting-Toomey and Chung (2022) advocated learning to make a distinction between inflexible (or mindless) stereotyping and flexible (or mindful) stereotyping. As the term suggests, inflexible stereotyping is rigid and stubborn, and it happens automatically. Because these stereotypes are deeply rooted in our mind, we tend to ignore information that goes against them. However, flexible stereotyping comes into play when we realize that categorizing is a natural tendency and we become more attentive and mindful. This means being open-minded, willing to learn new things, avoiding judgment, and understanding that intercultural interactions can be challenging (Samovar *et al.*, 2017).

—— Activities ————————————————————————————————

Comprehension Questions

1. Discuss the stereotypes of TCM listed in this section and indicate whether you agree with them.

2. Offer examples other than those mentioned in this section to explain the four dimensions of stereotypes.

3. On a scale of 1 to 5 (with 1 = least like me, and 5 = most like me), how would you rank yourself on the continuum of the mindlessness-mindfulness trait when communicating with a cultural stranger? Why do you see yourself that way? Can you offer three specific suggestions for self-change or growth?

4. What is the difference between inflexible and flexible stereotyping? In what way does flexible stereotyping facilitate TCM interculturalization?

5. Can you offer some examples to show racial/ethnic, linguistic, sexual, and/or religious stereotypes?

Survey

Stereotyping is everywhere. Stereotyping happens to almost everything. The following are common stereotypes of Americans (Chen, 2009a):

Americans are rich.

Americans drive big cars.

Americans talk a lot but say little.

Americans have superficial relationships.

Americans do not care about old people.

Americans think only about money.

Americans are outgoing and friendly.

Americans lack discipline.

Americans are disrespectful of age and status.

Americans are ignorant of other countries.

Americans are extravagant and wasteful.

Americans are loud, rude, boastful, and immature.

Americans are always in a hurry.

First, classify the common stereotypes toward Americans listed above into each dimension of stereotypes.

Next, do a survey among your fellow Chinese students and foreigners, asking them what they think about a variety of topics/people that interest you (some topics are listed in the table for your reference). Fill in the table below with the data and report to the class orally as well as in a written form. You may redesign the table if need be.

Targets	Direction	Intensity	Accuracy	Content
American people				
Chinese people				
Kung fu				
Chinese herbal medicine				
TCM physicians				

Translation

Translate the following text into English.

我们必须坚定历史自信、文化自信,坚持古为今用、推陈出新,把马克思主义思想精髓同中华优秀传统文化精华贯通起来、同人民群众日用而不觉的共同价值观念融通起来,不断赋予科学理论鲜明的中国特色,不断夯实马克思主义中国化时代化的历史基础和群众基础,让马克思主义在中国牢牢扎根。

——习近平总书记在中国共产党第二十次全国代表大会上的报告

Debate

Read the following statements.

Some claim social media sites and apps such as TikTok help mitigate stereotypes; others contend that in the era of "Internet Plus" where almost every netizen is a provider of information, social media only makes stereotypes worse.

What do you think? Form teams with classmates who share the same side, with

2-4 members on each side. Give alternate speeches for and against the topic.

Before reading this section, please consider the following questions:

1.Discuss with your partners the consequence(s) of blind loyalty to one's own cultural community.

2. What does it mean to be Chinese? Think of five adjectives to describe your understanding of being Chinese. Discuss with your group members and report to the class.

12.2 Ethnocentrism and TCM Interculturalization

"A Good Patient"

The following story takes place in an American hospital (Martin and Nakayama, 2022). Setsuko was a Japanese woman living in the US, and she had to spend several months in the hospital because of a chronic illness. She became extremely depressed, to the point of feeling suicidal. Whenever the staff asked her how she was doing, Setsuko answered that she was fine. Based on this lack of communication, the nursing and medical staff were unaware of her depression for weeks. It was not until she began to show physical symptoms of depression that she was offered a psychiatric consultation.

What was the problem with Setsuko? The problem was that, as a Japanese woman, Setsuko was culturally conditioned to be a good patient by not making a fuss or drawing attention to herself or embarrassing her family with complaints about being depressed. After all, mental disorder is an uncomfortable topic in Japan, so she always reported that she was fine. Although the psychiatrist tried to explain that in this context a "good patient" was expected to discuss and report any or all problems or symptoms, Setsuko still had trouble working to rethink of her cultural role as a good patient in order to receive better healthcare. In this case, both the healthcare providers and the patient struggled to negotiate a more effective communication framework to ensure better treatment.

Defining Ethnocentrism

Setsuko's problem, from the perspective of intercultural communication, is not a problem. Rather, it is a phenomenon, or a certain mindset. Technically speaking, it is **ethnocentrism**. This expression, coined by William Sumner, an American sociologist, derives from two Greek words: *ethnos*, meaning "nation" or "people" and *kentron*, meaning "center" (Gudykunst and Kim, 2003, p. 137). This denotes that ethnocentrism happens when one considers his or her own nation as the most important in the world. In other words, ethnocentrism occurs when we tend to relate to (谈论) and judge other groups based on the standards and values of our own group, such as our ethnicity, race, or culture. People with an ethnocentric mindset view individuals from other cultures as less important or inferior to their own group. Ethnocentric behavior can involve arrogance, vanity, and even contempt towards outsiders (Jackson, 2014).

Features of Ethnocentrism

By its very nature, culture tends to be ethnocentric. It influences people to see the world from a local perspective, which helps create distinct boundaries between different groups. Without instructive, comparative, intercultural knowledge, we tend to view the world solely through our own cultural lens. To fully appreciate the true essence of ethnocentrism, one has to become aware that ethnocentrism is at once favorable and unfavorable.

It should be noted at first that ethnocentrism is found almost in every culture in the world. Because we are ethnocentric, we tend to view our own cultural values and ways of doing things as more real, or as the right and natural values and ways of doing things. Examples of ethnocentric behavior or language abound. If a woman from Hmong, an ethnic group from the mountain areas separating Laos and Vietnam, gives birth to a new baby and asks the nurse or doctor to give her the placenta (胎盘), a Western medicine practitioner may find this request strange and will likely refuse such an "uncivilized" call. However, within the Hmong culture, the act of burying the placenta has extremely important cultural significance and is related to the migration of one's soul and to matters of life after death. In the TCM community, the placenta, known as "zi he che" (紫河车) in Chinese, is considered a kind of medicine, which is effective in dealing with deficiency-type panting or coughing. Burying the placenta, in the eyes of TCM, would be considered a waste of valuable medicine. These are just two examples of ethnocentrism.

Research also shows that ethnocentrism is not usually intentional. Like culture, it is learned at the unconscious level. For example, people who are born and raised in the US are exposed to numerous subtle cues that reinforce the idea of the US being the focal point of the world. A perfect example is the use of the term "American" to refer only to people from the US Citizens of other parts of North and South America are also "Americans". However, in daily conversation as well as in numerous books, "America" and "American" are often reserved for the US and its citizens respectively.

Ethnocentrism is not always harmful. It can help the members of the same culture associate and identify with the culture. Haviland *et al*. (2017) argued that to function effectively, a society must embrace the idea that its ways are the only proper ones, irrespective of how other cultures do things. This provides individuals with a sense of ethnic pride in and loyalty to their cultural traditions, from which they derive psychological support, and which binds them firmly to their group. Some scholars (e.g., Gudykunst and Kim, 2003) argue that when people see their own group as central and having the right standards, they are more likely to help their group when problems arise. In times of war, strong ethnocentric feelings make a country's military more committed to defeating enemies. In other words, strong ethnocentrism on some rare occasions may help foster patriotism (爱国精神).

Ethnocentrism, therefore, can benefit those within a particular group, but it often leads to negative outcomes for individuals outside of that group. The issue with ethnocentrism is that it frequently becomes an excuse for criticizing other cultures as inferior and exploiting them for one's own advantage. Excessive levels of ethnocentrism become problematic when they result in conflict and hostility with individuals from other groups. Extreme ethnocentrism becomes destructive when it is used to shut others out, provide the bases for derogatory (贬低的) evaluation, and reject change. It also becomes problematic with respect to effective communication with people from diverse cultural backgrounds. Ethnocentric mindsets lead to misconceptions of members of outgroups, causing us to make inaccurate interpretation about others' behavior, creating communicative distance, and even prejudice. Examples of misconceptions about TCM have already been discussed in the previous section.

Cultural Relativism: A Remedy

Intercultural communication specialists have been actively involved in reducing ethnocentrism ever since they began studying and immersing themselves in the lives of foreign peoples. Researchers argue for ethno-relativism, popularly known as **cultural relativism**, a concept pioneered by American anthropologist Franz Boas back to the turn of the 20th century. Simply put, cultural relativism is "the idea that one must suspend judgment of other peoples' practices in order to understand those practices in their own cultural context" (Haviland *et al.*, 2017, p. 42). By taking this approach, we can truly understand the values and beliefs underlying other cultures in addition to our own. This is also the rationale that TCM is transmittable across cultures. We should take into consideration the host/guest cultural factors while engaging in TCM intercultural activities and be aware of the negative impact of ethnocentrism. Instead of solely focusing on the Chinese perspective, we must incorporate local medical history, culture, and other elements in order to effectively reduce misunderstandings and tell the Chinese story well.

Activities

Comprehension Questions

1. How is the term "ethnocentrism" coined? What does it mean?
2. Chinese communication style is famous for its indirectness and implicitness. Is it an ethnocentric view or not?
3. What are some positive and negative consequences of ethnocentrism?
4. In what way does cultural relativism help reduce ethnocentrism?
5. How can we guard against ethnocentric viewpoints while engaging in TCM intercultural activities?

Case Study

Case 1

Baldwin, a communication specialist, is talking about the story of his student.

One of our students, Kyle, came back to the US from China after spending one semester there. At one point, he got into an argument with his family, because he claimed that, based on its consumption of a large portion of the world's energy resources and slowness to adopt recycling, the US was wasteful. His family claimed firmly that the US is not a wasteful culture. His father said, "If you liked China so much, why don't you just go back?" Kyle also claimed that acupuncture and tuina helped him recover from a terrible fever. His family once again argued against him. His mother said, "If this thing really works, why is it not approved?" Kyle tried to convince his mother that acupuncture is legal in most states, and it is also quite popular in China and other countries around the world. He tried to show his pictures to his family, and a relative told him, "You don't need to bring those out. No one really wants to see them."

Questions

1.Do you detect any ethnocentric argument held by Kyle and his family?

2.What suggestions can you offer to Kyle if he wants to get his message across

Case 2

Lisa is a 27-year-old woman who was born in Hong Kong but now lives in Sydney. She commented that:

"Western medicine is very good at doing surgery, but when it comes to diagnosing skin disorders and nose allergies, I find TCM better. I find the more Western medicine antibiotics you take, the higher the dose you will need. Chinese medicine, on the other hand, has fewer side effects which even a weak body can tolerate."

Lisa had complaints of various kinds; on the advice of her mother, she decided to try TCM. She realized her body had become weak under the influence of too many fried and cold foods. She used to have two to three bars of chocolate and sometimes 250 g of lollypops per day. Moreover, she said five out of ten foods in the Chinese vegetarian restaurant were sweet things like water-chestnut and tofu puddings, and she would have them all. She said, "My allergy is mainly from inside my body." She decided to abstain from fried, sweet and cold foods, and considered TCM as part of her food supplements.

Questions

1.What advantages does Lisa think that TCM has over Western medicine?

2.What misconception(s) does Lisa have toward TCM?

3.What suggestions can you offer to people like Lisa to help mitigate their misconceptions about TCM?

Action Point

As we have seen in this chapter, adjustment to a new culture can be quite daunting. See if your school has a second-language program to aid international students to your school. Get involved in giving language lessons. Try to conduct an in-depth talk with international students to find out their experience of working and studying in China. Explain their intercultural adaptation process by using the U-curve or W-curve model (For more information, please consult the next section of this chapter).

12.3　Culture Shock and TCM Interculturalization

A Trip to TCM World

Approximately a decade ago, a group of students from Butler University embarked on a cultural and TCM learning journey at Zhejiang Chinese Medical University. The overall outcome of this intercultural endeavor was highly positive, as evidenced by the reluctance of participants to bid farewell after their month-long stay in Hangzhou. Michael talked about his experience in China this way.

One month in Hangzhou sounds easy and exciting for me as an American student who travels so much around the globe. So, when I learnt that there was a new international exchange program to Zhejiang Chinese Medical University, I was thrilled and signed up in the first place. As usual, I prepared everything and rushed to LA airport with my schoolmates. I became even more eager when I got the news that one schoolmate directly came from the Republic of Korea because our group is indeed quite international. Everything went well. We safely arrived at Shanghai Pudong International airport and transferred to Hangzhou in a comfortable coach. Except for a little jet lag, I felt perfectly well. I even joked with my friends while some of our schoolmates seemed to be a little complaining about the long coach ride.

However, it turned out that the first night at the campus hotel was horrible. Firstly, we were told by the hotel attendant that Wi-Fi was not available. In order to use the internet service, we had to connect through cable. Then, after we tumbled to the internet with our laptop, we were asked to log on. I thought it was easy; yet there was Chinese everywhere, no English at all. Forget about the net, at least we could have a sound sleep. No way. The Asian mosquitoes bit so hard. The next morning, I was awake with two bumps on my left hand. They were so big that our team leader got worried. We rushed to the school infirmary but were told it was no big deal. They just gave me some antiseptic and referred me to the convenience store to buy a bottle of greenish Liushen Florida water. Oh, Gee. Fortunately, the Florida water worked. The worst thing happened when we were asked to order our lunch in the school cafeteria. Every dish seemed so odd. We even didn't know what they were made of. In the end, with the help of a Chinese girl, we just ordered eggs and cauliflower and Chinese noodles. We had expected to have a wonderful Chinese meal. But…That was really terrible.

Defining Culture Shock

Moving abroad can be an exciting experience. Many new impressions of unfamiliar surroundings and new people and activities, just like what Michael experienced when he first arrived at Hangzhou. However, all these exciting new experiences might also lead to a feeling of being a little bit lost. The worst thing could happen when you begin to feel terribly homesick and even have mental depression. In that case, you are experiencing **culture shock**, a term coined by Kalvaro Oberg to refer to a sense of "anxiety that results from losing all of our familiar signs and symbols of social intercourse" (Baldwin *et al.*, 2014, p. 251). This cultural impact usually takes place while one is moving from a familiar culture to an unfamiliar one.

The responses linked to culture shock can differ greatly among individuals. Culture shock can lead to either physical or mental reactions — or both — in individuals, such as feeling irritated, tired, disoriented (不知所措), rejected, or withdrawn (沉默自闭). However, different people experience culture shock to different degrees. Those with more exposure to diverse cultures tend to adapt faster. Our discussion in this section aims to prepare you to handle potential culture shock, rather than discourage you from exploring new cultures.

The U-curve Adaptation Model

Scholars have created different models to describe the stages of culture shock and adjustment that people undergo when entering a new culture. One of the well-known models is the **U-curve** adaptation model (Jackson, 2014).

The core concept is that sojourners (旅居者) typically go through predictable phases when adjusting to a new culture. The U-curve model consists of four stages, which have been labeled differently by various scholars. Sojourners initially feel excited and expectant (期待) (the honeymoon stage or initial euphoria),

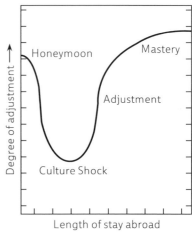

Fig. 12.3.1 The U-curve Adaptation Model

then face a phase of shock and disorientation (referred to as the bottom of the U curve), and eventually adapt to the new cultural environment (including adjustment or recovery, and mastery or adaptation stages). Although this framework is too simplistic and not applicable to every individual's experience, most sojourners tend to encounter these general stages at some point.

The W-curve Adaptation Model

Interestingly, sojourners may experience another round of shock after returning to their original cultural contexts, with difficulty in processing the old yet unfamiliar cultural norms and behavior. Therefore, the U-curve model is expanded to include this reentry experience, becoming a **W-curve** framework. In other words, the experiencing of intercultural adaptation moves through seven stages: honeymoon, hostility, humorous, in-sync, ambivalence, reentry culture shock, and resocialization stages (Ting-Toomey and Chung, 2022). The W-curve model applies especially to international students' experience abroad; it can also be used to predict the possible physical and/or psychological experience that a TCM culture facilitator might undergo in a strange environment.

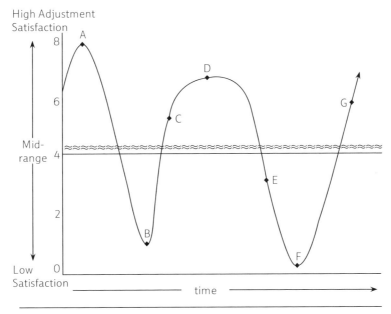

A: Honeymoon Stage
B: Frustration/Hostility Stage
C: Rebound/Humorous Stage
D: In-Sync Adjustment Stage

E: Ambivalence Stage
F: Re-entry Culture Shock Stage
G: Resocialization Stage

Fig. 12.3.2 The W-curve Adaptation Model

Let us imagine a situation where you are a TCM cultural ambassador and spend two years in South Africa participating in activities organized by the Confucius Institute for Chinese Medicine (CICM). While CICM is real, the experiences in this scenario are fictional and specifically fabricated to better explain the theory of culture shock. Now, let us go one by one.

Stage 1: **Honeymoon Stage**. During the honeymoon stage, individuals feel excited about their new cultural environment. It is the initial phase where everything seems fresh and exhilarating (激动人心的). You are excited to meet people in South Africa, eager to know them and share your understanding of TCM. You perceive local people and events through rose-colored (过于乐观) glasses. Nonetheless, you do experience mild confusion and perplexity about South Africa; you also feel lonely and homesick sometimes. Yet, it does not worry you much because you will always relate to your friends and family back in China through Wechat or other social media. Overall, you are enjoying your initial "friendly" contact with the locals. You are keen to explore a variety of possibilities of meeting new challenges, and you are confident in carrying out your mission of popularizing TCM in South Africa.

Stage 2: **Frustration/Hostility Stage**. As time goes by, however, your uneasiness and worry become more troubling. One day, you helped organize a Chinese cultural event where you were supposed to show your Chinese calligraphy together with a lecture on the colorful world of TCM. The whole program turned out to be a disaster. Among a small group of local participants who showed up, almost no one appreciated your endeavor. You experienced a major loss of self-esteem and self-confidence. You suddenly began to feel consciously incompetent and emotionally drained (精疲力竭). You are experiencing the hostility stage, and major emotional upheavals. This is the serious culture shock stage in which nothing works out smoothly. This stage can quickly follow the end of the honeymoon phase and catch you off guard (措手不及), bringing you back to reality sooner than anticipated. Many of these sojourners can either become very aggressive or totally withdrawn.

Eliza, a young woman from Thailand who had been studying in the US for six months, complained to her friends this way (Ting-Toomey and Chung, 2022, p. 125):

"This semester, you must talk to earn your participation points in the classroom. We have three parts of the grade in this class. One third is discussion participation, the other two-thirds is writing articles. So if you don't talk, you lose one third of your points. So you have to talk. Talking is so exhausting! And it's not just talk, you know, from the material. You need to say what you think about it. But in Thailand, you just participate or do your homework. That's ok. I want to go back to Thailand."

People in the hostility stage tend to constantly use their ethnocentric standards to compare and evaluate the local practices and customs. During this stage, some people manage to adapt and cope, while others may struggle. We sincerely hope that you navigate through this phase successfully. It is worth mentioning that sharing your concerns with friends in China can be a great source of support during this time.

Stage 3: **Rebound/Humorous Stage**. At this stage, you learn to laugh at your cultural mistakes and start to realize that there are pros and cons in each culture — just as there are both good and evil people in every society. That means you are able to compare both South African and Chinese cultures in realistic terms, and you no longer take things as seriously as in the hostility stage. You begin to socialize with the local people. And somehow, you find South Africans can be truly friendly and warm. Once again, you participated in a new cultural event. During this time, you made adjustments based on past mistakes and decided to focus less on Chinese philosophy. Instead, you organized plenty of hands-on activities that brought everyone joy. It was particularly wonderful that participants even had the opportunity to take part in tuina practice.

Stage 4: **In-Sync** (协调一致的) **Adjustment Stage**. During this stage, your satisfaction reaches a new high because you feel at ease in CICM. You have a strong sense of belonging to the community. As you become more involved in the community, the lines between outsiders and insiders blur, and you start to feel accepted by the residents. You are one of South Africans. You now can fully function as a qualified TCM cultural ambassador. We encourage you to seize this opportunity to effectively publicize TCM across diverse cultures.

Stage 5: **Ambivalence Stage**. Two-year stay at CICM is drawing to a close. You are packing your luggage and set about going back to China. No doubt, people in South Africa will miss you, and you will miss them too. You recall those awkward early days when you first arrived. It is a mix of sadness, nostalgia, and pride that fills your heart. You are not only reluctant to say good-bye, but also looking forward to sharing your intercultural stories with your family and old friends back home face to face. You finally say good-bye to your newfound friends and your temporarily adopted culture.

Stage 6: **Reentry Culture Shock Stage**. At the reentry culture shock stage, you face an unexpected confusion. Your friends or family maybe have no interest in hearing all your wonderful intercultural stories again. After all, you posted your moments with photos and short videos all the time. Everyone who cares has already given you a thumbs up. You may feel disappointed, dismayed, and of course frustrated. However, there is no need for concern. Most people who have traveled abroad have learned to adapt and persevere. They can use the strategies they developed to overcome challenges and move forward. Just stay positive and have faith in your friends and family.

Stage 7: **Resocialization stage**. You may quietly assimilate yourself back to your old role and behavior without appearing different from the rest of your friends and colleagues. However, more probably, instead of being a resocializer (重新回归原来的群体), it is possible for you to become a transformer, acting as an agent of change in China. In other words, you become an ambassador of both TCM and South African culture. You combine what you have learned in South Africa with the best parts of Chinese culture. By thinking creatively, understanding different perspectives, and using your cultural intelligence, you will solve problems and promote positive change in an inclusive learning organization. In other words, you become a competent TCM cultural ambassador, a concept that will be explored in detail in the next chapter.

Characteristics of Intercultural Adaptations

The W-curve adaptation model emphasizes the following characteristics (Ting-Toomey and Chung, 2022):

- There are peaks and valleys, or ups and downs in your intercultural experience. The adaptation process can go spiral. Progress, stagnation, and even regress (倒退) is common. Never assume that progress is inevitable. Sometimes, the conquered difficulties will reappear, even worse.
- In the new culture, it is crucial to stay conscious of our goals and monitor our progress. Achieving success in one set of goals can serve as a stepping-stone towards

accomplishing other goals.

• It is important to allow yourself sufficient time and personal space to adapt. Consider keeping a journal or vlog to express your daily emotions and miscellaneous thoughts.

• To thrive in a new culture, focus on building strong relationships and fostering connections with a wide range of people. Embrace opportunities to take part in major cultural events of the host culture. Most importantly, work on improving your ability to communicate effectively across cultures.

Chapter Summary

• Stereotype and ethnocentrism are two stumbling blocks to effective TCM interculturalization.

• Stereotypes can vary in four dimensions: direction, intensity, accuracy, and content.

• Learning to make a distinction between inflexible stereotyping and flexible stereotyping helps you overcome overgeneralization.

• Ethnocentrism, the mindset of using one's own cultural norms to evaluate everything else, is ubiquitous.

• Ethnocentrism can be positive within a particular group, but often leads to negative outcomes for outsiders.

• Moving to cultural relativism is a good way to mitigate ethnocentrism.

• Exploring a new culture can lead to feelings of anxiety and emotional strain, which can contribute to mental and physical exhaustion.

• According to the U-curve adaptation model, intercultural adaptation has four stages: honeymoon, culture shock, recovery, and mastery.

• According to the W-curve adaptation model, intercultural adaptation has seven stages: honeymoon, frustration/hostility, rebound/humor, in-sync adjustment, ambivalence, reentry culture shock, and resocialization.

Checklist	Yes	No
Cognitive: I have mastered the core information		
Behavioral: I have the ability of putting what I've learned into practice		
Affective: I am willing to carry out what I've learned		
Moral: I will take the ethical consideration into account during practice		

Chapter 13

Striving for Effective and Appropriate TCM Interculturalization

Chapter Objectives

After reading this chapter, you should be able to:

◆ Define intercultural communicative competence.

◆ Explain the difference between culture-specific and culture-general approaches to intercultural education.

◆ Weigh the pros and cons of different training models and methods.

◆ Recognize different levels of TCM interculturalization competence.

◆ Practice different techniques in intercultural training.

Key Terms

affective dimension	effective and appropriate
behavioral dimension	interaction model
Byram's Model	intercultural communication competence
case study	levels of competence
classroom model	moral dimension
cognitive dimension	role play
culture-general vs. culture-specific	simulation model
Dai and Chen's Model	TCM interculturalization competence

Quotes

"Media groups should build up their capacity in international communication, amplify their voices on the international stage, tell stories about China well, optimize strategic planning and build flagship media groups with strong global influence." (要加强国际传播能力建设, 增强国际话语权, 集中讲好中国故事, 同时优化战略布局, 着力打造具有较强国际影响的外宣旗舰媒体。)

——2016 年 2 月 19 日习近平主持召开党的新闻舆论工作座谈会并发表重要讲话

"Not having heard of it is not as good as having heard of it. Having heard of it is not as good as having seen it. Having seen it is not as good as knowing it. Knowing it is not as good as putting it into practice. Learning arrives at putting it into practice and then stops, because to put it into practice is to understand it, and to understand it is to be a sage." (不闻不若闻之, 闻之不若见之, 见之不若知之, 知之不若行之。学至于行之而止矣。行之, 明也; 明之为圣人。)

——《荀子·儒效》

"The world is a book, and those who do not travel read only one page." (天下犹如一部巨著, 未涉远行者, 只能窥见其中一页。)

——Augustine of Hippo

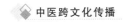
Before reading this section, please consider the following questions:

1. List five communication characteristics that you would like to develop if you were to visit another country as an exchange student.

2. How do you know whether you have communicated effectively and appropriately in intercultural interactions?

13.1　Gaining Intercultural Competence

Communication of TCM across cultures can be quite daunting in many ways, as experiential examples have illustrated throughout this book. In the previous chapters, we explored many different factors that play a role in human interactions, for example, at the social levels (such as value systems, worldviews, and outlooks, etc.), the sociocultural levels (such as our memberships in social groups, our social identities, and our roles in relationships), the psychocultural level (such as expectations, cognition, stereotypes and prejudices, and intergroup attitudes), and the environmental level (such as physical environment, situation, and psychological environment).

Now that we are approaching the end of this textbook and about to gain some hands-on experience in the journey of TCM interculturalization, a question that is often asked by our students is: How do I know whether I have become a competent TCM culture facilitator? Is there a useful tool to evaluate my intercultural competence? How can I improve my competence? What are some of the key skills and coping tactics that are necessary for a sojourner to survive in an intercultural setting? In this chapter, we are aiming to cope with these complex issues. Researchers in psychology, communication studies, foreign language teaching, and international politics have all attempted to offer their conceptualization and operationalization of intercultural communication competence. We try to explain the theoretical frameworks of intercultural communication competence that have taken place in several different academic fields with a focus on the communication studies and foreign language teaching research.

Terminologies and Definitions

Being a competent facilitator of TCM interculturalization is a worthy but often quite elusive goal. To become better communicators for TCM globalization, we have covered a lot of topics and discussed some issues that help us learn and make a change. What we desire to acquire is knowledge and experience that cannot be obtained by merely reading books. It takes time to become a good TCM physician, so does it to become a competent facilitator of TCM interculturalization. In this and following sections, we want to share with you ideas and offer you suggestions for improving your skills in communicating across cultures. However, as noted by Spencer-Oatey and Franklin (2009), several different terminologies are adopted by scholars from different fields with different focuses. For instance, Ruben's (1989) paper (Rnben, 1989) is entitled "The Study of Cross-cultural Competence". Yet, he began the paper with discussing intercultural competence. Obviously, for Ruben, these two terminologies are interchangeable. Michael Byram, a researcher in the field of foreign language teaching, traces the origin of communicative competence in the anglophone (讲英语) world to David Hymes' critique of Chomsky's linguistic competence. It follows that Byram prefers "intercultural communicative competence" to refer to an individual's ability to communicate and interact across cultures.

A great number of terms are used from different angles, indicating academic vigor, yet lacking semantic rigor (严谨). In this book, we use **intercultural communication competence (ICC)** or intercultural competence in general, and TCM interculturalization competence in specific. ICC seems to be a fairly simple concept—referring to communicating effectively across cultures. In fact, it is rather complicated. Researchers from different disciplines vary as to what constitutes ICC. Byram argued that communication is not just the exchange of information. More importantly, intercultural communicative competence "is focused on establishing and maintaining relationships" (Byram, 1997, p. 3). Accordingly, engaging in an intercultural interaction in a healthcare setting inevitably leads to the (dis)connection of interpersonal relationships. Given the complex relationship between language, culture, and intercultural communication, Byram coined "intercultural speaker" to refer to foreign language/culture learners who successfully build intercultural connections in their second language. Intercultural speakers are considered as competent, flexible communicators who can "engage with complexity and multiple identities" and "avoid stereotyping which accompanying perceiving someone through a single identity" (Byram *et al.*, 2002, p. 5).

Within the context of TCM interculturalization, both **culture-specific**（针对特定文化的）and **culture-general**（泛文化的）approaches should be taken into consideration in order to achieve ideal goals. Cultural-specific dimension encompasses a series of abilities of encoding and decoding verbal as well as non-verbal signals and behaviors specific to a given cultural group. For example, to be successful in running an acupuncture clinic in Germany, a TCM physician from China must be familiar with local communication styles, in addition to mastering medical skills. Meanwhile, he should also develop an intercultural awareness of core issues (for instance, culture shock, stereotype, prejudice, etc.) so he could cope with all kinds of encounters regardless of their specific cultural contexts. This is culture-general approach. Obviously, intercultural training should incorporate both culture-specific and culture-general aspects as broad intercultural competence cannot be obtained by only focusing on the abilities to cope with difficulties in a specific context.

For years, intercultural communication researchers have made huge effort to define the concept of ICC and identify its components. Spitzberg and Cupach (1984) have provided a systematic discussion of competence. First, they made a distinction between effectiveness and competence. Effectiveness refers to one's ability to accomplish tasks—that is, the "achievement of interaction goals" (p. 102). However, competence refers to being effective while at the same time displaying appropriate behavior (without violating communication norms). In other words, to be competent, one has to be both **effective and appropriate**. Second, Spitzberg and Cupach (1984) have identified three key dimensions of communication competence: knowledge, skills, and motivation.

Based on the above assumptions, Spitzberg (2015) has developed a well-recognized conceptualization of ICC. According to Spitzberg, ICC is "behavior that is appropriate and effective in a given context" (p.343). Here, context is broadly considered to incorporate cultural influences. Many intercultural communication specialists follow Spitzberg's definition, regarding appropriateness and effectiveness as two essential dimensions of competent communication. Kim (1991) offered a more detailed definition when she argued that ICC is "the overall internal capability of an individual to manage key challenging features of intercultural communication: namely, cultural differences and unfamiliarity, inter-group posture, and the accompanying experience of stress" (p. 256). Both Spitzberg and Kim inform us that being able to communicate TCM across cultures effectively and appropriately requires that correct mode of behavior be chosen based on sensible analysis of the context, both external and internal.

Seeing that TCM interculturalization can be understood as an intercultural activity with a focus on transmitting TCM across different cultural boundaries, we utilize ICC to describe the proficiency that encompasses not just effective verbal and non-verbal communication and appropriate behavior towards individuals from diverse cultural backgrounds, but also the ability to manage the psychological challenges and dynamic consequences that arise from such interactions. Likewise, **TCM interculturalization competence** refers to the ability to carry out TCM related cultural engagement with people of diverse cultural contexts effectively and appropriately.

Building on their empirical research and understanding of ICC, numerous specialists across the globe (e. g., applied linguists, interculturalists, communication specialists) have constructed models to outline ICC. We here offer two representative frameworks: Byram's model (1997) and Dai and Chen's ICC model (2015).

Byram's Model

Michael Byram is a prominent scholar in applied linguistics known for his research on intercultural communication and language learning. His conceptual framework (Byram, 1997) highlights the importance of incorporating culture in the teaching and learning of second languages. As illustrated in the diagram below, Byram draws on the research of both Hymes (1972) and Bachman (1990), expanding the communicative competence to include "linguistic competence, sociolinguistic competence, and discourse competence" in addition to intercultural competence.

The whole model consists of two parts. In the first part, Byram (1997) identified three language-related components as indicative of a second language speaker who possesses intercultural competence (referred to as an intercultural speaker or mediator):

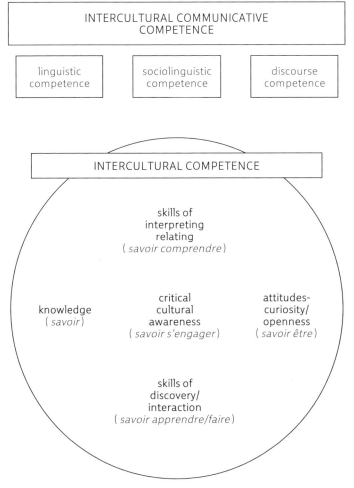

Components of Byram's Intercultural Communicative Competence

- Linguistic competence: the ability to understand the rules of a standardized language in order to effectively comprehend and express spoken and written language.
- Sociolinguistic competence: the ability to understand the intended or untended meanings through negotiation with the interactant, if need be.
- Discourse competence: the ability to use and adapt strategies for communicating through written or spoken texts that are aligned with the cultural norms of the interactant, or that are agreed upon as intercultural texts for specific purposes.

In the second part of Byram's model, five savoirs or components are outlined, which are associated with the cultural aspect of the intercultural speaker's proficiency. They are intercultural attitudes, intercultural knowledge, skills of interpreting and relating, skills of discovery and interaction, and critical cultural awareness. In this way, simply mastering grammatical rules and vocabulary is not sufficient for TCM culture facilitators to engage in a competent intercultural activity. Cultural learning is equally important.

Dai and Chen's Model

Communication specialists Chen Guoming and William Starosta (1998) have demonstrated that ICC includes three equally important and interrelated dimensions: (i) intercultural sensitivity (affective); (ii) intercultural awareness (cognitive); and (iii) intercultural adroitness (机敏) (behavioral). The affective dimension focuses on attitudes and emotions. The cognitive or knowledge dimension involves the understanding of cultural values and patterns, and the behavioral dimension deals with skills applied to fulfilling communication goals. This model is also widely used in ICC research.

However, as discussed in the previous chapters, intercultural communication in general, and TCM interculturalization in particular, is unbalanced in many situations, with one party dominating the other, and the other party being dominated. In other words, power, "a constraining force by which individuals, groups, and structures are able to achieve their aims and interests over/against the will of others" (Halualani, 2019, p. 32), must be taken into consideration when one is to explore the true essence of ICC.

Dai and Chen (2015) argued that genuine intercultural interaction becomes possible when individuals seek reciprocity and harmony, both of which are critical to the development of interculturality (文化间性), a space where diverse cultures encounter and adapt to each other. In this open and dynamic space, culturally different individuals endeavor to reduce cultural distance, negotiate shared meanings and mutually desired identities, and cultivate reciprocal relationships. Obviously, the tripartite (由三部分构成的) framework of "knowledge, skills, and motivation" is not conducive to this ideal outcome. In order to reach mutual understanding and harmonious co-existence, power must be constrained by morality. Therefore, moral dimension is to be included in defining ICC. The remaining portion of this section provides a description of each component in relation to TCM interculturalization, if necessary.

Components of Dai and Chen's Model

• Affective Dimension

The affective dimension refers to the emotional tendency or the willingness to engage in intercultural communication. This dimension serves as a driving force that motivates individuals to acquire knowledge and skills. Motivation is important, for it shapes how we acquire cultural knowledge and develop communication skills. Simply put, motivation refers to the underlying reason that can explain your verbal and non-verbal responses toward something. If you are highly motivated and have a positive attitude to the interactant, you are more likely to succeed in transmitting TCM across cultures. In other words, we cannot assume that people always want to communicate, or desire to know TCM. Sometimes, people lack high motivation because they come from large, more powerful groups who lack the incentive to know other cultures. Sometimes, people are afraid to engage interculturally because intercultural communication can be quite uncomfortable. As discussed previously, anxiety, uncertainty, and fear are common in intercultural interaction. We should not expect everyone in the world to enthusiastically embrace every aspect of TCM only after one or two casual encounters. Some TCM therapeutic methods like cupping, acupuncture and moxibustion are quite normal to insiders. Yet, they may be very intimidating (令人胆怯的) to newcomers. TCM culture facilitators should be patient in their engagement with people from diverse cultural backgrounds. Lastly, we should also know that there are intrinsic (内在) and extrinsic (外来) motivations. Since promoting TCM globalization is both a national and an individual effort, both the endorsement from the national administration and the embrace from the individual preference could serve as a strong driving force for communicating TCM across cultures, among which, your personal (intrinsic) motivation plays a critical role.

In order to obtain intercultural harmony, four affective elements are required, namely, open-mindedness, relational self-concept, active empathy (共情), and mutual appreciation. Open-minded people are highly motivated to take challenges. They are more willing to reformulate their self-concept in relation to people from different contexts. To promote mutual understanding and establish shared meaning in intercultural contexts, individuals with intercultural competence must actively cultivate empathy. Empathy has long been considered an important component of intercultural awareness. It refers to the ability to understand, vicariously (间接体验到地) experience, and/ or be sensitive to the feelings, emotions, and experiences of other people even though we have never experienced before. Active empathy requires the interactant to be willing to shift his perspective. Treating each participant on the same footing is needed so a harmonious intercultural relationship can be cultivated. In other words, mutual appreciation emphasizes the significance of intercultural interactants acknowledging the complementarity and correlation between both parties. This is helpful in guiding TCM culture facilitators in planning their cultural events, reminding them not to demean the local healthcare system.

• Cognitive Dimension

The cognitive dimension refers to intercultural awareness or understanding of cultural values and conventions. You need to learn about both your own and others' cultural values and conventions and identify the important differences between them. Throughout the textbook, we have talked about the requisite knowledge regarding cultural values, norms, and patterns of behavior. These knowledge enables us to achieve intercultural understanding. Furthermore, some highlights of TCM and its philosophical foundation are introduced so that TCM can be well understood by culturally different individuals, and Chinese stories, well received.

Here, we describe four essential cognitive abilities that aim to promote interculturality in interactions. These abilities are cultural knowledge, critical cultural awareness, cultural integration, and intercultural perspective. Cultural knowledge includes both one's own and others' culture. As Dai and Chen (2015) noted, knowing one's own culture, also known as self-knowledge, is a foundation for knowing other cultures. However, it is often easy to ignore the importance of knowing one's own culture. Frequently, we remain unaware of how others perceive us either due to a lack of effort in seeking such information or a lack of trust in the relationship, preventing people from openly sharing their perceptions. Correspondingly, having knowledge about how other individuals think and behave, known as other-knowledge, can significantly enhance your effectiveness as a communicator. Besides, language, values and customs, and the historical background of the counterpart's culture are vital aspects in this process of cultural learning. Linguistic knowledge deserves a further discussion here. Although English is now widely considered as a lingua franca and many

TCM classics are translated into English, it is still advisable to adapt to the participants in the intercultural activities related to TCM by using the local language. It can be expected that people from a foreign culture, say, Germany, would feel comfortable and may be more willing to negotiate once German language is used in discussing highlights of TCM such as five-phase theory.

Among the other three cognitive components, critical cultural awareness necessitates the capacity to reflectively evaluate both one's own culture and the culture of the counterpart. It helps the interactants beware of blindingly following suit. Cultural integration is the outcome of knowledge sharing and mutual criticizing. In other words, intercultural activities related to promoting TCM across cultures result in the interactant's knowing of elements of TCM in the first step, leading up to the acceptance of TCM practices around the globe. The final cognitive component, intercultural perspective, helps the participants transcend intercultural barriers like ethnocentrism to reach a joint action. Accordingly, competent TCM culture facilitators should encourage intercultural coordination with the participants, which helps develop cultural synergy, i.e., embracing TCM practice.

• Behavioral Dimension

The behavioral dimension refers to skills to perform intercultural communication tasks. It is the participant's ability to apply positive emotion and requisite knowledge to realistic communication. When you are capable of translating (转变为) communication theories into appropriate and effective behavior, you become a competent TCM culture facilitator. From the perspective of interculturality, four abilities are required to become a competent intercultural communicator: interaction skill, identity negotiation, rapport (和睦) building, and creative tension.

Communication scholars have identified certain universal behaviors that are relevant across different cultures and contexts in terms of interaction skills. These behaviors include active listening, adaptability, respect for others, and effective messaging (Martin and Nakayama, 2022). However, applying these behaviors in specific ways can be challenging. For example, while respect is important in all intercultural interactions, how it is expressed may vary depending on the culture and context. Both identity negotiation and rapport building highlight the dynamic interconnectedness between the participants in intercultural interaction. While the former emphasizes reciprocal relationships for cultivating intercultural harmony, the latter aims to achieve a harmonious and smooth relationship between participants, which is based on appropriate facework (面子保全策略), expectation and mutual sharing.

The last one is of special importance because it emphasizes the necessity of articulating one's own voice and defending one's own position. As mentioned before, TCM and Western medicine are strikingly different; there is a huge gap between the two systems of medical knowledge. They are rooted in different cultural soils, follow different logics, and operate via different mechanisms. It is ineffective or even wrong to apply Western tests to validating TCM. Therefore, when conflicts arise in TCM interculturalization, we need to work out new ways to solve the problem. Creative outcomes are likely obtained by exploring innovative ways to deal with the tension between TCM and Western medicine.

• Moral Dimension

The moral dimension refers to the ethical principles guiding intercultural interaction. In the previous chapters, we have covered four ethical principles that support positive relationships and interculturality in TCM interculturalization, namely, mutual respect, sincerity, tolerance, and responsibility, because it is so important to cultivate ethical facilitators for TCM globalization. While the four-principle ethics is popular in Western medicine,

Sun Simiao's "doctor's excellence and dedication" is widely acknowledged as an essential ethical norm of TCM.

From the perspective of interculturality, the moral dimension serves to regulate intercultural interaction, and facilitate the development of positive affect (情感), intercultural knowledge, and appropriate and effective behavior. Four ethical principles contribute to harmonious relationships and successful communication: mutual respect, sincerity, tolerance, and responsibility. These ethical principles are negotiated by culturally different individuals, and flexibly performed in intercultural situations. The addition of moral dimension to ICC framework addresses the gap in Western models and helps correct the Eurocentric (以欧洲为中心的) bias.

Four Levels of Competence

In this section, we discussed complexity of the terminology and what it means to be interculturally competent in today's diverse and connected world. We looked at two different models of intercultural competence with an emphasis on Dai and Chen's framework (2015). In demonstrating the complexity of competence, William Howell (1982) has identified four **levels of competence**: (i) unconscious incompetence; (ii) conscious incompetence; (iii) conscious competence; and (iv) unconscious competence. The development of lower-level competence facilitates attainment of higher-level competence. It is a long journey in which you start from being an inexperienced TCM culture facilitator to becoming a competent TCM cultural ambassador, contributing to the development of a global community of health for all.

Activities

Comprehension Questions

1.What benefits does the culture-general approach to studying ICC have compared with the culture-specific method?

2. What is your understanding of power? How does power play a role in TCM interculturalization?

3.What is interculturality? What is the ideal outcome of TCM interculturalization?

4.What is motivation? What factors can influence one's motivation for promoting TCM interculturally?

5.How does your personal attributes, such as gender, class, age, and other factors, impact your ability to communicate TCM effectively across different cultures?

Group Work

1.You are about to cooperate with someone from a different culture to organize a cultural event on "The Stories of Famous TCM Physicians". Create a list of methods for fostering alliance between yourself and him/her during a conversation. Consider various ways in which each of you can support one another. Pay attention to the precise communication techniques that can facilitate the development of mutual alliance. Finally, role-play your interaction in class.

2.Discuss with your group members to provide an illustration of how one can enhance one of the four dimensions (affective, cognitive, behavioral, and moral) of ICC. Please be detailed in your response. You should illustrate your point with a concrete example of TCM interculturalization. Finally, design and do a poster presentation with your partners.

Translation

Translate the following text into English.

　　坚守中华文化立场,提炼展示中华文明的精神标识和文化精髓,加快构建中国话语和中国叙事体系,讲好中国故事、传播好中国声音,展现可信、可爱、可敬的中国形象。

　　　　　　　　——习近平总书记在中国共产党第二十次全国代表大会上的报告

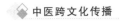

Before reading this section, please consider the following questions:

1. Have you ever attended any intercultural training course/seminar/workshop? Share your experience with your partner or search the internet to find some.

2. Aa a Chinese saying goes, "the master teaches the trade, but the perfection of the apprentice's skill depends on his own efforts." Which one plays a leading role in training for facilitating TCM interculturalization, the trainer or the trainee?

13.2 Evaluating Competence and Training for TCM Interculturalization

While Chinese travel around the world as tourists, students, businesspeople, or diplomats, those from other cultures also travel and work in China. As medical workers and other professionals, we must decide what communication practices work well in intercultural settings, especially in a healthcare context. As is mentioned before, successful intercultural adaptability and TCM interculturalization, to a great extent, is dependent on the sojourner's mastery of the host culture, communication skills and behavior, and moral constraints, i.e., sufficient amount of intercultural competence. No one is born with such competence. It requires systematic training and engaged (积极参与的) practice. Intercultural training programs are developed to improve interactional effectiveness by increasing your familiarity with customs of the host or guest cultures, with differences in perceptions, with the pool of meanings within the context, and with the use of varying nonverbal cues.

Evaluating Intercultural Communication Competence

Before getting trained, one is often curious about how good one's competence is. Besides, a reliable evaluation tool also provides a useful starting point to evaluate the effectiveness of intercultural training. An effective evaluation tool helps trainers maximize limited training resources. On the contrary, a poorly designed one has the potential to endanger the entire program.

Yet, proper evaluation is not easy to devise. The process of intercultural assessment involves a test to measure the participant's performance, attitudes, and amount of information about the host/guest culture. Usually, a holistic and systematic method is preferable to evaluate the overall performance, because this method is based on an underlying principle that each component plays an interconnected role in one's performance. However, evaluation tools that aim to measure the overall performance usually result in one condensed score. Such a global score may not be detailed enough to offer an elaborate understanding of each sub-branch of one's competence. Therefore, an independent evaluation tool focusing on one component may be a better choice if it is necessary to know more about that specific component.

Four evaluation methods are possible: observation, interview, portfolio (档案评估), and self-reported questionnaire, with the last one being the most frequently used. Some of the most popular evaluation tools are as follows.

• Cross-Cultural Adaptability Inventory developed by Kelly and Meyers (1987) which contains 50 items covering four dimensions, namely, emotional resilience, flexibility / openness, perceptual acuity, and personal autonomy.

• Cultural Intelligence Scale developed by Ang *et al.* (2007) which contains 53 items covering four dimensions, namely, metacognitive CQ, cognitive CQ, motivational CQ, and behavioral CQ.

• Generalized Ethnocentrism Scale developed by Neuliep (2002) which contains 22 items measuring one factor, i.e., degree of ethnocentrism.

• Revised Sociocultural Adaptation Scale developed by Wilson (2013) which contains 21 items measuring behavioral aspect of intercultural communication competence with five subscales:

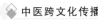

interpersonal communication, academic / work performance, personal interests and community involvement, ecological adaptation, and language proficiency.

Cultural Intelligence Scale

Similar to the concept of intelligent quotient, cultural intelligence (CQ, 文化智力) refers to one's capability to function effectively in culturally diverse settings. Ang *et el*. (2007) argued that the higher your CQ is, the better you adapt to the new culture. CQ can be further classified into four parts:

- Metacognitive Intelligence, which refers to control of cognition or the processes individuals use to acquire and understand knowledge,
- Cognitive Intelligence, which refers to knowledge structures,
- Motivational Intelligence, which refers to the mental capacity to direct and sustain energy at a particular task and recognize that motivational capabilities are critical to real world problem solving,
- Behavioral Intelligence, which refers to outward manifestations or overt actions.

While metacognitive CQ focuses on higher-order cognitive processes, cognitive CQ reflects knowledge of the norms, practices and conventions in different cultures acquired from education and personal experiences. Motivational CQ is about the capability to direct attention and energy toward learning and functioning in situations characterized by cultural differences. Finally, behavioral CQ measures the capability to exhibit appropriate verbal and nonverbal actions when interacting with people from different cultures.

The following table (Dai, 2018, pp. 217-219) is the evaluation tool that can help you assess your CQ.

The Cultural Intelligence Scale (CQS)

Read each statement and select the response that best describes your capabilities. Select the answer that BEST describes you AS YOU REALLY ARE (1 = strongly disagree; 7 = strongly agree)

Metacognitive CQ

· MC1. I am conscious of the cultural knowledge I use when interacting with people from cultural backgrounds.
· MC2. I adjust my cultural knowledge as I interact with people from a culture that is unfamiliar to me.
· MC3. I am conscious of the cultural knowledge I apply to cross-cultural interactions.
· MC4. I check the accuracy of my cultural knowledge as I interact with people from different cultures.

Cognitive CQ

· COG1. I know the legal and economic systems in other cultures.
· COG2. I know the rules (e.g., vocabulary, grammar) of other languages.
· COG3. I know the cultural values and religious beliefs of other cultures.
· COG4. I know the marriage systems of other cultures.
· COG5. I know the arts and crafts of other cultures.
· COG6. I know the rules for expressing non-verbal behaviors in other cultures.

Motivational CQ

· MOT1. I enjoy interacting with people from different cultures.
· MOT 2. I am confident that I can socialize with locals in a culture that is new to me.
· MOT 3. I am sure I can deal with the stresses of adjusting to a culture that is new to me.
· MOT 4. I enjoy living in cultures that are unfamiliar to me.
· MOT 5. I am confident that I can get accustomed to the shopping conditions in a different culture.

Behavioral CQ

· BEH1. I change my verbal behavior (e.g., accent, tone) when a cross-cultural interaction requires it.
· BEH 2. I use pause and silence differently to suit the different cross-cultural situations.
· BEH 3. I vary my rate of speaking when a cross-cultural situation requires it
· BEH4. I change my non-verbal behavior when a cross-cultural situation requires it.
· BEH 5. I alter my facial expressions when a cross-cultural interaction requires it.

Intercultural Training Models

The history of formal intercultural training can be traced back to the 1960s when Edward Hall was hired as a consultant and trainer at the Foreign Service Institute (FSI) of the US

Department of State. At FSI, he played a significant role in developing and delivering intercultural training programs for diplomats, foreign service officers, and personnel involved in international affairs. The training methods developed by Hall are still relevant in the intercultural communication training up till now. For example, Hall supported incorporating students' firsthand experiences in foreign countries into teaching materials and urged them to engage with individuals from different cultures in order to comprehend foreign cultures.

Taking into consideration objectives, experts have presented a range of models and techniques for intercultural training. Chen and Starosta (1999) have summarized six training models: the classroom model, the simulation model, the self-awareness model, the cultural awareness model, the behavioral model, and the interactional model. Specific training techniques are designed to deliver training, which include role playing, case studies, critical incidents, cultural assimilators, and simulations.

• The Classroom Model

Among the six training models, the classroom model may be the most popular approach used in intercultural training programs. It is also widely known as the university model because an increasing number of universities around the globe now offer intercultural communication or similar courses to students in order to prepare them with sufficient knowledge to cope with cultural variabilities. Lectures, films, readings, and different kinds of presentations are normally applied to this model to help participants know more about a culture.

One obvious advantage of the classroom model is its relatively fair demand on the trainers. It can be easily carried out in a physical building. Nowadays, with the prevalence of internet and smart classrooms equipped with advanced educational tools, a wide range of students can be trained wirelessly. Another strength is its ability to convey content knowledge to help participants understand a specific culture. Nevertheless, a clear limitation is the incapability to connect the disparity between the classroom setting and the actual firsthand experience in a different culture. In other words, this model solely instructs on "what to learn", neglecting the aspect of "how to act". Knowing the knowledge but not knowing how to perform or adapt behaviorally to it will not guarantee success in a new context. Besides, an instruction-based model may create a sense of simplicity and falsehood.

• The Simulation Model

The simulation model was developed in response to criticism of the classroom model. This model emphasizes the immersive (沉浸式) and experiential learning approach, where participants are actively engaged in an environment that closely mirrors a specific culture. The focus is on practical and interactive training to enhance participants' understanding and familiarity with the target culture. It is designed to help motivate participants in their interactions with people from different cultures and to increase their sensitivity to other cultural groups. Technically speaking, it aims to bridge the gap between reality and the classroom situation. Under a simulated context, participants are encouraged to encounter intercultural difficulties without concerns of creating real harm.

The simulation model has at least three advantages. Firstly, it is suggested that the real strength of simulations lies in their diversity (Salzman, 2020). They can reveal value differences, sources of intercultural faux pas, communication barriers, and the errors inherent in applying one's own judgments to a people who may in fact come from totally different social realities. Trainers can incorporate their hands-on experience in designing the simulation activities to help trainees become competent and confident to handle future difficulties if need be. Besides, simulations are training activities that may include game-like features such as goals, pay-offs (报酬), bonus, and constraints. A lot of features related to Massively Multiplayer Online Role-playing Games are borrowed into the simulation model. As a result, the simulation model is much more engaging (有吸引力) than a classroom model. Finally, the simulation model can save money, time, and energy. Though it is ideal for students to experience a true intercultural activity in a foreign context, say, sending a group of TCM students to engage with the local people in New Zealand under the supervision of an experienced mentor, this field trip (实地考察) is both time-consuming, effortful, and costly. Research shows that to be effectively immersed in a new culture, one has to spend at least 6-12 months in a host culture. It may require a substantial financial investment, let alone concerns over some unforeseeable dangers. On-line virtual simulation can greatly reduce such financial and temporal (时间上的) burdens.

However, this model has two weaknesses. First, it is difficult to truly recreate an overseas environment. Simulated reality should be as close to the target reality as possible to provide a true context, so the participants may not feel at a loss (不知所措) once they begin their real journey to a new culture. In other words, an inappropriate simulation procedure often leads to failure in living or working in the host culture (Chen and Starosta, 1999). Besides, it is still hard to claim that the model can satisfactorily teach the culture of the host nation: Due to the limited duration, typically ranging from a day to a few weeks, the training cannot possibly offer in-depth cultural knowledge. Therefore, combining the classroom model and the simulation model could enhance the intercultural adaptation process for learners, leading to greater effectiveness.

One more model that deserves our attention is the **interaction model** proposed by Gudykunst and his colleagues (Chen and Starosta, 1999). In the interaction model, participants have the opportunity to directly interact with members of the host culture. The underlying reason is that through direct interaction with people from the host culture in an intercultural training program, participants will experience increased comfort and ease when living and working in that particular cultural setting. Since almost ten years ago, several teachers from Zhejiang Chinese Medical University and other universities have begun to adopt this interaction model to train students both from China and other countries, which worked quite well (Xie, 2012). However, sometimes, students may idealize or distort their own culture and may not be able to present a real picture of it.

Each model has its strengths and weaknesses. Relying on only one model may not sufficiently help trainees boost their intercultural competence. Based on specific goals and realistic evaluation of training space available, a combination of two or more models is a better choice. Each one can offset (弥补) the shortcomings of the other and help enhance the training outcome. For example, to train a group of qualified TCM culture facilitators, a classroom model can help enrich the trainees' linguistic and non-linguistic knowledge. Then, the cultural awareness model (for more information, see Chen and Starosta, 1999) is adopted to deepen the understanding of self-knowledge and other-knowledge. Still a third method, say, the behavioral model (for more information, see Chen and Starosta, 1999) can be carried out to help trainees put theory into practice.

Delivering Methods of Intercultural Training

Once the training model is selected, what is equally important is to choose appropriate delivering methods. Some of the most frequently used methods include role play, case studies, critical incidents, cultural assimilators, and simulations.

• Role Play

Maybe role play is the most frequently used practice in an intercultural training program. During role-play exercises, participants are given specific roles and tasked with imitating real-life behaviors. Various problem-solving scenarios that reflect situations in the host culture can be created in a somewhat spontaneous manner. The participants assume the roles of themselves or others in a new situation (visiting doctors, interviewing, health management counseling, etc.) in an unrehearsed (未经排练的) manner and for a clearly defined purpose. The technique serves as an effective way to shift trainees from being mere observers to active participants.

In participating in role play, students can practice and learn intercultural communication skills; carry out certain actions or solutions in a specific situation; explore reactions and feelings; encourage involvement; and thus gain greater understanding of the thinking and behavioral patterns of people from different cultures. However, role play also suffers from some drawbacks. The most obvious weakness of role play is that it is heavily dependent on participants' efforts. Good preparedness is a requisite for successful role play. Poor preparation usually results in no development of the scenario, and hence no learning achievement. Besides, learning outcomes also depend on each participant's personality. Some participants may not take role play seriously — they may overact or act absurdly. Some participants may shy away from full engagement.

• Case Studies

Another frequently used technique is called case study, which originated in MBA courses. Case studies are simplified descriptions of complex cultural events. While the specific event described in the case study may never reoccur, semi-realistic situations allow us to effectively analyze and address the challenges it presents. Sometimes, cases can be constructed to reflect the trainees' situation which can make the case more focused. For instance, stories about culture shock that TCM culture facilitators may experience can be compiled into cases which then are used as training materials. These cases can be quite engaging. Trainees are quickly involved in the case, weighing different options and possible solutions or explanations.

However, some researchers argue that case studies also have some weaknesses. Firstly, it takes time to research and develop a well-suited case, let alone designing many cases related to TCM interculturalization. Besides, because cases are based on reality or adapted from realities, it can be quite frustrating (费解) for trainees with little or no intercultural experience. Lastly, cases usually aim to train the cognitive aspect of trainees' intercultural competence, and therefore, they should be complemented with other training methods if the overall competence is the goal.

Training is a necessity for TCM interculturalization. Proper training empowers TCM culture facilitators and ambassadors a real start in their future intercultural journey. It also offers an opportunity for students to practice what they have learned. Among many training models, the classroom model is the most widely used one. Under this model, a variety of training methods can be employed such as role play, case studies, and / or visual imagery (for more information, see Fowler and Yamaguchi, 2020) to enhance trainees' TCM interculturalization competence. With successful training, we can arrive at our destination all safe and sound.

Activities

Comprehension Questions

1. What are the strengths and drawbacks of self-reported survey used in evaluating intercultural competence?
2. What is cultural intelligence (CQ)? How is CQ measured?
3. What are the strengths and drawbacks of case studies in TCM interculturalization competence training?
4. In what way does a simulation model complement a classroom model?
5. What are the strengths and drawbacks of role play?

Role Play

Scenario

Mr. Wang, a Chinese of roughly 60 years old, is visiting a dentist in an American hospital for the first time. He went to the US a few months ago to visit his younger sister. He loves and believes in TCM very much. He can speak English, but with a foreign accent.

Assume one of the following roles:

Role A: The Patient

Your sister finally persuades you to see a dentist. You gum is bleeding. But you don't think it is a big deal. You already visited TCM physicians in China who gave you some prescriptions. You have heard about the bad attitude of dentists in the U.S. You don't think Western medicine could get you out of trouble. Your only purpose of seeing the dentist is to get some Chinese medicines from the hospital.

Role B: The Dentist

You have been a dentist for almost 15 years and treated bleeding gum for hundreds of patients. You enjoy talking to old people, though you think they are sometimes difficult to handle. You have never heard of any theory of TCM before. And you have received patients from other cultures, including Chinese. But none of them insisted on telling you the bleeding gum is caused by fire in the body.

In playing either of the roles, you have to act exactly as though this happened in a real situation, and you may say or do anything you feel that will be appropriate. Write a reflective report after you have finished your job.

Case Study

Case 1

Shelley Pollex is going to tell her experience with acupuncture in the US.

I started my first acupuncture treatments shortly after I finished chemotherapy and had begun taking my monthly Taxol, which is a drug known to cause neuropathy. My doctor had told me multiple times if the neuropathy got too bad in my hands and feet, they would stop my treatment. So I was going to do anything I could to keep it away! After a month of acupuncture treatments, my neuropathy was gone. I was astonished.

The first time I met Tina Berisha, I was instantly attracted to her personality.

Besides the physical benefits acupuncture has given me, I really enjoy the relaxation I get from each session, which typically lasts an hour. While most people imagine hundreds of needles, treatment usually only requires between five and twelve needles depending on what part of your body needs for that treatment. For me, the most important realization was that I really have to give my time and attention to that person for a whole hour. No phone, no distractions; just letting my mind and body go into that meditative state. Discovering acupuncture has truly been another positive to a scary, life-threatening diagnosis - and I'm all about finding silver linings.

Questions

1. What seems to bother Pollex? In what way was Pollex transformed after acupuncture?

2. What tips does Pollex offer to newcomers who are hesitant to do acupuncture?

Case 2

Brisbane-based engineer Geoffrey tried TCM for the first time after hurting his arm playing basketball. He details how he was treated by a TCM physician.

After several treatments, my arm still hurt. My pal recommended visiting a local acupuncture's clinic. With nowhere to go, I went to see the TCM physician. He led me into the treatment area. On the right were a row of empty patients' beds; on the left were a couple of old men with their heads cradled in some sort of harness attached to the wall. I guess it was therapeutic, but it looked like some torture. "Lie down. For you I think acupuncture."

He stuck eight needles into my arm, five of which I barely felt, three of which set my blood on fire, and attached electrical current to them. The feeling was strangely pleasurable. After 15 minutes, during which I managed to fall asleep, a stockier, younger man appeared. He disconnected the electricity, pulled out the needles, swabbed my thigh with alcohol, and then spread some cream that he extracted from a small green plastic jar onto my thigh.

"What is that?"

"Massage cream." Finally, some relief, I thought. Boy. I was wrong. For the next ten minutes, he used his body weight to lean into the strokes as he worked his palms up and down and across my arm unknotting the muscles. I lost count of the number of times I cried in pain. In the end, my whole body was quivering.

"Have you ever had cupping?" I assumed he was referring to the Swedish massage technique. "Sure." He lit a cotton ball that was on the end of some scissors, placed it inside a glass cup, removed it, and then stuck the cup on my arm, right on the area that he'd just flattened with his hands of steel. "Aggghhh... " but my objections were cut short as he stuck six more cups on any vacant arm. "Five minutes," and he vanished. When he reappeared, he quickly pulled the cups off, each one making a popping sound as it returned the thigh to its rightful owner. I got up to leave and he gently pushed me back down and spread some green paste onto my arm. "What is that?" I said. "Herbs." He wrapped my leg. "Come back in two days," and walked off.

The next day my arm felt better, and I have been back a couple of times. I have grown strangely fond of the whole process. After all, without the pain, what's the gain, right?

Questions

1. What impression does the clinic leave on Geoffrey?

2. Describe Geoffrey's emotional uneasiness when he saw some patients were in traction?

3. What do you think contributed to Geoffrey's attitudinal change in the end?

4. What suggestions can you offer to people who have never experienced acupuncture and tuina?

13.3　Tools of Evaluating Intercultural Communication Competence

The following are tools to evaluate your intercultural competence. The first is developed by Chen and Starosta (2000), the second by Wilson (2013).

Tool 1: Intercultural Sensitivity Scale

Below is a series of statements concerning intercultural communication. There are no right or wrong answers. Please work quickly and record your first impression by indicating the degree to which you agree or disagree with the statement. Thank you for your cooperation.

5: strongly agree

4: agree

3: uncertain

2: disagree

1: strongly disagree

Please put the number corresponding to your answer in the blank before the statement.

_____ 1. I find it is easy to talk with people from different cultures.

_____ 2. I am afraid to express myself when interacting with people from different cultures.

_____ 3. I find it is easy to get along with people from different cultures.

_____ 4. I am not always the person I appear to be when interacting with people from different cultures.

_____ 5. I am able to express my ideas clearly when interacting with people from different cultures.

_____ 6. I have problems with grammar when interacting with people from different cultures.

_____ 7. I am able to answer questions effectively when interacting with people from different cultures.

_____ 8. I find it is difficult to feel my culturally different counterparts are similar to me.

_____ 9. I use appropriate eye contact when interacting with people from different cultures.

_____ 10. I have problems distinguishing between informative and persuasive messages when interacting with people from different cultures.

_____ 11. I always know how to initiate a conversation when interacting with people from different cultures.

_____ 12. I often miss parts of what is going on when interacting with people from different cultures.

_____ 13. I feel relaxed when interacting with people from different cultures.

_____ 14. I often act like a very different person when interacting with people from different cultures.

_____ 15. I always show respect for my culturally different counterparts during our interaction.

_____ 16. I always feel a sense of distance with my culturally different counterparts during our interaction.

_____ 17. I find I have a lot in common with my culturally different counterparts during our interaction.

_____ 18. I find the best way to act is to be myself when interacting with people from different cultures.

_____ 19. I find it is easy to identify with my culturally different counterparts during our interaction.

_____ 20. I always show respect for the opinions of my culturally different counterparts during our interaction.

Notes

1. Items 2, 4, 6, 8, 10, 12, 14, 16, and 18 are reverse-coded before summing up the 20 items.

2. Behavioral Flexibility items are 2, 4, 14, and 18.

3. Interaction Relaxation items are 1, 3, 11, 13, and 19.

4. Interactant Respect items are 9, 15, and 20.

5. Message Skills items are 6, 10, and 12.

6. Identity Maintenance items are 8, 16, and 19.

7. Interaction Management items are 5 and 7.

Tool 2: Revised Sociocultural Adaptation Scale (SCAS-R)

Living in a different culture often involves learning new skills and behaviours. Thinking about life in [country], please rate your competence in each of the following behaviours (1 = Not at all competent; 5 = Extremely competent).

	1 Not at all competent				5 Extremely Competent
1. Building and maintaining relationships.	1	2	3	4	5
2. Managing my academic/work responsibilities.	1	2	3	4	5
3. Interacting at social events.	1	2	3	4	5
4. Maintaining my hobbies and interests.	1	2	3	4	5
5. Adapting to the noise level in my neighbourhood.	1	2	3	4	5
6. Accurately interpreting and responding to other people's gestures and facial expressions.	1	2	3	4	5
7. Working effectively with other students/work colleagues.	1	2	3	4	5
8. Obtaining community services I require.	1	2	3	4	5
9. Adapting to the population density.	1	2	3	4	5
10. Understanding and speaking [host language].	1	2	3	4	5
11. Varying the rate of my speaking in a culturally appropriate manner.	1	2	3	4	5
12. Gaining feedback from other students/work colleagues to help improve my performance.	1	2	3	4	5
13. Accurately interpreting and responding to other people's emotions.	1	2	3	4	5
14. Attending or participating in community activities.	1	2	3	4	5
15. Finding my way around.	1	2	3	4	5
16. Interacting with members of the opposite sex.	1	2	3	4	5
17. Expressing my ideas to other students / work colleagues in a culturally appropriate manner.	1	2	3	4	5
18. Dealing with the bureaucracy.	1	2	3	4	5
19. Adapting to the pace of life.	1	2	3	4	5
20. Reading and writing [host language].	1	2	3	4	5
21. Changing my behaviour to suit social norms, rules, attitudes, beliefs, and customs.	1	2	3	4	5

Notes

- Interpersonal Communication items: 1, 3, 6, 11, 16, 21, 13.
- Academic/Work Performance: 2, 7, 12, 17.
- Personal Interests and Community Involvement: 4, 8, 14, 18.
- Ecological Adaptation: 5, 9, 15, 19.
- Language Proficiency: 10, 20.

Chapter Summary

- The levels of competence are unconscious incompetence, conscious incompetence, conscious competence, and unconscious competence.
- Communication specialists have identified four individual components of intercultural communication competence: affection, cognition, behavior, and morality.
- Applied linguists have identified three dimensions of intercultural communicative competence: linguistic competence, sociolinguistic competence, and discourse competence.
- A competent TCM culture facilitator is both appropriate and effective in practicing TCM interculturalization.
- The classroom model is particularly prevalent in intercultural workshops.
- Four main methods, i. e., observation, interview, portfolio, and self-reported questionnaire are used in evaluating TCM interculturalization competence, with the last one being the most frequently used.
- Ideally, effective intercultural training programs aim to boost the overall competence of TCM interculturalization.
- Some of the most frequently used training methods in TCM interculturalization workshops include role play, case studies, simulations, among others.

Checklist	Yes	No
Cognitive: I have mastered the core information		
Behavioral: I have the ability of putting what I've learned into practice		
Affective: I am willing to carry out what I've learned		
Moral: I will take the ethical consideration into account during practice		

Chapter 14

Future of TCM Interculturalization: Challenges and Promises

Chapter Objectives

After reading this chapter, you should be able to:

- ◆ Probe into the essence of globalization and its impact.
- ◆ Review key concepts and elements in three fields, culture, TCM culture, and communication.
- ◆ Explore some possible opportunities and challenges for TCM interculturalization.
- ◆ Integrate the reality with the dreams to realize effective and appropriate TCM interculturalization.

───── Key Terms ──────────────────────────────────

globality   modernization of TCM

globalization   personal challenge

governmental challenge   promise

Quotes

"The practice of using the pandemic to pursue 'de-globalization' or clamor for 'economic decoupling' and 'parallel systems' will end up hurting one's own interests and the common interests of all." (利用疫情搞"去全球化",鼓吹所谓"经济脱钩""平行体系",最终只会损害本国和各国共同利益。)

　　——2020年11月17日习近平在金砖国家领导人第十二次会晤上的讲话

"When the way of virtue and justice prevailed, the whole world was one community. Then nobody was promoted but those of worth and talent. No doctrines were taught but those of sincerity and harmony, and they were followed in moral cultivation. Thus, men did not love only their own parents or treat only their own sons as their children. A life-long provision was made for the aged; employment was found for the able-bodied and, for the young, an environment in which they could mature. Widows, orphans, childless men, and those disabled by disease were sufficiently provided for. Males had their proper work, and females their homes." (大道之行也,天下为公,选贤与能,讲信修睦。故人不独亲其亲,不独子其子,使老有所终,壮有所用,幼有所长,矜、寡、孤、独、废疾者皆有所养,男有分,女有归。)

　　　　　　　　　　　　　　　　　　　　　　　　　　　——《礼记》

"Keep the kingdom small, its people few; make sure they have no use for tools that do the work of tens or hundreds. Nor let the people travel far and leave their homes and risk their lives. Boat or cart, if kept at all, best not to ride; shield and blade best not to show. Guide them back to early times, when knotted cords served for signs, and they took relish in their food and delight in their dress, secure in their dwellings, content in their customs, although a neighbor kingdom stood in view and the barnyard cries of cocks and dogs echoed from village to village, their folk would never traffic to and fronever to the last of their days." (小国寡民。使有什伯之器而不用;使民重死而不远徙;虽有舟舆,无所乘之;虽有甲兵,无所陈之。使人复结绳而用之。甘其食,美其服,安其居,乐其俗,邻国相望,鸡犬之声相闻,民至老死不相往来。)

　　　　　　　　　　　　　　　　　　　　　　　　　　——《道德经》

Before reading this section, please consider the following questions:

1. Do you know what post-modernism and globalization are? How are they similar or different from each other?

2. How do you interpret the idea of "traditional" in TCM? Does this term suggest that TCM is old-fashioned and no longer relevant? Do you think it self-contradictory to modernize TCM?

14.1   Globalization and TCM Interculturalization

Challenges and Opportunities

Congratulations to each and every one of you for your academic achievements thus far, as you have successfully reached the end of this book. While predicting the future is impossible, we can be certain that the world we inhabit tomorrow will differ greatly from the world we currently live in. We exist in a rapidly evolving world where humanity has made remarkable advancements in the past century, despite numerous wars. The 21st century has witnessed a sharp intensity in economic globalization and a swift transformation within the international political and economic landscape. The global order and systems of global governance have also undergone significant shifts. All of these factors demonstrate that we are currently situated in an era of profound development, transformation, and adjustment, experiencing the most extensive changes witnessed in a century, which President Xi Jinping has repeatedly emphasized on various occasions since the commencement of the 19th National Congress of the Communist Party of China. These circumstances highlight our interconnectedness with individuals whose cultural values and aspirations may differ significantly from our own.

Change brings about risks and challenges, particularly in the context of a vastly developing global landscape that encompasses intricate changes (SCIO, 2019). This results in the fundamental reconfiguration (重组) of the relationships between major nations and intellectual trends. As instability and uncertainty continue to surge, there is a corresponding decrease in trust, peace, and development. The world is facing a critical danger of regression into fragmentation (分裂) and potential confrontation. For example, as the largest and most influential economy in the world, the US has the responsibility of maintaining the existing world order. Yet, the American government withdrew from at least 17 international organizations such as UNESCO (in 2017), *Treaty on the Limitation of Anti-Ballistic Missile Systems*(《限制反弹道导弹系统条约》) (in 2002), *Trans-Pacific Partnership Agreement*(《跨太平洋伙伴关系协定》) (in 2017) etc. This irresponsible and erratic (反复无常的) behavior has set a bad example for other nations to follow. Furthermore, the outbreak of COVID-19 pandemic and its aftermath (后果) have further aggravated the decline in economic growth. These challenges pose a significant threat to the international order established after Second World War.

Change presents opportunities as well. A notable transformation is the rise of China and other emerging markets, which is significantly altering the international distribution of power. Western powers have dominated world politics and economic systems since the first industrial revolution. However, in recent decades, emerging markets and developing countries have experienced rapid growth by exploiting the historic opportunities presented by economic globalization. The newest expansion of BRICS reflects a totally different mentality in terms of how to co-exist in such a turbulent (动荡的) world in the spirit of openness, inclusiveness and win-win cooperation (Xinhua, 2023).

These big changes have led humanity to an important point. Having hope and confidence is crucial for overcoming difficulties and challenges. Understanding and managing the differences that arise from intercultural dynamics is essential for success in our rapidly changing world. The global promotion of traditional Chinese medicine (TCM) becomes even more significant as it aims to provide an alternative, equally effective and less expensive way of addressing health-related issues, which has the potential to benefit all individuals worldwide.

Demystifying Globalization

It is mentioned in Chapter 1 that we are currently living in a globalized community, as evidenced by the latest COVID-19 pandemic. The advancement of communication and transportation technologies, especially the widespread application of the internet, has significantly reduced physical distance between people, creating an intricate web of interdependence, thus the birth of globalization. The term **globalization** has been used since the 1960s to describe various aspects such as a process, condition, system, force, and age in both popular and academic literature. Steger (2003) suggested that it is more appropriate to use the term "**globality** to signify a social condition characterized by the existence of global economic, political, cultural, and environmental interconnections and flows that make many of the currently existing borders and boundaries irrelevant" (p. 7). He further argued that the term "globalization" should be used to refer to "a series of social processes that are believed to transform our current social condition into one of globality" (Steger, 2003, p. 8). In other words, globalization revolves around the changing ways in which humans interact; it is, therefore, the opposite to localization.

Some scholars argue that globalization does not exist as nation-states and national situations are still there, and nothing is truly new (Jameson, 1999). The recent closure of borders due to a global public health emergency serves as evidence to support this position. Others argue that globalization is not a new phenomenon, not because it does not exist, but because such processes have been ongoing for thousands of years. For instance, the trading route between the East and the West, known as the Silk Road, is a typical example that supports this position. Finally, while some researchers also agree with the second position, they maintain that the current degree of globalization is more intense than ever before. This is due to the accelerated advancements in technology, increased integration among people, and commercial interests.

Despite the notable differences of opinion, it is indeed possible to identify the fundamental characteristics of globalization (Steger, 2003). Firstly, globalization entails the establishment and proliferation (激增) of both new and existing social networks and activities that progressively transcend traditional political, economic, cultural, and geographical boundaries. The second characteristic of globalization is evident in the expansion and extension of social relationships and interdependencies. Thirdly, globalization involves the heightened intensity and acceleration of social exchanges and activities. Interestingly, the seemingly contradictory processes of globalization and localization are actually interconnected because the intensification of global social relations influences local events, and vice versa. Lastly, the formation and enlargement of social connections and interdependencies are not limited to objective, material aspects alone. Globalization also extends to the subjective realm of human consciousness. Notably, globalization can refer to individuals becoming increasingly aware of the growing manifestations of global interdependence and the rapid acceleration of global interactions. This highlights the significance and relevance of enhancing intercultural awareness for TCM culture facilitators who aspire to fulfill their tasks to the fullest extent.

Prospects of TCM Interculturalization

The profound impact of globalization has created opportunities for TCM practitioners, researchers, and TCM culture facilitators. In late 2021, the National Administration of TCM released the *Development Plan for Integrating High-Quality Traditional Chinese Medicine into the Belt and Road Initiative* (2021-2025). This plan emphasizes the promotion of TCM globalization, including international cooperation in developing TCM industrial parks and advancing Chinese materia medica. It serves as a guideline for future TCM development domestically and identifies potential areas for collaboration abroad because international collaborations and dialogues between TCM practitioners and Western medical workers are crucial for enhancing the quality of healthcare services on a global scale, with the aim of improving the quality of healthcare service for a global community of shared future.

As a result, more cooperative measures are to be taken at the governmental level and the individual level. Since 1997, China has embarked on an ambitious plan to modernize TCM (NHC, 2000) and has made significant investments in integrating TCM with Western science and medicine. This endeavor has yielded fruitful research results, including attempts to identify the active ingredients in compound prescriptions (中药复方) and conducting clinical trials on TCM practices. The **modernization of TCM** has resulted in two fundamental understandings: effective ingredients and mechanisms. These outcomes represent crucial progress in scientifically interpreting the significance of TCM.

The trend towards globalization will pose a direct challenge to higher education institutions as well. Colleges and universities must strive to provide an environment in which students can comprehend the nature of global society and acquire the skills necessary to communicate effectively with people from diverse cultures. As discussed in the previous chapter on TCM education, an increasing number of international students are pursuing university-level TCM studies in China. With the implementation of the Belt and Road Initiative, more students from participating countries will come to China. Designing a suitable curriculum for these students will be a challenging task.

Personally, the internet, a powerful technological innovation that connects people worldwide, enables individuals to have a closer global contact because in this virtual realm, we experience a truly borderless global village. Various popular social media platforms like Weibo, TikTok, YouTube, and Facebook bring together individuals who engage in lively discussions on a wide range of topics, both old and new. Within this dynamic atmosphere, personal anecdotes about the effective use of TCM can have a contagious impact. Many people share their short videos on TikTok, showcasing to the world their appreciation of Chinese culture, Chinese lifestyle, and TCM. They are TCM cultural ambassadors as well.

Responsibilities as Cultural Ambassadors

These are the things we believe we can and should do as ambassadors of TCM and Chinese culture. The path to success is never easy; it presents challenges and requires effort. There will be ups and downs. Yet, where there's a will, there's a way. If we are determined to achieve something, we will accomplish it, even if it seems difficult, frustrating, or impossible. The inclusion of TCM in the WHO's eleventh version of the *International Classification of Diseases* is not only a milestone for the ICD but also a crucial step for TCM. This significant achievement provides strong evidence for TCM practitioners and facilitators to promote TCM in other nations. However, this is only a small stride towards TCM interculturalization. We have much greater aspirations. Imagine a future where TCM and local healthcare systems stand side by side, where discussions no longer revolve around which one is superior, more scientific, effective, or efficient. People's responses to healthcare issues will become more tolerant and diversified. That day will come. Are you prepared to embrace it?

── **Activities** ────────────────────────────────

Comprehension Questions

1. Explain your understanding of globalization. What is the historical context of globalization in your culture? How does this global phenomenon impact your personal and professional life?

2. Choose a foreign country and study how globalization began to influence that particular nation.

3. Globalization should not be simplified solely as an increase in economic exchange between countries or as technological cooperation; it also affects culture. Discuss with your partners what one can do in face of global cultural homogeneity because of cultural globalization.

4. There are intense debates regarding the existence of globalization, as discussed in the second part of this section. Some individuals go so far as to claim that globalization is synonymous with Americanization, pointing to the widespread expansion of American brands worldwide. How do you respond to these arguments?

5. What is your perspective on the future of TCM interculturalization?

Group Work

1. This book explores intercultural challenges within the healthcare field, specifically focusing on TCM. Now, consider a different context such as business, education, nongovernmental organizations, or legal assistance, and identify potential cultural challenges. Present your findings to the class.

2. The phrase "think globally, act locally" is commonly seen as a symbolic statement that guides behavior in today's globalized world. It suggests that individuals and communities should consider a wider range of factors, ideas, and values beyond their immediate concerns when developing strategies for local activities. How does this slogan relate to combating global epidemics like COVID-19? And how does TCM contribute to the idea of thinking globally while acting locally? Have a discussion with your group members and share the outcomes with the class.

3. There are examples where TCM has been subjected to thorough preclinical investigation and proven in rigorous clinical trials to make a major contribution in delivering health benefits. Artemisinin therapy for malaria is a great example, but the success of artemisinin as an anti-malaria agent is attributable to a lengthy Chinese commitment to robust discovery research, including pharmacognosy and medicinal chemistry. Debates are going on surrounding two of the most popular TCM practices, i.e., Chinese herbal medicines and acupuncture. Have a discussion with your group members regarding one of the following concerns: the potential obstacles to globalizing Chinese herbal medicines or acupuncture, and then share the outcomes with the class.

Debate

Read the following statements.

Climate change presents one of the most significant challenges worldwide. It contributes to the rise in extreme weather events and consecutive hottest years. The loss of human lives due to these events serves as a vivid example of "loss and damage", which describes how people, especially the disadvantaged, are already suffering from the consequences of human-induced climate change. This change is primarily caused by emissions from a wealthy minority. The impacts of climate change, ranging from the submergence of low-lying island territories to the destruction of homes and businesses by cyclones, result in extensive and wide-ranging loss and damage. During the 2021 UN climate summit, a group mainly composed of developing nations representing the majority of the global population called on developed countries to offer funds for addressing loss and damage. However, this request faced opposition from major economies like the US and EU and was ultimately rejected.

First, discuss with your partners whether the world's rich nations must pay for climate damage, and then form teams with classmates who share the same side, with 2-4 members on each side. Give alternate speeches for and against the topic.

Before reading this section, please consider the following questions:

1. Does this textbook live up to what you were expecting?

2. How does this textbook stand out from other intercultural books? Are there any areas where you think this textbook could be improved?

14.2　Concluding Remarks

Possible Readers

Since we are reaching the very end of this textbook, it is time to reflect on our potential readers. People from various backgrounds and with different reasons come to read a book like this. Some are students, others are healthcare professionals. These readers come from different parts of the world or have diverse cultural backgrounds within a single nation. You might have opened this book because you have TCM skills and want to learn how to share them across cultures. Alternatively, you could be someone who feels they have not had a genuine intercultural experience before. Some readers may be looking for practical solutions for their work, while others are interested in blending TCM culture with global healthcare efforts. Regardless of who you are, one thing is certain: If you have enough time and know English well, you can definitely gain some valuable insights from this book.

Topics Addressed

This book discussed a few important themes. We started by looking at how culture and communication are intertwined, and we emphasized that it is not easy to fully grasp these concepts when it comes to TCM interculturalization. However, you do not need to worry because we also shared some Chinese insights on how communication works. Communication is a complex process involving both verbal and nonverbal cues. It serves various purposes, from expressing emotions to giving directions. It is fascinating to see how all these elements come together. For instance, we have a chapter dedicated to interlingual translation, where we discussed the potential loss of cultural aspects during the translation of TCM classics, partly because TCM classics are written in classical Chinese and rendering them into foreign languages involves crossing cultural boundaries.

However, we want to emphasize that the best way to promote TCM across cultures is by understanding the core concepts it is built upon. These underlying ideas include cultural values, beliefs, and norms that align with those values. In this book, we have introduced and examined various frameworks of such values. However, if you plan to work as a TCM culture facilitator or engage with people from specific cultures, please keep in mind that the information provided here is just a starting point. It should inspire you to conduct your own exploration and research into individual cultures. Otherwise, stereotyping and ethnocentrism are definitely going to impede your intercultural journey.

We focus on how people can get involved in communicating TCM across cultures, not just those from the government or organizations, but ordinary people too. There are many reasons why we should care about this topic and work together to make it happen. We do not want to force you to believe a certain way, but rather we hope this book helps you engage with the world around you and inspires you to make a positive impact on your own life and the lives of those around you.

However, we also recognize that we live in a world where material concerns such as school, work, and relationships take up a lot of our time. Therefore, while our main focus is on social action in the context of TCM interculturalization, we also wanted to provide information on practical matters like interpersonal relationships, intercultural adjustment and competence, and other relevant issues. Throughout the book, we explored TCM-related topics such as basic ethical considerations, core values, and features of TCM language. Our aim was to make this book useful both in professional settings and in everyday life.

Readers' Responsibilities

We have already shared some information on the current state of TCM in different countries and regions, including a short overview of national policies on TCM such as the Belt and Road initiative and TCM education for international students. However, we encourage you to keep exploring many complex aspects of TCM interculturalization, which is likely to help you take important steps towards effectively promoting TCM across cultures. Do not be afraid to get involved in TCM interculturalization, but always keep in mind that there is still so much more to discover and learn!

While the world has become more interconnected through globalization, countries still maintain their separate political identities. This has created a unique challenge where nations are economically dependent on each other but have differing political and national interests. Economic interdependency helps reduce the likelihood of major conflicts, but it also means that political disputes can only be resolved through dialogue. Chinese people treasure TCM; sharing it with the world is a sincere wish from China. However, it could be mistakenly seen as having ideological implications. As a result, the need for intercultural skills will continue to grow in your lifetime. Keeping this in mind, you are kindly asked to promote greater awareness, understanding, and effective communication across cultures with a focus on TCM and Chinese culture. We believe all of you can do it confidently, effectively, and appropriately in a harmonious way.

Activities

Comprehension Questions

1.Select five terms that have made an impact on you after reading the book. Describe each term using your own words, and then check the book to see if there are any discrepancies or new revelations.

2.In what way(s) is engaging TCM interculturalization both a civic and political endeavor?

3.Who do you think is the ideal reader of this book? And why?

4.What do you believe is the greatest difficulty in sharing TCM across cultures in today's globalized world? Provide potential solutions with real-life examples.

5.Please point out any shortcomings and/or potential improvements and send them to the chief editors of this book via email.

Translation

Translate the following text into English.

展望2035年,中医药融入更多共建"一带一路"国家主流医学体系,在国际传统医学领域的话语权和影响力显著提升,在卫生健康、经济、科技、文化、生态等方面的多元价值充分发挥,中医药高质量融入共建"一带一路"格局基本形成。

——《推进中医药高质量融入共建'一带一路'发展规划(2021—2025年)》

Chapter Summary

• Change brings about risks and challenges, particularly in the context of a vastly developing global landscape that encompasses intricate changes.

• Change brings opportunities; a notable transformation is the rise of China and other emerging markets, which is significantly altering the international distribution of power.

• The term globalization has been used since the 1960s to describe various aspects such as a process, condition, system, force, and age in both popular and academic literature.

• Globality is used to signify a social condition characterized by the existence of global economic, political, cultural, and environmental interconnections and flows that make many of the currently existing borders and boundaries irrelevant.

• Globalization should be used to refer to a series of social processes that are believed to transform our current social condition into one of globality.

- Regardless of who you are, one thing is certain: If you have enough time and know English well, you can definitely gain some valuable insights from this book.
- Chinese people treasure TCM; sharing it with the world is a sincere wish from China. However, it could be mistakenly seen as having ideological implications.
- Do not be afraid to get involved in TCM interculturalization, but always keep in mind that there is still so much more to discover and learn!

Checklist	Yes	No
Cognitive: I have mastered the core information		
Behavioral: I have the ability of putting what I've learned into practice		
Affective: I am willing to carry out what I've learned		
Moral: I will take the ethical consideration into account during practice		

References

[1] ADLER N J, GUNDERSON A, 2008. International dimensions of organizational behavior [M]. 5th ed. Mason, OH: Thomson South-Western.

[2] ALLPORT G W, 1954. The nature of prejudice [M]. New York: Macmillan.

[3] ALTARRIBA J, BASNIGHT-BROWN D, 2022. The psychology of communication: the interplay between language and culture through time [J]. Journal of cross-cultural psychology, 53(7/8): 860-874.

[4] ANG S, VAN DYNE L, KOH C, et al., 2007. Cultural intelligence: its measurement and effects on cultural judgment and decision making, cultural adaptation and task performance [J]. Management and organization review, 3 (3): 335-371.

[5] BACHMAN L, 1990. Fundamental considerations in language testing [M]. Oxford: OUP.

[6] BAILEY B, PEOPLES J, 2014. Essentials of cultural anthropology [M]. 3rd ed. Boston: Cengage.

[7] BAKER D, 2003. Oriental medicine in the Republic of Korea [M]//SELIN H. Medicine across cultures. London: Kluwer Academic Publishers: 133-153.

[8] BAKSHI D, MUKHERJEE B, BASU S, et al., 1995. Historical introduction of acupuncture in India [J]. Bulletin of the Indian Institute of History of Medicine, 25(1-2): 215-225.

[9] BALDWIN J R, COLEMAN R R, GONZÁLEZ A, et al., 2014. Intercultural communication for everyday life [M]. Malden, MA: Wiley Blackwell.

[10] BEAUCHAMP T L, CHILDRESS J F, 2013. Principles of biomedical ethics [M].

7th ed. Oxford: OUP.

[11] BIRDWHISTELL R, 1970. Kinesics and context [M]. Philadelphia: University of Pennsylvania Press.

[12] BOND M H, 1991. Beyond the Chinese face: insight from psychology. Oxford: OUP.

[13] BURGOON J K, GUERRERO L K, FLOYD K, 2010. Nonverbal communication [M]. London: Routledge.

[14] BURKE K, 1984. Permanence and change: an anatomy of purpose [M]. 3rd ed. Berkeley: University of California Press.

[15] BYRAM M, 1997. Teaching and assessing intercultural communicative competence [M]. Clevedon, UK: Multilingual Matters Ltd.

[16] BYRAM M, GRIBKOVA B, STARKEY H, 2002. Developing the intercultural dimension in language teaching [M]. Strasbourg: Council of Europe.

[17] CHEN G M, 2009a. Foundations of intercultural communication [M]. 2nd ed. Shanghai: ECNU Press.

[18] CHEN G M, 2009b. Toward an I Ching model of communication [J]. China media research, 5(3): 72-81.

[19] CHEN G M, STAROSTA W J, 1998. Foundations of intercultural communication [M]. Boston, MA: Allyn and Bacon.

[20] CHEN G M, STAROSTA W J, 2000. The development and validation of the intercultural sensitivity scale [J]. Human communication, 3(1): 3-14.

[21] CHEN J, 2002. BRICS [EB/OL]. [2023-06-11]. https://www.investopedia.com/terms/b/brics.asp.

[22] CHEN Y, WANG X F, LIU C, 2019. The spread of traditional Chinese medicine in Britain and its enlightenment [M]//SUGUMARAN V, XU Z, P S, et al. Application of intelligent systems in multi-modal information analytics. New York: Springer: 686-692.

[23] CHOI J H, CHUNG M J, OH D H, 2012. Classification of Sasang constitutional body types using immunostimulatory activities of constitution-specific herbal extracts in human primary immune cells [J]. Journal of medicinal food, 15(9), 824-34.

[24] DAI X D, CHEN G M, 2015. On interculturality and intercultural communication competence [J]. China media research, 11(3): 100-113.

［25］DANIELSON B L, LAPREE A J, Odland M D, et al., 1998. Attitudes and beliefs concerning organ donation among native Americans in the upper Midwest [J]. Nursing, 8(3): 153-156.

［26］DAWSON P M, 1925. Su-Wen, the basis of Chinese medicine [J]. Annals of medical history, 7(1): 59-64.

［27］EIPPERLE M K, ANDREWS M A, 2020. Influence of cultural and health belief systems on health care practices [M]//ANDREWS M M, BOYLE J S, COLLINS J W. Transcultural concepts in nursing care. 8th ed. Philadelphia: Wolters Kluwer: 75-92.

［28］ELAHEE S F, MAO H J, SHEN X Y, 2019. Traditional Indian medicine and history of acupuncture in India [J]. World journal of acupuncture - moxibustion, 29(1): 69-72.

［29］FANG T, FAUREB G O, 2011. Chinese communication characteristics: a yin yang perspective [J]. International journal of intercultural relations, 35(3): 320-333.

［30］FDA, 2020. Botanical drug development: guidance for industry [EB / OL]. [2023-07-17]. https://www. fda. gov / regulatory-information / search-fda-guidance-documents/botanical-drug-development-guidance-industry.

［31］FDA, 2023. Dietary supplements [EB/OL]. [2023-07-17]. https://www.fda.gov/ food/dietary-supplements.

［32］FENG Y L, 1966. A short history of Chinese philosophy [M]. New York: The Free Press.

［33］FOWLER S M, YAMAGUCHI M, 2020. An analysis of methods for intercultural training [M]//LANDIS D, BHAWUK D P S. The Cambridge handbook of intercultural training. 4th ed. Cambridge: CUP: 192-257.

［34］FROMKIN V, RODMAN R, HYAMS N, 2014. An introduction to language [M]. 10th ed. Boston: Wadsworth.

［35］GALANTI G, 2015. Caring for patients from different cultures [M]. 5th ed. Philadelphia: University of Pennsylvania Press.

［36］GASIOROWSKI-DENIS E, 2016. Serving South Africa the Chinese way [EB/OL]. [2023-04-04]. https://www.iso.org/news/2016/03/Ref2065.html.

［37］GEERTZ C, 1973. The interpretation of cultures [M]. New York: Basic Books.

［38］GENETTI C, 2019. How language works [M]. Rev. ed. Cambridge: CUP.

[39] GHEBREYESUS T A, 2022. WHO director-general's opening remarks at the WHO press conference [EB/OL]. [2022-05-09]. https://www.who.int/director-general / speeches / detail / who-director-general-s - opening-remarks-at-the-who-press-conference-13-April-2022.

[40] GIBBONS S, 2016. Could ancient remedies hold the answer to looming antibiotics crisis? [EB/OL]. [2023-04-13]. https://www.nytimes.com/2016/09/ 18 / magazine / could-ancient-remedies-hold-the-answer-to-the-looming-antibiotics-crisis.html?_r=2.

[41] GILLMORE M, 2001. The hospital: a foreign culture [J]. International journal of childbirth education, 16(1): 18-22.

[42] GILLON R, 1994. Medical ethics: four principles plus attention to scope [J]. British medical journal, 309:184-188.

[43] GUDYKUNST W B, Kim Y Y, 2003. Communicating with strangers: an approach to intercultural communication [M]. 4th ed. Boston: McGraw Hill.

[44] GUMPERZ J J, COOK-GUMPERZ J, 2012. Interactional sociolinguistics: perspectives on intercultural communication [M]//PAULSTON C B, KIESLING S F, RANGEL E S. The handbook of intercultural discourse and communication. Malden, MA: Wiley-Blackwell: 63-76.

[45] HALL B J, COVARRUBIAS P O, KIRSCHBAUM K A, 2018. Among cultures: the challenge of communication [M]. 3rd ed. New York: Routledge.

[46] HALL E T, 1959. The silent language [M]. Garden City, NY: Doubleday.

[47] HALL E T, 1966. The hidden dimension [M]. Garden City, NY: Doubleday.

[48] HALL E T, 1976. Beyond culture [M]. Garden City, NY: Doubleday.

[49] HALL E T, 1983. The dance of life [M]. Garden City, NY: Doubleday.

[50] HALUALANI R T, 2019. Intercultural communication: a critical perspective [M]. Solana Beach, CA: Cognella Academic Publishing.

[51] HAN S Y, KIM H Y, LIM J H, et al., 2016. The past, present, and future of traditional medicine education in the Republic of Korea [J]. Integrative medicine research, 5(2):73-82.

[52] HARRINGTON N G, 2015. Health communication: an introduction to theory, method and application [M]//HARRINGTON N G. Health communication: theory, method and application. New York: Routledge: 1-27.

[53] HARRISON L E, KAGAN J, 2006. Developing cultures: essays on cultural

change [M]. London: Taylor and Francis.

[54] HAVILAND W A, PRINS H E L, MCBRIDE B, et al., 2017. Cultural anthropology [M]. 15th ed. Boston: Cengage.

[55] HEAD K J, COHEN E L, 2015. Factors affecting the patient [M]//Harrington N G. Health communication: theory, method and application. New York: Routledge: 181-211.

[56] HERZBERG F, MAUSNER B, SNYDERMAN B B, 2017. The motivation to work [M]. New York: Routledge.

[57] HILPERT M, 2007. Chained metonymies in lexicon and grammar: a cross-linguistic perspective on body part terms [M]//RADDEN G, KÖPCKE K M, BERG T, et al. Aspects of meaning construction. Amsterdam: John Benjamins: 77-98.

[58] HOEBEL E A, FROST E L, 1976. Cultural and social anthropology [M]. New York: McGraw-Hill.

[59] HOFSTEDE G, 1984. Culture's consequences [M]. Beverly Hiss, CA: Sage.

[60] HOFSTEDE G, HOFSTEDE G J, MINKOV M, 2010. Cultures and organizations: software of the mind [M]. New York: McGraw Hill.

[61] HOWELL W S, 1982. The empathic communicator [M]. Belmont, CA: Wadsworth.

[62] HSU E, 1999. The transmission of Chinese medicine [M]. Cambridge: CUP.

[63] INFANTE D A, RACER A S, WOMACK D F, 1990. Building communication theory [M]. Prospect Heights, IL: Waveland Press.

[64] JACKSON J, 2014. Introducing language and intercultural communication [M]. London: Routledge.

[65] JAMESON F, 1998. Notes on globalization as a philosophical issue [M]// JAMESON F, MIYOSHI M. Cultures of globalization. Durham: Duke University Press: 54-77.

[66] JANDT F E, 2018. An introduction to intercultural communication: identities in a global community [M]. 9th ed. Thousand Oaks, CA: Sage.

[67] JIAO L, LIU Y, CHEN Z., et al., 2011. Local and international TCM education comparison [J]. International journal of TCM, 33(3): 257-259.

[68] KAPLAN R B, 1966. Cultural thought pattern in intercultural education [J]. Language learning, 16: 1-20.

［69］KIM Y Y, 1991. Intercultural communication competence: a systems-theoretic view [M]//Ting-Toomey S, Korzenny R. Cross-cultural interpersonal communication. Newbury Park, CA: Sage: 259-275.

［70］KLUCKHOHN F K, STRODTBECK F L, 1961. Variations in value orientations [M]. Evanston, IL: Row, Peterson.

［71］KROEBER A L, KLUCKHOHN C, 1952. Culture: a critical review of concepts and definitions [M]. Cambridge, MA: The Museum.

［72］KROUT M H, 1954. An experimental attempt to produce unconscious manual symbolic movements [J]. Journal of general psychology, 51: 121-152.

［73］LAN F L, 2015. Metaphor: the weaver of Chinese medicine [M]. Germany: Verlag Traugott Bautz GmbH.

［74］LASS R, 2015. Lineage and the constructive imagination: the birth of historical linguistics [M]// BOWERN C, EVANS B. The Routledge handbook of historical linguistics. Oxford: Routledge: 45-63.

［75］LEININGER M, MCFARLAND M R, 2002. Transcultural nursing: concepts, theories, research, and practice [M]. New York: McGraw-Hill.

［76］LEWIS M, TAMPARO C D, 2007. Medical law, ethics, bioethics: for the health professions [M]. 6th ed. Philadelphia: F. A. Davis Company.

［77］LI R F, HOU Y L, HUANG J C, et al., 2020. Lianhuaqingwen exerts anti-viral and anti-inflammatory activity against novel coronavirus [J]. Pharmacological research, 156(June): 104761.

［78］LIN Y T, 1998. The importance of living [M]. Beijing: Foreign Language Teaching and Research Press.

［79］LITTLEMORE J, 2015. Metonymy hidden shortcuts in language, thought and communication [M]. Cambridge: CUP.

［80］LIU C, 2015. Traditional medicine enters UK market [EB/OL]. [2023-05-03]. https://www.chinadaily.com.cn/business/2015-03/03/content_19699320.htm.

［81］LUSTIG M W, KOESTER J, 2010. Intercultural competence: interpersonal communication across cultures [M]. 6th ed. Boston: Allyn and Bacon.

［82］MAGNER L N, KIM O J, 2018. A history of medicine [M]. 3rd ed. Boca Raton, FL: CSC Press.

［83］MARTIN J, NAKAYAMA T, 2018. Experiencing intercultural communication

[M]. 6th ed. New York: McGraw Hill.

[84] MARTIN J, NAKAYAMA T, 2022. Intercultural communication in contexts [M]. 8th ed. New York: McGraw Hill.

[85] MCLUHAN H M, 1964. Understanding media: the extensions of man [M]. 2nd ed. New York: New American Library.

[86] MEEUWESEN L, VAN DEN BRINK-MUINEN E, HOFSTEDE G, 2009. Can dimensions of national culture predict cross-national differences in medical communication? [J]. Patient education and counseling, 75: 58-66.

[87] MEHRABIAN A, WIENER M, 1967. Decoding of inconsistent communications [J]. Journal of personality and social psychology, 6(1):109-114.

[88] MEYER H, 2010. Framing disability: comparing individualist and collectivist societies [J]. Comparative sociology, 9: 165-181.

[89] MHRA, 2020. Guidance on new provisions for traditional herbal medicinal products and homeopathic medicinal products [EB/OL]. [2023-06-17]. https://www.gov.uk/guidance/guidance-on-new-provisions-for-traditional-herbal-medicinal-products-and-homoeopathic-medicinal-products.

[90] MILLER K, 2005. Communication theories: perspectives, processes, and contexts [M]. 2nd ed. Boston: McGraw Hill.

[91] NAUGLE D K, 2002. Worldview: the history of a concept [M]. Grand Rapids, MI: Wm. B. Eerdmans Publishing Co.

[92] NCCIH, 2020. NCCIH Strategic Plan FY 2021-2025: mapping a pathway to research on whole person health [EB/OL]. [2023-04-17]. https://www.nccih.nih.gov/about/nccih-strategic-plan-2021-2025.

[93] NEULIEP J W, 2002. Assessing the reliability and validity of the generalized ethnocentrism scale [J]. Journal of intercultural communication research, 31: 201-215.

[94] NEULIEP J W, 2018. Intercultural communication: a contextual approach [M]. 7th ed. Los Angeles: Sage.

[95] NI M S, 2011. The yellow emperor's classic of medicine [M]. Boston: Shambhala Publications, Inc.

[96] OGDEN C K, RICHARDS I A, 1923. The meaning of meaning [M]. London: Routledge Kegan Paul.

[97] PAYER L, 1989. Medicine and culture: notions of health and sickness in

Britain, the United States, France, and West Germany [M]. London: Victor Gollancz.

[98]PEI M, 1965. The story of language [M]. Rev. ed. New York: Mentor Books.

[99] PURNELL L D, 2013. Transcultural health care: a culturally competent approach [M]. 4th ed. Philadelphia: F. A. Davis Company.

[100] QURESHI B, 1994. Transcultural medicine: dealing with patients from different cultures [M]. 2nd ed. Boston: Springer.

[101]RICHMOND V P, MCCROSKEY J C, HICKSON M L, 2012. Nonverbal behavior in interpersonal relations [M]. 7th ed. New York: Allyn and Bacon.

[102] RUBEN B D, 1989. The study of cross-cultural competence: traditions and contemporary issues [J]. International journal of organizational behavior, 13: 229-240.

[103] SALZMAN M B, 2020. Intercultural simulations: theory and practice [M]// LANDIS D, BHAWUK D P S. The Cambridge handbook of intercultural training. 4th ed. Cambridge: CUP: 258-280.

[104] SAMOVAR L, PORTER R, MCDANIEL E, et al., 2017. Communication between cultures [M]. 9th ed. Boston: Cengage.

[105] SEEBERG V, 1984. Book reviews [J]. Journal of applied gerontology, 3(1): 108-112.

[106] SHEEHAN M P, ATHERTON D J, 1992. A controlled trial of traditional Chinese medicine plants in widespread non-exudative atopic eczema [J]. British journal of dermatology, 126(2): 179-184.

[107]SHIRAEV E B, LEVY D A, 2017. Cross-cultural psychology: critical thinking and contemporary applications [M]. 6th ed. New York: Routledge.

[108] SPENCER-OATEY H, FRANKLIN P, 2009. Intercultural interaction: a multidisciplinary approach to intercultural communication [M]. New York: Palgrave Macmillan.

[109] SPITZBERG B H, CUPACH W R, 1984. Interpersonal communication competence [M]. Beverly Hills, CA: Sage.

[110]SPITZBERG B H, 2015. A model of intercultural communication competence [M]//SAMOVAR L A, PORTER R E, MCDANIEL E R, et al. Intercultural communication: a reader. 14th ed. Boston: Cengage: 343-354.

[111]STEGER M B, 2003. Globalization: a very short introduction [M]. Oxford: OUP.

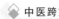

[112] THIN N, 2010. Environment [M]//Barnard A, Spencer J. The Routledge encyclopedia of social and cultural anthropology. 2nd ed. London: Routledge: 231-234.

[113] TING-TOOMEY S, CHUNG L C, 2022. Understanding intercultural communication [M]. 3rd ed. New York: OUP.

[114] TROMPENAARS F., HAMPDEN-TURNER C, 1998. Riding the waves of culture. New York: McGraw Hill.

[115] TSAI D F C, 1999. Ancient Chinese medical ethics and the four principles of biomedical ethics [J]. Journal of medical ethics, 25(4): 315-321.

[116] UN, 2022. Report of the Secretary-General on the work of the organization [R/OL]. [2023-08-11]. https://www. un. org / annualreport / files / 2022 / 09 / SG-Annual-Report-2022_eBook-PDF_EN.pdf.

[117] UNCTAD, 2023. Global trade update (June 2023) [EB / OL]. [2023-08-30]. https://unctad.org/system/files/official-document/ditcinf2023d2_en.pdf.

[118] UNESCO, 2020. UNESCO annual report 2021 [R/OL]. [2022-06-13]. https:// en.unesco.org/sites/default/files/unesco_annual_report_2021.pdf.

[119] UNSCHULD P U, 2003. Huang Di nei jing su wen: nature, knowledge, imagery in an ancient Chinese medical text [M]. Berkeley: University of California Press.

[120] UNSCHULD P U, TESSENOW H, 2011. Huang Di nei jing su wen: an annotated translation of huang di's inner classic - basic questions (Vol. 1) [M]. Berkeley: University of California Press.

[121] VULCHANOVA M, VULCHANOV V, FRITZ I, et al., 2019. Language and perception: introduction to the special issue "speakers and listeners in the visual world" [J]. Journal of cultural cognitive science, (3): 103-112.

[122] WANG Y Y, 2019. The scientific nature of traditional Chinese medicine in the post-modern era [J]. Journal of traditional Chinese medical sciences, 6(3): 195-200.

[123] WATZLAWICK P, BEAVIN J H, JACKSON D D, 1967. Pragmatics of human communication [M]. New York: Norton.

[124] WHO, 2013. WHO traditional medicine strategy: 2014-2023 [EB/OL]. [2023-05-11]. https://www.who.int/publications/i/item/9789241506096.

[125] WHO, 2019a. WHO Global Report on traditional and complementary

medicine [R / OL]. [2023-05-11]. https://www.who.int / publications / i / item / 978924151536.

[126] WHO, 2019b. World health assembly update [EB/OL]. [2023-05-11]. https://www.who.int/news-room/detail/25-05-2019-world-health-assembly-update.

[127] WHO, 2022. WHO international standard terminologies on traditional medicine [M / OL]. [2023-07-15] https://www.who.int / publications / i / item / 9789240042322.

[128] WILSON J, 2013. Exploring the past, present and future of cultural competency research: the revision and expansion of the sociocultural adaptation construct [D]. Wellington, New Zealand: Victoria University of Wellington.

[129] WINES W A, NAPIER N K, 1992. Toward an understanding of cross-cultural ethics: a tentative model [J]. Journal of business ethics, 11: 831-841.

[130] WISEMAN N, 1998. A practical dictionary of Chinese medicine [M]. Boulder, NV: Paradigm Publications.

[131] XIE Z F, 2010. Contemporary introduction to Chinese medicine [M]. Beijing: Foreign Languages Press.

[132] XINHUA, 2021. South Africa launches center to teach traditional Chinese medicine [EB/OL]. [2023-03-26]. https://www.xinhuanet.com/english/africa/2021-04/13/c_139877896.htm.

[133] XINHUA, 2022. Acupuncture: a bridge of friendship between India and China [EB/OL]. [2023-03-26]. http://www.china.org.cn/arts/2022-03/25/content_78130028.htm.

[134] YE X, 2016. Traditional Chinese medicine in the UK in the past forty years: an interview with Professor Bo-ying Ma [J]. Journal of integrative medicine, 14 (2): 77-83.

[135] YIN H H, 1992. Fundamentals of traditional Chinese medicine (Shuai Xuezhong trans) [M]. Beijing: Foreign Language Press.

[136] YOU L S, LIANG K, AN R, et al., 2022. The path towards FDA approval: a challenging journey for traditional Chinese medicine [J]. Pharmacological research, 182(August):1-2.

[137] YU W J, MA M Y, CHEN X M, et al., 2017. Traditional Chinese medicine and constitutional medicine in China, Japan and the Republic of Korea: a

comparative study [J]. American journal of Chinese medicine, 45 (1): 1-12.

[138]YULE G, 2020. The study of language [M]. 7th ed. Cambridge: CUP.

[139]ZHANG R X, 2018. Li Shizhen and the spirit of investigation of things and the extension of knowledge [J]. Chinese medicine and culture, 1(3): 116-120.

[140] ZHENG C M, LEE J, 2016. Traditional Chinese medicine: surging international interest and a shifting educational landscape in China [R/OL]. [2022-01-17]. https://wenr.wes.org/2016/12/traditional-chinese-medicine-surging-international-interest-shifting-educational-landscape-china.

[141]ZHU G S, YAN H, CHEN L Y, et al., 2019. Historical evolution of traditional medicine in Japan [J]. Chinese medicine and culture, 2(1):36-43.

[142]包惠南,包昂,2004. 中国文化与汉英翻译 [M]. 北京:外文出版社.

[143]编委会(Editors),2018. 易学百科全书 [Z]. 上海:上海辞书出版社.

[144]编委会(Editors),2021. 中华思想文化术语 历史卷 [M]. 北京:外语教学与研究出版社.

[145]编委会(Editors),2023. 中医药行业发展蓝皮书(2022年)[M]. 北京:中国中医药出版社有限公司.

[146]蔡昉,2018. "一带一路"手册 [M]. 北京:中国社会科学出版社.

[147]柴可夫,2007. 中医基础理论 [M]. 北京:人民卫生出版社.

[148]陈忠,张翼宙,2020. 医学类专业课程思政教学实录 [M]. 北京:中国中医药出版社.

[149]陈积敏,2018. 正确认识"一带一路" [N]. 学习时报,2-26.

[150]陈骥,何姗,唐路,2019. 中医典籍《伤寒论》英译历程回顾与思考 [J]. 中国中西医结合杂志,39(11):1400-1403.

[151]崔瑞兰,2017. 医学伦理学 [M]. 北京:中国中医药出版社.

[152]崔钰,冷文杰,李富武,等,2020. 美国各州中医针灸立法管理现状 [J],中医药导报,17(1):157-160.

[153]戴晓东,2018. 跨文化能力研究 [M]. 北京:外语教学与研究出版社.

[154]董静怡,张宗明,陈骥,等,2022. 基于跨文化传播视角的英美澳中医药立法对比研究 [J]. 浙江中医药大学学报,46(4):468-472.

[155]范骏,张晶滢,2020. 从日本中世医书看中医与密教的融合 [J]. 医学与哲学,41(12):77-81.

[156]郭剑华,2002. 中医在南非的发展概况 [J]. 实用中医药杂志,18(10):55-56.

[157]郭沫若,1947. 春天的信号 [N]. 文汇业刊,第一期.

［158］国家卫健委（NHC），2000. 中共中央、国务院关于卫生改革与发展的决定［EB/OL］.［2023-06-10］. http://www.nhc.gov.cn/wjw/zcjd/201304/743ba60a223646cd9eb4441b6d5d29fa.shtml?eqid=e66e184700027fd100000004644a548f.

［159］国家中医药管理局（NATCM），2016. 中医药"一带一路"发展规划（2016-2020 年）［EB/OL］.［2022-02-11］. https://www.yidaiyilu.gov.cn/wcm.files/upload/CMSydylgw/201703/201703200329031.pdf.

［160］国家中医药管理局（NATCM），2021. 推进中医药高质量融入共建"一带一路"发展规划（2021-2025 年）［EB/OL］.［2022-02-11］. https://www.gov.cn/zhengce/zhengceku/2022-01/15/content_5668349.htm.

［161］国家中医药管理局（NATCM），2022. 2021 年全国中医药统计摘编［R/OL］.［2022-03-24］. http://www.natcm.gov.cn/2021tjzb/%E5%85%A8%E5%9B%BD% E4%B8%AD% E5%8C% BB% E8%8D% AF% E7%BB% 9F% E8%AE% A1%E6%91%98%E7%BC%96/others/main-bookindex.htm.

［162］国务院（State Council），2016a. 中医药发展战略规划纲要（2016—2030 年）［EB/OL］.［2022-02-11］. https://www.gov.cn/zhengce/content/2016-02/26/content_5046678.htm.

［163］国务院（State Council），2016b. "健康中国 2030"规划纲要［EB/OL］.［2022-02-11］. https://www.gov.cn/zhengce/2016-10/25/content_5124174.htm.

［164］国务院新闻办公室（SCIO），2019. 新时代的中国与世界［EB/OL］.［2023-06-10］. http://www.scio.gov.cn/ztk/dtzt/39912/41838/index.htm?eqid=c4ca3b1b000e9b850000000364591a30.

［165］何文娟，梁凤霞，2016. 巴西中医针灸发展概况［J］. 上海针灸杂志，35(12)：1488-1490.

［166］洪蕾，陈建萍，2016. 中医药文化学［M］. 北京：科学出版社.

［167］侯建春，鲍燕，2012. 中医药在南非［J］. 世界中西医结合杂志，7(3)：259.

［168］胡丽雯，2017. 俄将种人参等草药出口中国［EB/OL］.［2023-03-05］. https://www.chinanews.com/business/2017/02-14/8148985.shtml.

［169］iFeng，2006. 20 年间"汉医"变"韩医"［EB/OL］. https://news.ifeng.com/history/200610/1025_25_23767_1.shtml.

［170］贾春华，2014. 基于隐喻认知的中医语言研究纲领［J］. 北京中医药大学报，37(5)：293-296.

[171]贾平凡,2022. 我在南非的大学里教中医 [N]. 人民日报海外版,12-19.

[172]贾玉新,(英)BYRAM M,贾雪睿,等,2019. 跨文化交际新视野 [M]. 北京:外语教学与研究出版社.

[173]江幼李,2017. 道家文化与中医学 [M]. 北京:中国中医药出版社.

[174]教育部(MOE),2019. 来华留学生简明统计 [M] 北京:教育部国际合作与交流司出版.

[175]教育部(MOE),2020. 教育部关于规范我高等学校接受国际学生有关工作的通知 [EB/OL]. [2022-01-18]. http://www.moe.gov.cn/srcsite/A20/moe_850/202006/t20200609_464159.html.

[176]兰凤利,2004.《黄帝内经素问》的译介及在西方的传播 [J]. 中华医史杂志,34(3):180-183.

[177]兰昊,熊淋宵,陈锋,2023. "一带一路"倡议下中医药文化在俄罗斯传播的现状、问题及对策 [J]. 世界中医药,18(14):2098-2102.

[178]李灿东,万朝义,2021. 中医诊断学 [M]. 第5版. 北京:中国中医药出版社.

[179]李经伟,余瀛鳌,蔡景峰,等,2009. 中医大辞典 [Z]. 2版. 北京:人民卫生出版社.

[180]李世娟,2015. 中医古籍东传对朝(韩)医学理论的影响 [J]. 中国中医基础医学杂志,21(6):677-680.

[181]李孝英,邝旖雯,2021. 从中医典籍外译乱象看中国传统文化翻译的策略重建 [J]. 外语电化教学,(5):26-33.

[182]李孝英,赵彦春,郭虹园,2023. 中医药文化负载词内涵挖掘及英译认知研究——以"阴""阳"为例 [J]. 外语教学理论与实践,3:90-96.

[183]李宇轩,谢粤湘,2021. 基于丰厚翻译理论探讨中医翻译中"文化缺省"现象的补偿机制 [J]. 中医药导报,27(4):225-228.

[184]李照国,刘希茹,2005. 黄帝内经(中英对照) [M]. 北京:世界图书出版公司.

[185]李振吉,2007. 中医基本名词术语中英对照国际标准 [M]. 北京:人民卫生出版社.

[186]梁漱溟,1999. 东西文化及其哲学 [M]. 北京:商务印书馆.

[187]林声喜,2001. 中医针灸在美国第一个州立法经过 [J]. 中国针灸,21(8):458-460.

[188]林子强,2016. 澳洲维州中医立法的昨天、今天与明天 [J]. 中国中医药信息杂志,13(4):1-2+36.

[189]蔺紫鸥,2019. 中国的全球发展贡献者形象更加鲜明 [EB/OL]. [2022-05-

19]. https://www.gov.cn/xinwen/2019-10/19/content_5442165.htm.

[190]刘保延,邓良月,2014. 世界针灸:国际针灸应用调查与分析 [M]. 北京:科学技术出版社.

[191]柳莺莺,周亚东,2023. 美国中医药立法现状及我国应对策略 [J]. 世界中医药,18(09):1352-1355.

[192]马伯英,2010. 中国医学文化史 [M]. 上海:上海人民出版社.

[193]马慧敏,张树剑,2023. 卜弥格《医学的钥匙》探微 [J]. 医学与哲学,44(1):73-77.

[194]全国人大(NPC),2016. 中华人民共和国中医药法 [Z/OL]. [2022-07-15]. http://www.npc.gov.cn/npc/c12435/201612/b0deb577ba9d46268dcc8d38ae40ae0c.shtml.

[195]山东中医药大学(SDUTCM),2023. 2023年山东中医药大学国际学生招生简章 [EB/OL]. [2023-04-13]. https://gjjiaoyu.sdutcm.edu.cn/info/1158/1774.htm.

[196]邵培仁,姚锦云,2014. 传播模式论:《论语》的核心传播模式与儒家传播思维 [J]. 浙江大学学报(人文社会科学版),44(4):56-75.

[197]邵晓秋,温金童,2009. 外籍医生与抗日根据地的卫生建设 [J]. 兰州学刊,188(5):214-217.

[198]沈潇,2020. 中医典籍英译中的文化缺省与补偿对策研究 [J]. 临床医药文献电子杂志,7(14):184.

[199]石慧,张宗明,2022. 针灸在美国本土化的历程、特色与成因探究 [J]. 自然辩证法研究,38(1):104-110.

[200]石强,2018. 中医四诊技能实训 [M]. 北京:中国中医药出版社.

[201]孙俊芳,2012. 中医语言的文化特点及翻译对策 [J]. 中国中医基础医学杂志,18(10):1151-1153.

[202]滕金聪,张宗明,2021. 古丝绸之路视域下中医药在印度的传播及现代意义 [J]. 世界中医药,16(4):677-681.

[203]田代华,2023. 黄帝内经素问 [M]. 北京:人民卫生出版社.

[204]王传军,2019. 他用中医学在澳大利亚"起死回生" [N]. 光明日报,10-28.

[205]王琦,2021. 中医体质学 [M]. 北京:中国中医药出版社.

[206]王蕊,2022. "一带一路"民心相通与我国高质量发展测度研究 [J]. 价格理论与实践,(2):59-62+200.

[207]王若瞳,2021. 中国—巴西医疗卫生合作历史、现状及前景 [J]. 文化创新比

较研究,(29):142-145.

[208]王天芳,2007. 中医诊断学［M］. 北京:人民卫生出版社.

[209]王天芳,2016. 针灸在美国的多元化发展［M］. 北京:中国医药科技出版社.

[210]王文,2023. "一带一路"金融合作十年回望［J］. 中国金融,(13):29-31.

[211]王新华,2016. 中医学［M］. 北京:科学出版社.

[212]王银泉,2023. 法国汉学家、加拿大裔美国生理学家与《黄帝内经》首部英译本［J］. 中医药文化,18(2):105-126.

[213]魏辉,巩昌镇,田海河,等,2017. 美国中医教育访谈录(一)［J］. 中医药导报,23(14):1-5.

[214]吴连胜,吴奇,1997. 黄帝内经(汉英对照)［M］. 北京:中国科学技术出版社.

[215]吴永贵,戴翥,熊磊,2013. 英美中医教育的现状及思考［J］. 云南中医学院学报,36(1):80-82.

[216]习近平,2014. 习近平谈治国理政［M］. 北京:外文出版社.

[217]习近平,2017. 习近平谈治国理政(第二卷)［M］. 北京:外文出版社.

[218]习近平,2018. 习近平谈"一带一路"［M］. 北京:外文出版社.

[219]习近平,2020. 习近平谈治国理政(第三卷)［M］. 北京:外文出版社.

[220]习近平,2022a. 习近平谈治国理政(第四卷)［M］. 北京:外文出版社.

[221]习近平,2022b. 在复兴之路上坚定前行［M］//金冲及. 复兴文库(第一篇). 北京:中华书局.

[222]夏瑾文,2017. 英国中医发展现状调查［N］. 中国青年报,1-19.

[223]夏林军,2016. 匈牙利中医概况和中医立法后的思考(一)［J］. 中医药导报,22(8):1-7.

[224]谢苑苑,2012. 中外学生混编模式下的《跨文化交际》课程对提升跨文化交际能力的实验研究［J］. 浙江中医药大学学报,36(11):1241-1244+5.

[225]新华社(XINHUA),2017. "一带一路"国际合作高峰论坛圆桌峰会联合公报［EB/OL］. [2022-02-13]. https://www.gov.cn/xinwen/2017-05/15/content_5194232.htm.

[226]新华社(XINHUA),2023. 习近平在金砖国家领导人第十五次会晤上的讲话［EB/OL］. [2023-09-13]. https://www.gov.cn/yaowen/liebiao/202308/content_6899768.htm.

[227]徐靖婷,张宇鹏,张逸雯,等,2023. 基于《难经》与《素问》两种脉法异同探析《难经》理论来源［J］. 中国中医基础医学杂志,29(3):352-353+384.

[228]薛妍,2015. 理查德·霍加特的文化价值论思想探析［D］. 太原:山西大学.

[229]闫婕,张瑛莹,马玉梅,2020. Hofstede 文化价值取向研究的新进展与应用[J].河南工业大学学报(社会科学版),36(5):100-105.

[230]颜春明,涂延,何洁,等,2021.葡萄牙中医药全面立法的回顾、解读与启示[J].浙江中医药大学学报,45(4):413-419.

[231]杨渝,陈晓,2020.《黄帝内经》英译文本分类述评[J].中医药文化,15(3):35-45.

[232]杨宇洋,2018.中俄主要药品管理法规比较研究[D].北京:中国中医科学院.

[233]杨宇洋,张文彭,朱建平,等,2012.俄罗斯及前苏联针灸发展历史与现状[J].中国针灸,32(10):928-932.

[234]于敦海,2023.守望相助,共同浇灌中马友谊的健康之花[EB/OL].[2023-09-07]. http://switzerlandemb.fmprc.gov.cn/zwbd_673032/wjzs/202308/t20230829_11134788.shtml.

[235]张大庆,2021. 20 世纪初美国的中西医论争[J].中国科技史杂志,42(3):322-334+318.

[236]张光霁,张庆祥,2021.中医基础理论[M].4 版.北京:人民卫生出版社.

[237]张建斌,2021.中国针灸在俄罗斯的传播模式与跨文化调适[J].中医药文化,16(4):298-304.

[238]张建华,周尚成,潘华峰,2023.中国中医药传承创新发展报告(2022)[M].北京:社会科学文献出版社.

[239]张其成,1999.中医文化学体系的构建[J].中国中医基础医学杂志,5(5):52-54.

[240]张其成,2018.中医药文化核心价值"仁、和、精、诚"四字的内涵[J].中医杂志,59(22):1895-1900.

[241]张益嘉,2021. 16 世纪前中医针灸在日本的传播及其原因[J].文化遗产,(6):45-51.

[242]赵俊卿,2008.《难经》首部英译本评述[J].中医研究,25(5):61-63.

[243]郑晓红,王旭东,2012.中医文化的核心价值体系与核心价值观[J].中医杂志,53(4):271-273.

[244]中国外文局编辑,2014.习近平谈治国理政(第一卷)(英文版)[M].北京:外文出版社.

[245]中国外文局编辑,2017.习近平谈治国理政(第二卷)(英文版)[M].北京:外文出版社.

[246]中国外文局编辑,2020. 习近平谈治国理政(第三卷)(英文版)[M]. 北京:
外文出版社.

[247]中国外文局编辑,2022. 习近平谈治国理政(第四卷)(英文版)[M]. 北京:外
文出版社.

[248]中国新闻社(CNS),2021. 华人业者看好中医药海外发展潜力[EB/OL].
[2022-03-24]. https://www.chinanews.com/hr/2021/07-21/9525150.shtml.

[249]朱勉生,阿达理,鞠丽雅,2018. 中医药在法国的发展史、现状、前景[J]. 世
界中医药,13(04):1013-1019+1024.